THE ETHICS OF BIOMEDICAL RESEARCH

The Ethics of Biomedical Research

An International Perspective

BARUCH A. BRODY, PH.D.
Baylor College of Medicine and Rice University

New York   Oxford
OXFORD UNIVERSITY PRESS
1998

Oxford University Press

Oxford   New York
Athens   Auckland   Bangkok   Bogota   Bombay
Buenos Aires   Calcutta   Cape Town   Dar es Salaam
Delhi   Florence   Hong Kong   Istanbul   Karachi
Kuala Lumpur   Madras   Madrid   Melbourne
Mexico City   Nairobi   Paris   Singapore
Taipei   Tokyo   Toronto   Warsaw

and associated companies in
Berlin   Ibadan

Library of Congress Cataloging-in-Publication Data
Brody, Baruch A.
The ethics of biomedical research :
an international perspective / Baruch A. Brody.
p.   cm.
Includes bibliographical references and index.
ISBN 0-19-509007-1
1. Medicine—Research—Moral and ethical aspects.
2. Human experimentation in medicine—Moral and ethical aspects.
3. Medical ethics.
I. Title.   [DNLM: 1. Research.   2. Ethics, Medical.
W 20.5 B8645e 1998]   R852.B76   1998
174'.28—dc21   DNLM/DLC   for Library of Congress   97-41328

9 8 7 6 5 4 3 2 1

Printed in the United States of America
on acid-free paper.

To my grandchildren,
Azriel and Akiva

PREFACE

This book summarizes the results of more than a decade of my research. Portions of that research appeared as a book, *Ethical Issues in Drug Testing, Approval, and Pricing*, published by Oxford in 1995. The current book takes a broader look at a larger set of ethical issues raised by scientific research on animal and human subjects. It also emphasizes, in a way that my earlier book only indicated, the emergence of an international dialogue about research ethics. This dialogue has resulted in the adoption of extensive official policies in many countries on this broader set of ethical issues. This fascinating development has not received adequate attention in the scholarly literature.

When I first began working on this book, I was not fully aware of the extent of this material. Much of it is not published in the indexed literature, so even finding out about it is not an easy task. I made an extensive effort to locate all of the official material from the international organizations and from the policy-making bodies of the research intensive countries in North America, western Europe, and the Pacific Rim. These are, after all, the main centers for biomedical research. The search uncovered thousands of pages of material, much of it of a very thoughtful nature. This book deals with the issues of research ethics through an analysis of the official policies in this area that had been adopted by July 1, 1997.

There is another set of ethical issues related to scientific research that this book does not address, although they too have attracted much official attention throughout the research-intensive parts of the world. These are questions related to scientific integrity in the conduct and publication of scientific research. I hope to return to these questions in a companion volume to this book.

My interest in these ethical issues and in the official policies relating to them was stimulated by my extensive practical involvement with them. I prepared two background reports on the ethical issues related to patenting the results of biotechnology and one background report on the ethical issues related to the new reproductive technologies for the Congressional Office of Technology Assessment. I headed the NASA Bioethics Policy Task Force. I have served on many Data Safety and Monitoring Boards for the National Institutes of Health; currently, I serve on such boards for the NHLBI, the Eye Institute, and the AIDS Clinical Trials Group. I am thankful to all of these agencies for giving me the opportunity both to serve and to learn. As I argued in my 1995 Presidential Address to the Society for Health and Human Values, this type of practical learning is crucial for understanding the complexities of the issues of research ethics.

Special thanks are due to my research assistant, Maureen Kelley, for her extraordinary help with this project. Her efforts extend beyond the usual help expected of research assistants, such as help in finding material and in copyediting the manuscript. She has continually challenged earlier versions of this manuscript on a wide variety of intellectual issues. I believe that this has resulted in a much more thoughtful analysis.

Finally, the dedication of this book to my first two grandchildren is an acknowledgment of the joy they continually provide to Dena and myself.

Houston, Tex.   B. A. B.
June 1997

CONTENTS

THE ETHICS OF BIOMEDICAL RESEARCH

INTRODUCTION

The Emergence of Research Ethics Policies

In February of 1997, the world was stunned to learn that a Scottish research group, headed by Ian Wilmut, had created a living lamb, Dolly, through cloning from an adult cell. The immediate reaction was a combination of wonder at this new scientific advance and of ethical concern about this new technological capacity. The ethics of research on cloning humans attracted particular concern. Throughout the world, political leaders (such as President Clinton of the United States, President Santer of the European Commission, and President Chirac of France) called upon their bioethics advisory committees to advise them about whether new official policies were needed to deal with this new issue of research ethics.[1] These political leaders took for granted that new issues of research ethics were of concern to their governments and that there might be a need for new official ethics policies to be developed by official bioethics advisory boards.

It is not surprising that they could take this for granted. Such official policies on research ethics have become very common. To give just one example, the Committee of Ministers of the Council of Europe, in November of 1996, approved a Convention on Human Rights and Biomedicine. This Convention contained four articles directly related to research and several other articles indirectly related to research. As Maurice DeWachter[2] has pointed out:

> Finally, we must remember that the convention should be read as a legal not an ethical document. . . . On the other hand, the text is a mix of law and ethics, both in being clearly informed by ethical principles and in explicitly incorporating ethics into specific rules for certain fields of biomedicine.

3

The same could be said about many other already adopted official policies relating to research ethics and about those official policies that may emerge in response to the issue of human cloning research.

This book analyzes the issues of research ethics through a review of official national policies that respond to ethical questions about most aspects of research involving subjects, both animal and human. Most of these policies have emerged in the past thirty years (1967–96), although a few date back to the late nineteenth century. As the review will show, these official policies have identified a large number of issues and have developed ethically informed responses to them. They serve therefore as a splendid springboard for an analysis of the issues of research ethics.

There are both a large number of issues and a significant number of responses to each of the issues. Since my goal is to analyze the issues, not just describe official policies, I will offer a preliminary evaluation of the official responses. In that evaluation, emphasis will be placed on whether particular policies have paid attention to the relevant values that have been discussed in the course of the policy development process and on whether those values have been properly balanced. My assumption is that the best official policies are those that have properly balanced the many relevant values that have been identified.

Such an analysis, focusing on each issue separately and looking only at the balancing of the values explicitly identified in the policy development process, is obviously incomplete. What is also needed is a more systematic analysis focusing on questions of origins, of comprehensiveness, of convergence, and of evaluation. Why have so many official policies been adopted to deal with questions of research ethics? How comprehensive are they? Do the policies agree or disagree? Finally, and most crucially, do they represent real moral insight into the issues of research ethics or just a compromise among those values that have found official acceptance? These broader questions will be discussed in Chapter Ten.

The rest of this introduction will briefly describe the topics to be covered in the nine main chapters and say something about the main sources of the official policies.

The Book's Coverage

Chapter One examines issues related to the use of animals in research. It identifies five major positions on the legitimacy of their use and shows that the official policies are based on one of two positions, the human priority position or the balancing of interests position. It shows how these two positions structure the policies by which animals are protected, what protections are required, and what balancing of interests must occur. Finally, two special issues, transgenic animals and xenografts, are considered.

Chapter Two covers issues related to the use of human beings in research. It reveals a remarkable consensus in the official policies about general principles, with some disagreement in details, about such questions as: when must research be independently reviewed, what standards of informed consent and favorable risk/benefit ratio must be met, whom should be chosen as subjects, and how should confidentiality be protected. The issue of compensation for research harms receives special attention because there is less of a consensus about it.

Chapter Three deals with issues raised by epidemiological research, where one is collecting and analyzing information about human subjects rather than experimenting on them. Emphasis is placed on the treatment in the official policies of three concerns: protecting confidentiality, minimizing invasions of privacy, and obtaining consent where appropriate. Cross-cultural studies raise some further concerns, which are examined. Special attention is paid to these issues in connection with policies about genetic studies on stored tissue samples and about HIV seroprevalence studies. Finally, ethical issues in the new area of interventional epidemiology are given a preliminary analysis.

Chapter Four discusses ethical issues relating to genetic research. A separate analysis is offered of the policies governing genetic engineering, gene therapy, the use of the results of the genome project, and the patenting of genes. While each of these areas has been very controversial, it is shown that there is an increasing consensus in the official policies that the ethical issues in genetic research should be dealt with by applying the standard principles of research ethics.

Chapter Five examines ethical issues related to reproductive and fetal research. Three main issues are considered: research on fetuses in utero, the use of fetal tissue in research, and research on preimplantation zygotes. Issues related to research on pregnant women are examined in a later chapter. It is shown that these are among the most contentious areas of research ethics; the attempt to forge official policies that constitute moral compromises on these issues has been far from successful, although there has been more success on the fetal tissue issue than on the preimplantation zygote issue.

Chapter Six deals with ethical issues related to research on vulnerable subjects. The official policies cover three groups of vulnerable subjects: children, mentally infirm adults, and prisoners. We examine the special protections offered under these policies and consider the question of whether or not these special protections may sometimes have been excessive and may have resulted in these groups losing the benefits of being research subjects.

Chapter Seven identifies the main features of controlled clinical trials, the most important contemporary form of clinical research on human subjects, and raises a series of ethical issues related to these features. Among the issues considered: when it is appropriate to commence such a trial, what type of control group should be employed, how should randomization be conducted when there is subject opposition to being randomized, what burdens for protecting blinding are acceptable, what end points should be chosen, and what type of interim monitoring mechanisms and stopping rules should be employed. It is noted that official policies, while strongly favoring controlled clinical trials, do not really address these issues, so they are analyzed in light of the broader professional literature.

Chapter Eight addresses ethical issues raised by the drug and device approval policies. The first part of the chapter analyzes the ethical foundations of these policies themselves. The second half of the chapter raises research ethics issues related to these policies, including the conduct of phase I trials, monitoring for safety in the research process, extrapolating research results from one population to another, and the use of surrogate end points.

Chapter Nine examines issues related to gender and underrepresented minorities in the research process. Among the issues considered are including women and members of various minority groups in clinical trials, including women of childbearing potential in clinical trials, and including pregnant women in clinical trials. Recent changes in official policies are presented and analyzed.

The Sources of the Official Policies

These national policies have at least four sources. Some of them are found in national legislation, some in regulations and/or guidelines issued by governmental agencies that fund the research in question, some in reports issued by commissions created by national governments, and some in guidelines and/or reports issued by major national professional organizations. Often, they were issued in response to international policies formulated by a wide variety of international organizations. Many of these policies are reprinted in the appendices to this book.

At the international level, it is clear that three efforts have played and/or are playing a major role in stimulating the continuing development of official policies on research ethics. The first is the World Medical Association's Declaration of Helsinki (1964; latest revision, 1996, Appendix 1.2), which remains the fundamental international statement on research involving human subjects. That organization has also issued other influential statements, including a 1989 statement on fetal tissue research (Appendix 1.3) and a 1992 statement on the Human Genome Project (Appendix 1.4). The second is the collaborative efforts of the World Health Organization and the Council for International Organizations of Medical Sciences, which resulted in the publication of international guidelines on research involving human subjects (1982, revised in 1993, Appendix 1.8), on research involving animals (1984, Appendix 1.6) and on epidemiological research (1991, Appendix 1.7). The third is the International Harmonization effort carried out by the major drug/device regulatory agencies, whose recent reports (most importantly, 1996 Guidelines for Good Clinical Practice, Appendix 1.5) are just now beginning to stimulate needed policies. Although none of these efforts constitute official policies, they have certainly stimulated and will continue to influence the development of such policies at the national level.

In the United States, the most important sources of official policies are the regulations and reports issued by such agencies as the Department of Health and Human Services (DHHS), the National Institutes of Health (NIH), which funds a major portion of biomedical research, and by the Food and Drug Administration (FDA), which reviews and evaluates research in deciding whether to approve new drugs and devices for sale. The most important regulations are regulations dating back to the 1960s (revised many times) on the clinical research needed to support drug/device approval (portions of which are Appendices 3.4 and 3.5), 1981 regulations (supplemented in 1983 and revised in 1991) on research on human subjects (Appendix 3.1), 1985 regulations (revised in 1986) on the care and use of laboratory animals (the governing principles of which are Appendix 3.3), 1994 regulations (replacing regulations from the 1970s and 1980s) on safety in research involving genetic engineering and on gene therapy,[3] 1993/1994 regulations on the inclusion of women and minorities in research (Appendices 3.6 and 3.11), and 1995 regulations on emergency research (Appendix 3.7). These regulations are supplemented by a number of major reports, some of which have been implemented and others of which have not. These include a 1994 report on preimplantation zygote research (Appendix 3.9), a 1995 report on genetic research on stored tissue samples,[4] and a 1997 report on genetic testing.[5] They are also supplemented by a number of important NIH internal policies such as the 1986 policy on research involving impaired human subjects (Appendix 3.8) and the 1996 policy on patenting human genomic sequences (Appendix 3.10). None of this denies a role to legislation as a source of official policies on research ethics in the United States. In addition to creating the statutory basis for the above-described regulations, legislation has played a significant role in the formulation of official policy on the use of fetal tissue (allowed by 1993 legislation, Appendix 3.11) and on the inclusion of women and minorities in clinical research (mandated by 1993 legislation, Appendix 3.11). It has also played a continuing role in the debate on preimplantation zygote research. There are also important reports from various professional groups. But it is clear that the regulations and reports issued by the major federal agencies are the source of most of the operative official U.S. policies on research ethics.

A similar picture emerges when one looks at Canada and Australia. In Canada, the main source of official policies has been guidelines issued by funding agencies and quasi-official bodies. Two of the most important of these are the 1993 guidelines on the care and use of research animals issued by the Canadian Council on Animal Care (Appendices 4.9 and 4.10) and the 1990 Canadian Federal Center for AIDS guidelines on seroprevalence research (Appendix 4.11). In addition, replacing earlier guidelines dating back to the 1970s, the three councils that fund research issued in March of 1996 the draft of a very comprehensive code dealing with a large number of issues related to research involving human subjects.[6] A revised version of that draft appeared late in the spring of 1997.[7] The most important legislative activity is the 1996 act on reproductive research,[8] but this is really an exception to the general practice of formulating official policies in guidelines. In Australia, the main sources of official policies are guidelines from the Australian National Health and Medical Research Council on human experimentation (the latest version, issued in 1992, Appendix 4.12, contains supplements on vulnerable subjects, clinical trials, and reproductive and genetic research) and on the care and use of research animals (1990).[9] Reproductive research provides once more the main example of legislative activity, with legislation from Victoria, from 1984 and from 1995, being the main examples of legislative contributions to official policies on research ethics.[10]

The picture in western Europe is quite different. With the exception of Great Britain, which will be discussed below, legislation is the main source of official bioethics policy there.

Before turning to particular countries, we should consider crucial transnational European legislation on research ethics. There are two sources of transnational European legislation, the Council of Europe and the European Union (formerly known as the European Community). The Council of Europe, the group with more members but with less legal authority, has been particularly active in the area of research ethics. Its Committee of Ministers issued a 1990 recommendation (Appendix 2.2) to member states on adopting legislation on research involving human subjects and a 1992 recommendation (Appendix 2.5) to member states on adopting legislation on genetic testing and screening. Its Parliamentary Assembly adopted a 1982 recommendation on genetic engineering[11] and 1986 and 1989 recommendations on the use of fetuses and embryos in research (Appendix 2.4). In 1996, it adopted a convention on human rights and biomedicine (the sections on research are in Appendix 2.3). The European Union, with fewer members but with far more legal authority, has also been active in the area of research ethics. Its Council issued a 1986 directive on the use of animals in research (Appendix 2.1), three very important 1990 directives (modified in 1994) on genetic engineering,[12] and a 1995 directive on privacy of personal data, which included important policies on the use of such data in epidemiological research.[13] It extensively debated a proposed directive on patenting the results of biotechnological research but was unable to agree on a final directive. The work of these two transnational European groups constitutes a major legislative effort to fashion official bioethics policy. There are also some nonlegislative European transnational policies. One good example is the 1988 recommendations of the European Medical Research Councils on human gene therapy (Appendix 2.6). But these are clearly far less important than the legislative efforts.

Although France has an extremely active and influential official national ethics committee, official bioethics policy, including research ethics policy, is set through legislative action. There is 1987 legislation on animal experimentation,[14] 1988 legislation on human research (Appendix 4.8), and 1994 legislation on reproductive and genetic research.[15] Germany has been far less active in research ethics, but legislation has been central to such formulation of official policy as has occurred. There is 1986 legislation on animal research,[16] 1990 legislation on reproductive and genetic research (Appendix 4.7), and a first modest legislative effort on research involving humans incorporated into the 1994 revisions of the German Drug Law.[17]

Great Britain provides an excellent example of official research ethics policy being formulated in a wide variety of sources. There is important legislation including 1986 legislation on animal research (replacing legislation ultimately dating back to 1876, Appendix 4.3) and the 1990 Human Fertilization and Embryology Act governing reproductive research (Appendix 4.4). There are important official guidelines including 1992 guidelines from the Medical Research Council on research on human subjects[18] and on the use of vulnerable subjects (Appendix 4.2), 1994 gene therapy guidelines from the Gene Therapy Advisory Committee,[19] and a 1993 code of practice from the Human Fertilisation and Embryology Authority.[20] The official research policy incorporated in these legislative acts and guidelines has been greatly influenced by a series of official reports, including the 1984 Warnock Report, which considered reproductive research,[21] the 1989 Polkinghorne Report, which considered the use of fetal tissue in research (Appendix 4.5), and the 1992 Clothier Report, which considered gene therapy (Appendix 4.6). Finally, there are extremely influential reports issued in 1990 (Appendix 4.1) and 1996[22] by the Royal College of Physicians and by the recently constituted Nuffield Council on Bioethics.[23]

Japan's efforts in this area are relatively recent (Appendix 4.13), although it is now an active partner in the International Harmonization Effort. It remains to be seen which pathways for the development of research policy in Japan will predominate.

This review of the existing sources clearly substantiates the claim that the formulation of such policies has been a widespread activity in the past thirty years. We turn in the next nine chapters to an analysis of the content of this international regulation of research on subjects.

animals. This is, of course, exactly what is called for by the human priority position.

According to another (the "balancing") position, animal interests, although not as important as human interests, are sufficiently important that they can sometimes take precedence over human interests. This is true when the benefits to humans from some research is modest while the sufferings and losses to animals is great. In such cases, according to the balancing position, we should give up the potential benefits and not perform the research; merely attempting to minimize the considerable suffering and losses, as called for by the human priority position, is not enough. The balancing position leads, on at least some occasions, to animal interests impacting upon whether research is performed, and not just on how it is performed. As we shall see below, this position has also had some impact on official national policies.

According to the last of the human welfare positions, the "equal consideration" position, animal losses and suffering count as much as the equivalent human losses and sufferings, although the differences between species may mean that some experiments on animals would cause less losses or less sufferings than the same experiments on humans. This means that any evaluation of experiments on animals needs to consider the impacts on all affected equally and are morally licit only when the gains for human beings are sufficient to outweigh the suffering and losses to the animals. This is the position advocated by Peter Singer in 1975 in his book *Animal Liberation*,[16] a book that has had a tremendous role in strengthening the opposition to the use of live animals in research. In that book, Singer argued that suffering was equally bad regardless of the species that suffered; a failure to accept this was considered speciesism, a form of discrimination akin to racism or sexism. Those following this position have sometimes suggested that the painless killing of those animals (including at least some mammals) that did not have a conscious awareness of themselves as distinct entities was less problematic. If this was done as part of a research project that produced sufficient benefit, it might be a legitimate example of animal research. The same is true for the killing of animals bred for research who would be replaced with other animals bred for the same purposes. Still other animal research, even on animals that had a conscious awareness of themselves, would be justified if the losses to the animals were outweighed by the gains to humans, counting all interests equally. This position is, therefore, less restrictive on human research than the animal rights position, which does not ever allow aggregate human gains to outweigh losses to research animals, although it is certainly far more restrictive on animal research than any of the other animal welfare positions. It should be noted, however, that many recent authors have suggested that the animal rights position should be modified by allowing that animal rights are not absolute and can be overridden by sufficient benefits from the research, benefits that fall short of those involved in Regan's ''lifeboat'' cases of extreme necessity. This would bring the animal rights position closer to agreement with the equal consideration version of the animal welfare position.

In short, we have one position (human dominion) that places no moral constraints on animal research, two (human priority and balancing) that place constraints while accepting the basic legitimacy of animal research, and two (equal consideration and animal rights) that challenge the basic legitimacy of most animal research. The following table summarizes these various positions:

	Human Dominion	Human Priority	Balancing	Equal Consideration	Animal Rights
Animals have rights	No	No	No	No	Yes
Animal interests count	No	Yes	Yes	Yes	Yes
Animal interests can outweigh human interests	No	No	Yes	Yes	Yes
Equality for animal interests	No	No	No	Yes	Yes

In the next section, we will see how either the human priority or the balancing position lies behind the national policies on animal research that have emerged in most countries, all of which accept that animal interests count but none of which accept that they deserve the same consideration as human interests. These approaches face serious intellectual challenges, both in defending their assigning greater significance to human interests and in defining their differing views on how animal interests count; we will return to these issues in the final section of the chapter. Nevertheless, in a world in which humans consume animals for food, it is not surprising that only these two positions have been adopted as the basis for official policies.

National Policies on Animal Research: A Cross-National Comparison

The development of policies regulating animal research is now a common practice in research-intensive countries. As just indicated, these policies attempt to implement the animal welfare position either in the form of the human priority position or in the form of the balancing position. In this section, we will review these policies, identifying the issues on which they agree as well as those on which they disagree.

Our analysis in the first two sections makes it easier to identify the crucial issues faced by any policy designed to implement the animal welfare approach. They are:

1. Which animals are protected, and are some animals given more protection than others?
2. How are the policies enforced?
3. What requirements are imposed to replace the use of animals where possible?
4. What requirements are imposed to reduce the number of animals used?
5. What requirements are imposed to minimize pain and discomfort in the conduct of research?
6. What requirements are imposed to minimize pain and discomfort in the living conditions of research animals?
7. Is there a requirement to balance the losses to the animals against the gain to humans from the research?

In looking at the policies in place in each country, we will focus on these seven issues.

We will begin with Great Britain, given that the first act governing animal research implementing an animal welfare position was passed there in 1876. British animal research is currently governed by the Animals (Scientific Procedures) Act of 1986 (Appendix 4.3), which replaced the 1876 legislation. The earlier act had not addressed many crucial issues, including the care of animals outside of the actual research, the number and type of animals used, the consideration of alternatives to the use of animals, and the balancing of the gains of the research against the losses to the animals. By the 1979 general election, all major parties, in response to considerable public concern, had agreed that new legislation was needed.

The 1986 act protects all living vertebrates, although cats, dogs, primates, and equidae are given greater protection in that they cannot be used in any research for which other animals are suitable and available. In addition, mice, rats, guineapigs, hamsters, rabbits, dogs, cats, and primates must be obtained from designated breeding or supplying establishments. The Act is enforced by the Secretary of State through a set of inspectors and independent assessors who recommend the issuance of personal licenses authorizing individuals to do certain types of research and the issuance of project licenses authorizing particular research projects. No research that may have the effect of causing pain, distress, or lasting harm to a protected animal can be performed unless the investigator has a personal license and unless the project has a project license. Before a project license is issued, the investigator must show that it is not feasible to achieve the results by use of alternatives to vertebrates. The personal license requires that pain and distress in the research be minimized consistently with the purposes of the research and that research animals be humanely killed at the end of the research if they are likely to continue to suffer or undergo adverse effects. The project license specifies where the research will be conducted, and such establishments must have a person responsible for day-by-day management of the animals and an expert who advises on animal health and welfare. A Home Office Code has regulated the housing and care of animals in such establishments. Finally, the Act specifies the purposes for which animals are legitimately used and requires that the Secretary "weigh the likely adverse effects on the animals concerned against the benefit likely to accrue as the result of the programme to be specified in the licence" (Appendix 4.3, section 5.4).

This last clause is particularly important. To begin with, it indirectly authorizes a reduction in the number of animals used, for the weighing will be more favorable to the research if fewer animals suffer the adverse effects. More importantly, however, it clearly shows that the British policy is based on the balancing position, as opposed to the human priority position. All of the other provisions summarized above maintain the priority of needed research and merely call for minimizing losses to animals when that is compatible with carrying on the research. It is only this last provision that would stop research when the gains to humans are not sufficient to justify the losses to the animals, and that is what is called for by the balancing approach.

In 1991, the Institute of Medical Ethics published a report on the meaning and implementation of the 1986 act.[17] One of the most important chapters was devoted to the question of how this balancing should be carried out. No algorithm was provided, but the Working Party developed a detailed scheme for rating proposed research in the light of likely benefits from the research and likely costs to the animals. Their analysis is an important contribution to the development of the balancing approach.

The rest of Europe also actively developed animal research policies in the 1980s. Central to these efforts was a directive issued in 1986 by the European Communities (Appendix 2.1). The Directive protects all living vertebrates, and it mandates that animals with the lowest degree of neurophysiological sensitivity be used, thereby offering greater protection to primates, cats and dogs, and so forth. In general, only animals bred for use in research should be used, and no exceptions can be given to this principle in the case of dogs and cats. Each member country is required to set up an authority to supervise animal research. The minimum number of animals must be used, and it must be demonstrated that there are no feasible alternatives to the use of those animals. In the conduct of the experiments, anesthesia must be used where possible, pain must be limited if that is not possible, and it must be ensured that "in any event the animal is not subject to severe pain, distress or suffering" (Appendix 2.1, section 8.3). This last clause is later modified by the provision that experiments producing severe prolonged pain will not be allowed unless the authority is satisfied "that the experiment is of sufficient importance for meeting the essential needs of man or animal" (Appendix 2.1, section 12.2). How that is to be reconciled with the earlier provision is unclear. In any case, if necessary to prevent post-research pain or suffering, the animals should be euthanized. Living conditions should be structured so that the animals receive housing, freedom of movement, food, water, and care appropriate to both their health and well-being, and restrictions imposed that limit their satisfying their physiological and ethological needs are to be limited to the absolute minimum. There is no explicit provision for a general balancing of human gains and animal losses, although such a balancing seems to be suggested in the above-mentioned clause authorizing experiments that produce severe prolonged pain.

Because there is no general balancing rule, the European Directive seems to be based on the human priority position, rather than the balancing position that is the basis for the 1986 British Act, despite the provision limiting experiments that produce severe prolonged pain. In any case, as can be seen from the above summary, the European version of the human priority position is very strict in protecting animal welfare within the constraints of human priority. In addition, the Europeans have funded a major center, the European Center for the Validation of Alternative Methods (ECVAM), which is responsible, among other things, for developing and/or validating alternative methods for testing the toxicity of cosmetics. The goal had been to complete the development/validation process before a ban on animal testing went into place in 1998, but problems in validation have led to a delay in the ban at least until 2000.[18]

Most of the European countries, whether or not members of the European Union, have adopted legislation in keeping with the Directive. There are some differences. Some countries (Sweden, the Netherlands) require research to be approved by institutional or multi-institutional ethics committee, others (Germany, Switzerland) require regional governmental approval, while others (France) require approval at a national level (Ministry of Agriculture). More crucially, the countries vary on how close they come to the British adoption of a complete balancing position. The following provision of the German statute comes close: "Experiments may be carried out on vertebrates only if the pain, suffering, or harm which they can be expected to inflict upon the animals is ethically justifiable in relation to the purpose of the experiment."[19] The Swiss 1981 statute calls for a general balancing approach. Moreover, it prohibits research producing severe pain that cannot be alleviated, regardless of the benefits to be obtained from the research, going beyond the balancing approach. Nevertheless, the Directive, with its partial commitment to balancing, seems to be the impetus for much of the European legislation.

We turn from the European policies to the policies in the United States. There are two different regulatory schemes in place in the United States, one administered by the Public Health Service (PHS) through the NIH and the other by the Department of Agriculture. Both were strengthened in 1985–86. In part this was a result of public pressures arising from controversies such as the controversy mentioned above over the University of Pennsylvania's program to study whiplash damage in baboons, a program whose videotapes were stolen and then made public by animal activists. In part, however, this was part of an international trend that produced the revisions to the U.K. Act and the European Directive.

The PHS's regulations issued in September of 1986[20] reflect both an extension of its own activities, which go back to 1971, and a 1985 congressional mandate that required by law what had been until then just an internal PHS policy. The regulations explicitly define their role as implementing and supplementing the "Interagency Principles for the Utilization and Care of Vertebrate Animals Used in Testing, Research, and Training"(Appendix 3.3). These principles, which clearly embody the human priority position, emphasize the humane care of animals both during the research and while they live in research facilities, but also talk about using alternative methods, choosing the right species, and minimizing the number of animals used. At no point do they introduce any balancing considerations.

The PHS regulations cover all vertebrates used in research, training, experimentation, or testing funded by the PHS. Most crucially, the regulations are primarily enforced by local institutional animal care and use committees (IACUCs), whose activities are overseen by the Office for Protection of Research Risks at the NIH. These committees (which must contain a research scientist; a veterinarian; a non-scientist such as a clergyman, ethicist, or lawyer; and an individual not affiliated with the institution) are responsible (1) for reviewing both the institution's program for humane care and use of animals and the institution's animal facilities to ensure that they are in accord with the National Research Council's *Guide for the Care and Use of Laboratory Animals* (1985, revised in 1996[21]) and (2) for reviewing all research protocols involving animals to ensure that they are in accord with NIH policy. Proposals from investigators must justify both the use of animals and the species and number employed, and the evaluation of this justification is the main mechanism for replacing or reducing animal research. Unless sound research considerations require otherwise, procedures must minimize discomfort, distress, and pain; and sedation, analgesia, or anesthesia must be used when there is more than momentary slight pain or distress. At the end of the research, animals that would otherwise experience severe or chronic pain or distress must be euthanized. The living conditions of research animals must be appropriate for their species and contribute to their health and comfort. The *Guide* and supplementary documents specify conditions for housing, sanitation, veterinary care, and the environment. As noted above, there are no balancing provisions. In short, the PHS regulations are very much like the European Directive except for avoiding any references to balancing and for employing as a specific enforcement mechanism the IACUC.

In 1993, the U.S. Congress strengthened the commitment to the 3R program, which is central to the human priority position. In the 1993 NIH Revitalization Act,[22] Congress directed the NIH to develop a plan for research into methods of research that do not require animals (replacement research), into methods of research that employ fewer animals or nonmammalian marine life (reduction research), and into methods of research that produce less pain or distress (refinement research). The plan should provide for validating these new methods, for encouraging their use, and for training researchers in their use. It remains to be seen what will result from this new mandate, as a similar mandate in the 1985 Health Research Extension Act produced few results.

The second U.S. regulatory scheme is enforced by the Department of Agriculture and grows out of the 1985 version of the Animal Welfare Act.[23] In one respect, it is broader than the PHS regulatory scheme; in other respects, it is less encompassing; and in many respects, it is very similar. It is broader in that it regulates research on animals, regardless of whether the research is funded by federal funds. It is less encompassing in that the statute explicitly applies only to warm-blooded animals and is interpreted not to apply to birds, rats, and mice. That interpretation was challenged in the courts, but the challenge was ultimately dismissed on procedural grounds,[24] so the interpretation remains in place. It is very similar in many ways, because it also mandates enforcement by IACUCs, regulates the conditions under which research animals live (with extra provisions for dog exercise and primate physical environment adequate to promote psychological well-being), requires that research pain is minimized by appropriate use of anaesthetic or analgesic drugs and by euthanasia, and calls upon the principal investigator to consider alternatives. It does all of this despite a specific provision that the Secretary has no authority to regulate the actual conduct of research. As a result, the officially sponsored *Institutional Animal Care and Use Committee Guidebook*[25] guides committees to satisfy the very similar requirements of the two regulatory schemes.

This system of using local committees to supervise animal research was actually invented by the Canadians in 1968 when the Canadian Council on Animal Care (CCAC) was created by a coalition of researchers, academic and commercial research sponsors, and humane societies. That system continues in effect today, with the local committees enforcing nationally developed guides in a process that is monitored by a CCAC Assessment Program. The national standards (Appendix 4.9) are very strongly in the human priority camp, with an emphasis on the 3Rs, but some forms of extreme suffering are treated as unacceptable, no matter what the research rationale. They are also noticeable for extending their protection to some invertebrates such as cephalopods that are judged to have nervous systems as well developed as those of some vertebrates, and for developing an extremely useful system for categorizing the invasiveness of animal experiments as a guide to the deliberations of the local committees.

More generally, the system is notable for its involvement of nearly all groups with an interest in the issue, ensuring much less controversy than exists in other countries.

Australia is the major example of a country using the local committee approach that has adopted the balancing position. Animal research in Australia is governed by an *Australian Code of Practice for the Care and Use of Animals for Scientific Purposes*, whose fifth edition was issued in 1990.[26] Several states have mandated by legislation that researchers follow that code, which has several notable features. Although the code is formally confined to vertebrates, investigators are encouraged to apply it to "higher order invertebrates."[27] The local committees must contain at least one representative from an animal welfare organization. There is a strong preference for animals bred in captivity. Most crucially, and somewhat analogously to the British Act, one of the standards for approval is that "experiments using animals may be performed only after a decision has been made that they are justified, weighing the scientific or educational value of the experiment against the potential effects on the welfare of the animals."[28] It is this standard that represents the Australian commitment to the balancing position.

Having reviewed the policies in place in the major research countries, let us now summarize what we have learned about the seven questions we asked at the beginning of the section. On the whole, the policies apply to research involving all vertebrates. The U.S. regulations, however, do not apply to privately funded research involving cold-blooded vertebrates or birds, mice, and rats. Many of the policies require, where possible, the use of specially bred research animals, and primates, dogs, and cats are offered extra protections by some policies. The policies are enforced in the United Kingdom and France by a national agency, in Germany and Switzerland by local agencies, and in Sweden, the United States, Canada, and Australia by local institutional committees. All of the policies are committed at least in theory to encouraging researchers to consider alternatives to the use of animal subjects and to minimize the use of animals when they are required. All certainly emphasize minimizing animal suffering both in the conduct of research and in the living conditions of the research animals. Finally, some (Great Britain, Switzerland, Australia, and perhaps Germany) explicitly endorse the general balancing principle of forbidding research when the gains to humans are not sufficient to justify the sufferings of the animals, others (those following the European Directive) do so at least in cases where there is severe pain or distress, and some (primarily, the United States) involve no explicit balancing principle. As a conclusion, we can say then that the international policies agree that animal interests count, but not equally with human interests, and disagree as to whether animal interests can sometimes outweigh human interests.

Two Special Cases: Transgenic Animals and Xenotransplantation

In recent years, two types of research involving animals have raised considerable controversy. One involves the creation of transgenic animals and the other involves transplanting animal organs to critically ill human recipients. In this section, I will examine these controversies to see what additional issues are raised by them. Do these two controversies illustrate the need to amplify currently existing national policies, or are the issues raised in these controversies resolvable by reference to the already existing policies on animal research?

The issue of research on transgenic animals was brought to public attention when the U.S. Patent Office issued on April 12, 1988, a patent for a transgenic nonhuman animal whose germ cells and somatic cells contain an activated oncogene sequence that causes an increased propensity for the animal to develop cancerous tumors.[29] These Harvard oncomouses can be used to test in smaller amounts materials suspected of being carcinogenic and can also be used to test the efficacy of substances that might confer protection against the development of cancers.

This example illustrates the use of transgenic animals as disease models. A second use of transgenic animals is to produce valuable and expensive pharmaceuticals in their milk. A third use is the modification of animals (e.g., pigs, sheep) to produce animals with more desirable features such as being lower in fat and cholesterol.

The issuance of the patent in 1988 was based on an earlier announcement in 1987 by the U.S. Patent Office[30] that "nonnaturally occurring nonhuman multicellular living organisms, including animals" would be patentable subject matter under U.S. Patent law.

The European Patent Office, the central office for patents in the European Union, operates under the European Patent Convention that allows the patenting of life forms if they are novel, inventive, and applicable in industry, providing that the patents are not contrary to public order and that they do not cover plant or animal varieties per se. Under this approach, the European Patent Office also eventually issued a patent for the Harvard oncomouse.[31]

The debate over these patents and over the creation of transgenic animals took a different path in the United States and in Europe. In the United States, there were calls for a moratorium and a discussion of the issues by a variety of figures, but these were not heeded, and the Patent Office issued additional patents in 1992 and in subsequent years. However, in 1995 the issue was rekindled by a strong statement of opposition issued by a large number of religious leaders.[32] The results of that debate remain to be seen. In Europe, the debate centered around the attempt, starting in 1988, to draft a European Union Directive on the Legal Protection of Biotechnological Inventions, a Directive that also attempted to address other issues, including the highly controversial issue of patenting human parts and genes. By early 1995, that attempt failed when the European Parliament rejected the latest version.[33] It remains to be seen what will happen to the debate in Europe as new attempts are being made to revise the Directive.

What issues were raised in this controversy? Some, about the legitimacy of interfering with genetic integrity and about the patentability of what is living, are issues about genetic biotechnology in general, and will be discussed in Chapter Four. Others, however, relate primarily to animals, and they are our concern here.

One of the animal-specific issues relates to patentability. A concise statement of it is found in a 1995 statement by Methodist Bishop Kenneth Carder, who said, ''The patenting of life forms reduces life to its marketability. Gone is the fundamental principle that life is a gift that ought to be shared and nurtured.''[34] A number of observations seem in place: (1) Whatever the merits of this claim in connection with the patenting of human genes or parts, it seems questionable when dealing with animals whom we market for food on an everyday basis. Why may we own, market, and slaughter for food individual animals, but not own and market for use in research animal types? (2) The current policy consensus on research on animals is clearly based on one or another version of the idea that important-enough human interests take precedence over animal interests. There is a significant human interest in the patenting of transgenic animals. Commercial sponsors of research will not fund research on transgenic animals unless they can benefit from that research by having the exclusive ownership of its results offered by patents. Unless society is prepared to pay directly for this research, we will lose its potential benefits if we adopt a non-patenting policy. Why then should respect for animal life suddenly take precedence? In short, unless the proponents of the ban on patenting animal life forms are really calling for a far broader revolution in our attitude toward animals, a revolution that extends much beyond this patenting issue, the basis for their proposed ban on patenting is unclear.

The other animal-specific issue is directly related to the animal research questions that have been the main focus of this chapter: can we be sure that the development of transgenic animals will not impose undue suffering on animals? Early transgenic pigs carrying human growth gene suffered, for example, from many health problems (e.g., defective vision, lethargy, and arthritis). Similar concerns about animal suffering were raised by the Harvard oncomouse and were discussed in the decision of the European Patent Office.[35] This issue should be resolvable by a continued application in this area of the general policies on animal research. This is what the European Patent Office did for the Harvard oncomouse, noting the importance of the research (thereby justifying it even according to the balancing approach) and the fact that fewer animals need to be used in testing when oncomouses are used (thereby justifying it according to the 3R aspect of the human priority approach). Naturally, such an analysis might lead to a different conclusion when the research to be advanced by use of the transgenic animals is less important and/or involves no reduction in animal use. There is, however, one problem specific to the United States that needs to be examined. Much research on transgenic animals is non-federally funded research carried on in the labs of private biotechnology firms. As such, it is not governed by the PHS regulations, but only by the Department of Agriculture regulations. As noted above, however, it interprets its regulations to not apply to mouses, so there are animal welfare grounds for being concerned about some of the research on transgenic animals in the United States. This provides a good example of why the U.S. needs to modify its current regulatory schemes to cover all vertebrates in all research settings, which is standard in the policies of all of the other major research countries. If that is done, there would seem to be no animal-specific issue raised by research on transgenic animals that cannot be resolved by appeal to current national policies, whether based on the balancing or the human priority approach.

The second special issue, xenotransplantation research, was intensely discussed in 1995–96. The acute shortage of human organs, resulting in the death of more than three thousand patients on the waiting list in 1994, motivated this interest. On the one hand, advances in controlling rejection and in producing transgenic animals whose organs are less vulnerable to being rejected increased the likelihood of success. On the other hand, past failures of xenografts, including the failure of a transplant of a baboon heart into Baby Fae in 1984 and of baboon bone marrow into a patient with AIDS in 1995, argued for great caution.

As a result, several groups undertook to prepare in 1995–96 reports analyzing both the scientific and ethical issues of xenotransplantation research. In the United States, a report from the Institute of Medicine was issued in 1996.[36] In Great Britain, the Nuffield Council on Bioethics (funded in part by the Medical Research Council) issued a report in early 1996. Another report was issued later in 1996 by a more official government group.[37]

Four crucial ethical issues are clearly identified in the more extensive British reports. The issues and their recommendations are:

1. The ethics of using animals as sources of organs—this seems as acceptable as using animals in research in general; their use as a source for organs should be governed by the standard policies governing animal research.
2. The choice of species—as part of following those policies, nonprimates should be the source of organs for clinical use and, if possible, for the research. The use of transgenic pigs engineered to reduce the risk of rejection is acceptable once further research has validated that the risk is moderate.

3. Independent approvals—research protocols for xenotransplantation must be approved by the usual independent review of research protocols involving animal subjects (discussed in this chapter) and human subjects (discussed in the next chapter). Special attention must be paid to a realistic and full informed consent process. In addition, approval should be obtained from a special national authority that should review, among other things, the minimization of the risks of transmitting pathogens from the animal sources to the human recipients.

4. Choice of subjects—xenotransplantation should begin by using consenting adult patients. Extension of the protocols to cover children and incompetent adults should follow only after successes have been achieved. Those who receive xenotransplants should not be excluded from later receiving human organs if they meet the usual clinical criteria.

As one reviews the animal-related components of these recommendations, one sees that they clearly rest on the standard policies for animal research. The only new animal-related issues are the creation of transgenic pigs and the transmission of pathogens. In dealing with the former, the British reports relied on the growing acceptance, already discussed, of transgenic animals. In dealing with the latter, it adopted the requirement that this new promising research should proceed only after careful assessment of risks by a national panel. As we shall see in Chapter Four, a similar approach was adopted both in Great Britain and in the United States for early research protocols on gene therapy.

Because the United States in 1996 was eliminating that national review of gene therapy protocols, it was not surprising that the Institute of Medicine rejected that proposal. It proposed instead the development of a set of national regulations to be enforced by IRBs in their review of xenotransplantation research protocols, a national advisory committee to monitor results and to suggest changes in the regulations, and a national register of recipients and contacts to facilitate checking for the emergence of new diseases.

In this section, we have reviewed two special cases of research involving animals that have attracted considerable attention. Each raises important ethical concerns, but the animal related ethical concerns raised by both seem manageable within the framework created by currently existing policies.

Conclusion

Research on animals is extensively regulated under the official national policies of the research-intensive countries. One of the reasons for the development of these policies has been revelations of questionable cases that have provoked considerable public concern. This has been the pattern from the concerns in the nineteenth century raised by the public demonstrations given by Magendie and Bernard to the concerns in the 1980s raised by primate research, by the Baby Fae case, and by the Harvard oncomouse. Another reason for the development of these policies is greater concern about animal suffering encouraged by utilitarian and animal rights thinkers, which led to the rejection of the human dominion position.

The national policies that have emerged embody, however, neither the utilitarian equal consideration position nor the animal rights position. Instead, because they all accept that animal interests count, they all adopt the major demands of the human priority position (animal use be replaced where possible, be reduced in extent to the minimum required, and be refined to limit animal suffering both in research and in general living conditions). Many, because they believe that animal interests can sometimes outweigh human interests, also adopt some components of the balancing position, insisting that some research should not be allowed because the burdens it imposes on animals are excessive in comparison to the benefits from the research to humans. We have here an example of an incomplete international consensus, with the major agreement being that animal interests count but not equally with human interests and the major disagreement being over the question of whether the moral status of animals requires a balancing approach.

To an unusual extent, the national policies have been formulated in legislation. This is certainly true for the European Union and for such countries as France and Germany. But it is also true for Great Britain (the 1986 Act) and the United States (the 1985 Animal Welfare Act and the 1993 NIH Reauthorization Act).

Two preliminary evaluative points. First, one aspect of the current U.S. policy, its exclusion from regulation of privately funded research on many vertebrates, is dissonant with all other national policies, has little justification (why should private research on these animals be exempt from regulation when publicly funded research is covered?), and gives rise to particular concerns in the area of research on transgenic animals. It needs to be changed. Second, without entering into a full discussion of the moral status of animals, it is fair to say that the adoption of official policies embodying the human priority position or the balancing position are the only options for societies that accept as legitimate such practices as raising animals for food. Of the two, the balancing position seems more consistent. After all, the policies of limiting animal suffering adopted under the human priority position impose considerable costs on research. Consider, as just one example, the costs of improving the living conditions of research animals. Those funds could have been used instead to fund more research, but we have decided to give a higher priority to protecting animal interests. It seems inconsistent to not give those interests the same priority in cases where the harm to animals from the research is great and the benefits to humans from the research relatively small. It is hard to see how this demand of the balancing position can justifiably be resisted. Further reflection is required to decide whether we should adopt the British general balancing approach or the more limited balancing of the European Directive. Moreover, the question of how to balance interests across species, especially when the interests of one are given some—although not absolute—priority, requires additional reflection. But some balancing of interests seems appropriate even for societies that reject the equal consideration position, and it is to be hoped that it will be incorporated into the national policies not yet containing a balancing component. Whether more is required as a result of a fundamental rethinking of the status of animals is an issue to which we shall return in Chapter Ten.

Chapter two

RESEARCH ON HUMAN SUBJECTS

Basic scientific research often requires research on human subjects and/or on materials drawn from human beings. In addition, basic research often leads to clinical applications, and this involves, as an intermediary step, research on the safety and efficacy of possible clinical applications. A certain amount of that research can be done with animal models, and that is one of the reasons why the animal research discussed in Chapter One is so important. But there comes a time when research on human subjects is required. Basic and clinical research on human subjects must therefore be encouraged if we are to achieve scientific advances and reap their benefits. At the same time, such research often gives rise to ethical dilemmas. In this chapter, we will identify those dilemmas and see how the various official policies have attempted to deal with them in a way that allows needed research to continue while avoiding ethical abuses.

A Historical Introduction

The development of ethical reflection in this area has been greatly influenced by a series of revelations about the inappropriate use of human subjects in research. The most famous of these revelations occurred during the trial in Nuremberg of Nazi physicians for experiments carried on during World War II using unconsenting concentration camp victims as subjects and subjecting them to great pain and suffering, disfigurement, and death. Although these revelations shocked the conscience of humanity and led to some of the earliest international statements of ethical principles governing research on human subjects, they could be dismissed by other researchers as an aberration of the Nazi period that had no relevance to the research efforts of reputable decent researchers. The same attitude could not be adopted to a series of revelations in the United States in the 1960s and the 1970s. Some were primarily noted in an article by Henry Beecher in the *New England Journal of Medicine*.[1] Others (most notably, the Jewish Chronic Disease Hospital case, the Willowbrook case, and the Tuskegee syphilis study) attracted independent attention. Together, they illustrated the need for appropriate standards for conducting research on human subjects even outside the setting of regimes that promoted systematic denials of human rights and they greatly influenced the actual development of official policies on this topic.

Beecher said in his 1966 article that he was concerned that the growing availability of research funds after World War II, combined with the need to publish research results to get that funding and to advance professionally, would put pressure on ambitious young researchers that might lead them to perform unethical experiments. His article described 22 examples from a larger sample of 50 he collected. I will cite just two of his examples to illustrate the nature of the problems he found. One involved a placebo controlled trial of chloramphenicol for typhoid fever after its effectiveness had been recognized. Of the patients who received the placebo 22.9% died as opposed to 7.97% of the patients who received the active drug. Another involved the use of healthy institutionalized subjects to demonstrate the suspected toxicity of a drug. Most developed the expected hepatic dysfunction. Those with the worst results were hospitalized and underwent liver biopsies that demonstrated liver damage. After their liver function test results returned to normal, four were given the drug again, leading in three cases to renewed liver dysfunction. Beecher's own conclusions were that (1) no research should be performed without informed voluntary consent of the subjects, and nobody would have given informed voluntary consent to participate in these dangerous experiments; (2) the gains anticipated from the experiment must be commensurate with the risks, and they were not in these cases, given the losses to the subjects. As a way of enforcing these standards, he suggested that editors should not publish results from studies that did not follow them.

Two of the other studies Beecher mentioned, both of which involved institutionalized patients, acquired independent notoriety. One (the Jewish Chronic Disease Hospital case)[2] involved the injection of live cancer cells into patients in a chronic disease hospital, to study the rate of rejection, without informing the patients that they were being injected with cancer cells. Even if the injection posed no risks to the patient, the research was done without their consent. The second (the Willowbrook case)[3] involved injecting isolated strains of hepatitis virus into the inhabitants of a state institution for mentally retarded children in an attempt to understand the natural history of hepatitis and to test the effects of gamma globulin. Questions were raised both about the safety of the experiment for the children and about the voluntariness of the parental informed consent. These examples suggested to many that special care was needed to protect vulnerable subjects (the institutionalized, children, mentally retarded individuals) from the risks involved in research.

A final example that attracted considerable attention was the Tuskegee syphilis study.[4] This study, begun in the 1930s and involving poor black sharecroppers, evolved into an observational study of the consequences of untreated syphilis, and continued even after effective treatments for syphilis became available. The untreated subjects were systematically discouraged from receiving those treatments. In no way did they understand the nature of, and consent to participate in, this study. It illustrated once more the need for informed consent, for ensuring that the gains were commensurate with the risks, and for protecting vulnerable subjects. Because this study was more epidemiological than interventional, it also illustrated the need for policies governing that type of human research. Policies on epidemiological research will be discussed in Chapter Three.

These U.S. scandals may have attracted the most attention, but they were certainly not unique. One year after Beecher's article was published, M. H. Pappworth[5] published *Human Guinea Pigs*, in which he alleged similar problems in British research. In Canada, much attention was focused in the 1960s on the Halushka case, in which a subject in a study who had not received adequate information about what was involved in the study suffered serious injury after use of a new drug and invasive monitoring.[6] In New Zealand, investigations in the 1980s[7] focused on research in the 1960s and 1970s in which women with cervical cancer in situ were left untreated to study the natural history of the disease. As was expected, many developed invasive carcinoma from which some died. Questions were raised both about the appropriateness of the research and about the consent process. Abuse of subjects in research was, unfortunately, an international phenomenon.

As a result of these revelations, many official policies governing research on human subjects were developed. I will not offer a complete analysis of each of them, but rather a historical review of the development of the common themes that unite them, which will serve as an introduction to the issues that will be considered in the rest of this chapter.

The Nuremberg Code (1949, Appendix 1.1) is a series of ten principles that were articulated as part of the judgment in Nuremberg against some of the physicians who led the Nazi research on concentration camp inmates. Recent scholarship[8] has shown, by examining the relation between those principles and earlier German codes of research ethics and between those principles and the opinions of experts on research ethics used by the court, that the principles were not as original as sometimes suggested. Nevertheless, they had a great deal of influence. The principles articulated the requirement that there be informed voluntary consent from the subject before the experiment begins and during the continuation of the experiment and the requirement that there be appropriate benefits and risks. This latter requirement means that the amount of harm should not be too great, that the harm should be minimized, and that the benefits should be sufficient to outweigh the minimized harms associated with the research. These two substantive principles have been central to all subsequent official policies.

The Declaration of Helsinki (Appendix 1.2), adopted by the World Medical Association in 1964 after several years of work, and modified several times (1975, 1983, 1989, and 1996) since then, was designed to meet the threat that inappropriate research posed both to the integrity and the reputation of the research enterprise. It added three major influential points to the Nuremberg Code. The first was a conceptual distinction between clinical therapeutic research (research "whose aim is essentially diagnostic or therapeutic for a patient") and nontherapeutic biomedical research (research "which is purely scientific and without direct diagnostic or therapeutic value to the person subjected to the research"). The former type of research is justified by its benefit to the patient and the latter type is justified so long as the interest of society does not take precedence over the well-being of the research subject. Although this distinction has rightly been criticized by some, particularly because therapeutic research often involves a placebo control group that does not get the intervention in question, it remains influential in official policies. The second was the advocacy in 1975 of an institutional mechanism to ensure that its principles were followed. The mechanism, which had already been adopted to some degree in various countries, was the submission of the research protocol by the investigator to an "independent committee for consideration, comment and guidance." Such an independent review might notice problems that had been overlooked by the researchers who had a personal interest in the success of the research project. Unfortunately, the Declaration of Helsinki was not sufficiently explicit about the final authority of that independent review. The third was an explicit provision for proxy consent by family members when the subject could not consent. The importance of this provision will emerge more clearly in later chapters when we discuss research on special subjects.

In the United States, the Food and Drug Administration and the National Institutes of Health had been active in formulating policies about research ethics in the 1960s, including policies mandating independent review. But in 1974, as a result of increasing congressional concern about research ethics, fueled in part by the revelations about the Tuskegee study and other controversial research studies, Congress created the National Commission for the Protection of Research Subjects of Biomedical and Behavioral Research. It was charged with identifying the basic ethical principles underlying research on human subjects and with recommending requirements for legitimate research. In a 1979 report called the Belmont Report (Appendix 3.2), it identified as the basic principles the principle of *respect for persons* (treating individuals as autonomous agents and protecting persons with diminished autonomy), the principle of *beneficence* (minimizing harms and maximizing benefits), and the principle of *justice* (fairness in the distribution of the benefits and burdens of research). These three principles were perceived as leading to the fundamental requirements on legitimate research using human subjects. The principle of respect for persons led to the requirement of informed consent, the principle of beneficence led to the requirement of an appropriate risk/benefit ratio, and the principle of justice led to the requirement of an equitable selection of research subjects. Many official policies have explicitly identified these three principles as the moral basis of the policy.

In a series of seventeen reports, these principles and requirements were applied by the U.S. National Commission to a large number of questions. The recommended applications, after considerable discussion and modification, were incorporated in 1981 into parallel regulations from the FDA[9] and the NIH (Appendix 3.1). In 1991, these were adopted by fifteen agencies as a common federal rule (Appendix 3.1). These regulations will be analyzed in detail below. For now, it suffices to say that they go beyond Nuremberg and Helsinki in that they require in most cases advanced approval of research by independent committees (called Institutional Review Boards), they spell out the conditions required for obtaining informed consent and the information that must be provided under those conditions, and they add two other requirements, the requirement of an equitable selection of research subjects and the requirement of provisions to protect the privacy of subjects and the confidentiality of research data. There are also special regulations, which will be analyzed in other chapters, governing research on fetuses and pregnant women, on prisoners, and on children.

As late as the mid-1980s, this approach to research on human subjects had not been incorporated into the official policies of many European countries, and practice varied considerably both between countries and within countries. As a result, the Council of Europe began a process of developing European guidelines in 1985. They were adopted by its Committee of Ministers as recommendations to the member states for legislation in early 1990 (Appendix 2.2). In addition, the European Union published in 1990[10] guidelines about good clinical trials on medicinal products, guidelines that must in general be followed if the trials can be used to support an application for the approval of a new drug; those guidelines contain a section dealing with issues of research ethics. These two documents, taken together, constitute a common European approach to accepting the principles of the Declaration of Helsinki, a commitment that was strengthened in 1996 when it was incorporated into a broader Convention on Biomedicine adopted by the Council of Europe (Appendix 2.3). This common approach adopted in 1990 has been supplemented in Great Britain by two reports from the Royal College of Physicians, one (1996) on ethics committees[11] and one

(1990) on research involving patients (Appendix 4.1), by 1992 guidelines from the Medical Research Council,[12] and by 1993 National Health Service Guidelines on Local Research Ethics Committees.[13] In France, it has been adopted and supplemented by national legislation passed in 1988 and amended in 1990 (Appendix 4.8). German legislation in 1994 adopted some of it.[14] The Nordic countries adopted it in common guidelines in 1989.[15] While there are some disagreements about details, all of this additional European material is in accord with, and often supplements, the common European approach.

The above-outlined approach was also adopted by the Medical Research Council of Canada in its 1978 guidelines (revised in 1987) for Research Ethics Boards[16] and in the 1996 and 1997 drafts of a Code of Conduct for Research Involving Humans.[17] In 1992, consolidating earlier work, the National Health and Medical Research Council of Australia issued an important statement incorporating it with important supplements on specific problem areas (Appendix 4.12). With slight modifications in its policies related to informed consent, it was also adopted in 1989 by the Japanese Ministry of Health and Welfare in its guidelines for drug trials.[18]

Two final documents deserve special mention. The first is the 1993 revision by the World Health Organization (WHO) and the Council for International Organizations of Medical Sciences (CIOMS) of their 1982 international guidelines for human research (Appendix 1.8). Much of the material is familiar. But it introduces a new set of issues raised by research done by investigators from more developed countries on human subjects in less developed countries. Proposals are put forward on how to deal with informed consent in a way that is culturally sensitive and how to avoid exploitation of less developed countries in the research process. As biomedical research on human subjects becomes a truly international enterprise, these issues will increase in importance, and we will discuss them below. The second is the 1996 draft Guideline for Good Clinical Practice from the International Conference on Harmonization (Appendix 1.5), which is a joint effort of the European Union, Japan, and the United States to develop a common approach to the research leading to the approval of new drugs. It contains extensive ethical standards for the conduct of research on human subjects, and its official adoption would represent a common set of official policies on research on human subjects. When we discover disagreement in the current official policies on a specific topic, we will consult this draft Guideline to see if an agreement has been reached.

A clear-cut consensus has emerged in all of these official policies about the basic conditions for the licitness of research on human subjects. Procedurally, such research needs to be approved in advance by a committee that is independent of the researchers. Substantively, informed voluntary consent of the subjects must be obtained, the research must minimize risks and involve a favorable risk-benefit ratio, there should be an equitable non-exploitative selection of subjects,

and the privacy of the subjects and the confidentiality of the data must be protected. These substantive standards are rooted in fundamental moral commitments to respect for persons, to beneficence, and to justice.

This statement of the consensus suggests many issues that need further careful
analysis. Some of the issues relate to special groups of research subjects (zygotes
and fetuses, members of vulnerable groups such as children and mentally infirm
adults, and members of various groups such as women and minorities often
underrepresented in research) and will be discussed in other chapters. Others
relate to the details of the consensus as it applies to research subjects in general,
and those issues will be the focus of our attention in the rest of this chapter.
These issues include: What is research? Are there any forms of research that
are licit without conformity to the above standards? What should be the composition, function, and authority of the independent review group (the IRB, the
Research Ethics Committee/Board)? How should informed voluntary consent be
obtained? What information must be provided to the research subjects? How
should benefits and risks be assessed? How can one avoid injustices and exploitation in the selection of subjects? How can the protection of privacy and
confidentiality be reconciled with adequate data preservation and review? What
compensation, if any, should be provided to those subjects injured in the research process?

The Major Issues

What Is Research? Physicians always have the right to try innovative therapeutic approaches if justified by the patient's condition and if the patient voluntarily consents to the treatment after being properly informed. Doing this does
not require the physician's obtaining approval in advance from an independent
review committee. However, such an independent review is required in advance
if the treating physician is engaged in research, even therapeutic research. Given
that both innovative therapy and therapeutic research involve nonstandard treatments and given that both are attempts to aid the patient, how shall we distinguish therapeutic research that requires advance independent review from
providing innovative therapies that does not? Researchers who are also treating
patients have long recognized that these different roles are not always easy to
differentiate. Does that mean that independent review is required in every such
case? Or is it only required if the treatment of the patient and the collection of
the data is part of an organized research plan?

The Belmont Report struggled with this problem and finally offered the following definitions: Practice constitutes "interventions that are designed solely
to enhance the well-being of an individual patient or client and that have a
reasonable expectation of success" whereas research constitutes an activity "de-

signed to test an hypothesis, permit conclusions to be drawn, and thereby to develop or contribute to generalizable knowledge'' (Appendix 3.2, section A). Recognizing that by these definitions innovative therapeutic innovations by physicians/researchers need not constitute research requiring independent advance review, unless it is part of a plan to collect data that will contribute to knowledge, it went on to insist that major innovations should be incorporated into formal research projects that would then require independent review.

These definitions, while helpful, leave many ambiguities about the most difficult case, the innovative physician/researcher who keeps careful records about the outcome of the therapeutic innovations. The British Royal College of Physicians attempted to address this issue by emphasizing the motive of the physician and by making it clear that systematic and formalized retrospective collection of data (in a chart review study or by use of a registry) certainly turns the project into research.[19] The former suggestion is less helpful, because motives are often difficult to disambiguate, even by the physician in question. The latter is more helpful, because it provides an objective, publicly observable differentiation between pure innovative treatment and treatment combined with research. The Royal College also emphasized the position that it is really best if these innovative therapeutic interventions become the subject of formal research before they become part of regular practice. In New Zealand,[20] this is now the formal policy of the Department of Health, which requires that all innovations be formally approved by independent review, ending the distinction between innovative therapies and medical research. It remains to be seen whether this will limit the introduction of innovative therapies.

Whatever definition of research is adopted, the ethical standards should remain the same regardless of the sponsorship of the research or the purposes for which the research is conducted. This is unfortunately not true in the United States, where the standards contained in the regulations apply only to federally sponsored research, to research intended for submission to the FDA to support drug or device approval, and to research conducted at institutions that apply the standards to all research. Legislation was introduced[21] in 1997 to close this gap.

What Research Can Be Carried Out Without Meeting All of the Standards? It is important to differentiate two very different questions that have been raised under this heading. The first is whether there are forms of research on human subjects that can be carried out legitimately without any independent review of the research and without any consent from the human subjects involved. The second is whether there are forms of research on human subjects that require independent review before they can be carried out but that do not require for their legitimacy obtaining consent from the subjects involved.

An example of the first type of question relates to those forms of research (e.g., interviews, chart reviews) that seem to pose few risks to the subjects. Can such forms of research be carried out legitimately without going through the whole process of independent review? This question will be extensively analyzed in Chapter Three, as it is one of the central issues in the ethics of epidemiological research.

An example of the second type of question relates to medical research in emergency situations where there is no time to obtain consent and/or no competent individual from whom to obtain consent. Under what conditions, if any, can these types of research be carried out legitimately without obtaining informed consent? Consider, as one case, the 1994–95 trials of thrombolytic therapy[22] on patients presenting with an acute ischemic stroke. The therapy in question had the potential of causing serious harms due to intracerebral hemorrhages but it also had the potential for producing great benefits in limiting the damage caused by the stroke. Research was needed to see which effect would be more important. But the therapy had to be administered shortly after the onset of symptoms, so there was little time for obtaining informed consent even if the patient was capable of giving that consent or even if the patient was accompanied by a surrogate who was capable of giving that consent. Some of the trials attempted to obtain valid consent prospectively but others did not.

A number of points are clear. To begin with, if the patient's treating physician wishes to treat the patient in an innovative fashion, independent of any research effort, then independent review is not required and informed consent need not be obtained in those cases in which the usual emergency exception to obtaining consent to a therapeutic intervention applies. Of course, as noted above, the physician may well be advised to incorporate this innovation into a research protocol. Second, if research is involved, advanced independent review of the research plan must be undergone; there is, after all, no reason not to have such research protocols reviewed in advance. Third, if meaningful prospective consent from the patient or a family member can be obtained either for the commencement or the continuation of the research, it should certainly be obtained. The question is what to do about planned research that has been independently reviewed and approved but for which consent cannot be obtained.

One approach, favored by some of the researchers[23] in this area, attempts to justify the research by obtaining retrospective approval (often called deferred consent) from the patients/subjects or from their families. These researchers appeal to studies that show overwhelming approval, but doubts have been cast both on those studies and upon the rationale of using retrospective approval to justify earlier enrollment. In what sense is the patient's deferred consent relevant to justifying the earlier research given that their refusal would be irrelevant because the research has already been done? A second approach was advocated by the U.S. Office for Protection from Research Risks of the NIH[24] According to this approach, research without valid prospective consent in the emergency setting is legitimate only if it involves no more than minimal risks, does not adversely affect the rights and welfare of the subjects, and could not otherwise practicably be carried out. On this approach, both therapeutic and nontherapeutic research could be approved without consent, because it is the innocuousness of the research that justifies it. However, research could not be carried out without prospective full consent, no matter what the possible benefit to the patient, if the risks are more than minimal or if other subjects (e.g., those who can consent or who are accompanied by family members who could consent for them) could be found. Arguing for a liberalization of this approach, a coalition of critical care researchers[25] proposed that emergency research should be acceptable even if the incremental risks are more than minimal as long as these incremental risks (those greater than the risks of receiving the standard treatment for the condition in question) are still likely in the judgment of the independent review board to be acceptable to the vast majority of potential patients. They called this approach the appropriate incremental risk approach. The N.I.H. approach, and maybe even the proposed liberalization, would have difficulty justifying the stroke research because the intervention in question posed far more than minimal risks. A fourth approach, adopted by the Council of Europe (Appendix 2.2, section 8), emphasizes that such research can proceed without consent providing that it is "intended for the direct health benefit of the patient." On this account, it is the benefits to the subject/patient that justify research without consent. The following table summarizes these approaches:

Justification	Advocated By
Retrospective consent	Some researchers
Minimal risk	OPRR
Appropriate incremental risk	Coalition of researchers
Benefits to subjects	Council of Europe

The most reasonable approach seems to be that all of these values (the benefits to the subject/patient, the risks of the research, the possibility of getting some degree of consent beforehand and more later, and the possibility of finding other subjects) need to be considered in deciding whether or not to approve the research protocol. The U.S. Food and Drug Administration adopted such a multifactorial approach in 1996 (Appendix 3.7). Emergency research without consent is justified only if certain substantive and procedural requirements are satisfied.

The substantive requirements are that:

1. The need is great because the subject's condition is life-threatening and the available treatments are unsatisfactory.

2. The risks to the subjects are reasonable in light of the potential benefits to the subjects.
3. Consent cannot be obtained because of the subject's condition and the time constraints and because potential subjects cannot be identified in advance.

The procedural requirements are that:

1. The research must be carried out under an approval from the FDA as well as the usual IRB approval.
2. The research must be monitored by an independent data and safety monitoring board.
3. Community consultation is obtained.
4. Subjects and/or their surrogates will be informed about the research as soon as possible and given the opportunity to discontinue further participation.

There is certainly room for clarification of these requirements, but their adoption seems to be a reasonable way to avoid exploiting nonconsenting subjects while not denying them a chance to obtain needed benefits. A similar approach, with fewer formal details, was adopted in the 1997 proposed Canadian Code.[26] Unfortunately, this approach is not incorporated into the International Harmonization Guidelines for Good Clinical Practice (Appendix 1.5), which simply calls upon the independent review committees to ensure that emergency research protocols meet ethical and regulatory requirements.

The Composition and Functions of the Independent Review Panel. The review committees (the IRBs or Research Ethics Committees/Boards) are supposed to be independent of the investigators who are proposing the research being reviewed. However, they often consist of colleagues at the same institution or in the same field. Do they really have the required independence? If outsiders are added to provide more independence, can they have sufficient expertise to meaningfully participate? Is there a need for interdisciplinary input, and if so, what disciplines should be represented? Should these committees consider the scientific merits of the proposed research or just the human subjects issues? Are these committees merely responsible for reviewing the research protocols or do they have some responsibility for post-approval monitoring of the actual conduct of the research? Finally, how do differences in the system of independent review affect the quality of that review?

Institutional Review Boards and Research Ethics Committees/Boards are meant to provide independent review of research. But the notion of independence is crucially ambiguous. Does it merely mean independence from the particular researchers, so that other researchers in the same institution can compose the committee that does the review? Or does it also involve at least some measure of independence from the institution and from the research perspective, in which case the membership of the committee must be far broader? These problems are particularly pressing in countries where nearly all the independent review of research is carried out by committees created by the institutions in which the research is conducted. It is less pressing in countries such as the Scandinavian countries in which much independent review is regionalized.

Most of the national regulations have moved in the direction of the stronger notion of independence. In the United States (Appendix 3.1, section 46.107), Institutional Review Boards must contain at least one member who is not otherwise affiliated with the institution and at least one member from a nonscientific background (a lawyer, ethicist, or clergyman). These specific requirements were adopted in the 1996 draft of the International Harmonization Guidelines for Good Clinical Practice (Appendix 1.5, section 3.2.1), so they represent the emerging international standard. In addition, in the United States, the membership is supposed to possess sufficient racial and cultural diversity and sensitivity to community attitudes. The 1996 Royal College of Physicians Guidelines[27] and the 1997 proposed Canadian Code[28] also emphasize gender diversity as well as independence. However, only in Denmark and New Zealand do the lay members constitute one half of the committee. Some recent scholars[29] have advocated this full independence, with the lay members being seen as patient/subject representatives, but others have doubted whether this is really necessary.

Two major questions have been raised about the functions of the independent review panel. Before approving the research protocol, should they consider its scientific validity or should they only focus on the standards designed to protect the subjects (adequate informed consent, minimization of risk, etc.)? Do they have a role in monitoring the actual conduct of the research afterwards? In many traditional discussions, support is expressed for independent review being confined to the ethical issues and for the panel receiving post-approval reports from the investigators but not doing any actual monitoring. To some degree, these limitations reflect a realistic assessment of the capacities of the panels combined with a trust that funding sources will adequately review scientific merit and that investigators will conduct their research in accordance with the protocols they submit. Recent official policies have reversed direction on these issues. The Council of Europe (Appendix 2.2, principle 11) makes it clear that bad science cannot be the basis for ethical research; and CIOMS, in its Guidelines,[30] explicitly assigns to independent review committees the role of reviewing the scientific merits of the proposed research. The Royal College of Physicians, in its 1996 Guidelines,[31] accepts that role but insists that protocols should be rejected on scientific grounds only when adequate needed expertise has been obtained. The 1996 proposed Canadian Code of Conduct is the clearest statement of this expanded conception of the role of independent review, emphasizing the importance both of the review of the scientific merits of the research and of more active monitoring where appropriate.[32] That emphasis is *not* present in the 1997 revised version, where both approaches are accepted as legitimate.[33]

There are few data about whether this more expanded role improves the ethical quality of research. More generally, there is little information about the quality both of independent review of research and the ways in which different structures impact upon that quality. Two U.S. reports in 1996, one summarizing data from studies done for the Advisory Committee on Human Radiation Experiments[34] and one published by the Government Accounting Office,[35] are disturbing. The former documented, among other issues, significant concerns about the consent process in protocols that had been approved by IRBs; the latter raised concerns about the capacity of national agencies to oversee the functioning of local IRBs. Nevertheless, these findings are very preliminary. In truth, we know little about the actual quality of the independent ethical review of research, and even less about how that quality varies both with different structures and different functions of the independent review committee.

Under What Conditions Should Consent be Obtained? What requirements, if any, should be imposed on the process of obtaining consent to maximize the voluntary and informed nature of the consent? When, if ever, do financial rewards for participating in research become so great that the resulting consent is really being obtained coercively? Should there be independent witnesses who confirm that the consent is both voluntary and informed? Who should obtain the subject's consent? Should it be the investigator, who is in the best position to fully inform the patient but who may be biased in favor of the subject's agreeing to participate? Should it be the patient's treating physician, who has less of that bias but who is less informed about the research? Under what conditions is it appropriate to use research nurses and other research personnel to obtain consent?

The question of the conditions under which consent to participate in research is obtained is very important. If the conditions are inappropriate, the consent may be uninformed or nonvoluntary and therefore irrelevant no matter what information is provided. The United States regulations (Appendix 3.1, section 46.116) recognize this point and stipulate that consent shall be obtained only "under circumstances that provide the prospective subject or the representative sufficient opportunity to consider whether or not to participate and that minimize the possibility of coercion or undue influence." Unfortunately, however, little is said in these regulations about what are those circumstances in which consent should be obtained. The guidelines from the U.K. Royal College of Physicians (Appendix 4.1, section 17) are more helpful on this issue. They emphasize the importance of giving potential subjects time to think about participation, encouraging subjects to consult their family/friends and their own physician about participation, and asking subjects to fill out a consent form that explicitly asks them whether they are satisfied with the information they have received. While not perfect solutions, all of these measures seem helpful in making the informed consent process more meaningful.

One question about coerciveness that has attracted a lot of attention is the question of payments to research subjects for participation. There is no question that reimbursement for actual expenses is legitimate. The question that has been controversial is that of additional payments to induce volunteers to participate. Those who approve of them see these payments as legitimate compensation for the bother and discomfort of participation. Those who object to them see them as making participation so attractive that the potential subjects are coerced to participate (in philosophical terminology, these are called coercive offers) or are exploited in their participation. The U.S. regulations do not discuss these issues. A recent discussion by the Office for Protection from Research Risks of the NIH recommends being explicit in the consent form about payments and making them proportional to the inconvenience, but draws no conclusions about the difficult question of the coerciveness or exploitativeness of substantial payments to induce subjects to participate in more risky research. Their best suggestion is that "IRBs might consider whether only the destitute agree to volunteer."[36] The British Royal College of Physicians accepts the legitimacy of payments but cautions Research Ethics Committees to be satisfied that the payments "should not be such as to persuade patients to volunteer against their better judgement" (Appendix 4.1, section 41). The Council of Europe is somewhat stricter, opposing inducements but allowing "a modest allowance" for inconveniences suffered (Appendix 2.2, principle 13.1). The French statute has the most elaborate rules, allowing volunteers to participate in only one nontherapeutic trial at a time and setting (by regulation) a limit on compensation (Appendix 4.8, section 209–15). All of these rules seem to be excessively paternalistic. If the independent review panel has already concluded that the risk-benefit ratio of the research is acceptable (otherwise, the research could not be approved), how can the large payment harm the subject? And in what way are large payments for acceptable research coercive or exploitative?

Some have expressed a preference for the principal investigator being the person who obtains the subject's consent to participate, but that preference is not mandated in any of the regulations and it is not clear that such a preference is justified or practical. In very large studies, where many subjects are being enrolled, such a requirement is impractical. Moreover, although the principal investigator may be the person most knowledgeable about the study, others (research nurses, house officers) may know the potential subjects better, may have more time to devote to obtaining truly informed and voluntary consent, and may have fewer conflicts of interest in enrolling subjects. It seems more important for the investigator to attend to the conditions under which consent is obtained than to actually obtain it; attending to those conditions is, after all, "ascertaining the quality of the consent," and that is the personal obligation imposed on investigators by the Nuremberg Code (Appendix 1.1, section 1). As part of fulfilling that responsibility, the investigator may want to consider the suggestion that voluntariness is increased if the final consent is obtained by a health care professional on whom subjects have no dependency for their care.

What Information Should be Provided as Part of the Consent Process? What types of information need to be provided to each of the subjects? Must the information be provided in writing and must a written consent be obtained? How can one best convey relevant information in a manner that is both accurate and understandable by subjects who have a wide variety of educational backgrounds and who are often unfamiliar with the basic concepts both of clinical research and of the area of medicine in question? How shall informed consent be handled in a society in which written individual agreement is not part of the normal social norms?

There is broad agreement about the items of information that should be provided in the consent process, although there are modest differences in the actual requirements in the various official policies. The most recent policies—the CIOMS Guidelines (Appendix 1.8), the International Harmonization Guidelines (Appendix 1.5), and the 1997 draft Canadian code[37]—are the most complete and thoughtful. Taken together, they require that the following information be provided:

1. the purpose and the research nature of the project;
2. the duration of the subject's participation, the treatment and procedures the subject will undergo (with a clear specification of which are experimental), and the subject's responsibilities;
3. the risks of harms and discomforts that might result from participating in the research;
4. the possible benefits to the subject or to society from the research;
5. the alternatives to participating in the research;
6. the right to not participate and to stop participating at any time without penalty or loss of benefits to which the subject is otherwise entitled;
7. the measures to protect confidentiality;
8. the anticipated payments, if any, to the subject and the anticipated expenses, if any, that will be borne by the subject;
9. the compensation and treatment available for injuries sustained in the research;
10. the identity of a contact person to discuss questions about the research;
11. the circumstances under which the subject's participation will be terminated;

12. the assurance that new information relevant to participation that becomes available during the research will be provided to the subject;
13. the names of the sponsors of the research and the ownership of any commercial results.

All of these seem appropriate if the consent is to be informed, and providing them ensures that all official requirements are met, even if not every official policy requires that every one of these items be discussed.

Can this information be withheld when it is judged harmful for the patient/subject to receive it? Two policies most clearly allow this. One is the French statute (Appendix 4.8, section 209–9), which allows information about the prognosis to be withheld from research subjects in those exceptional circumstances when, in the sick person's own interest, the diagnosis has not been disclosed. The other is the Japanese regulations[38] which allow for consent to research related to malignant tumors based on an explanation of the symptoms rather than the provision of a diagnosis.

Should the information be provided in writing or is an oral explanation as good or better? Does the subject need to sign a document consenting to participate or is an oral consent adequate? With one exception (involving research such as questionnaires where the primary concern is confidentiality and the only linkage to the subject is the signature on the consent form), the U.S. regulations require that the subject sign a consent form. These regulations allow for the required information to be presented in writing as part of the consent form or for the required information to be presented orally and for the subject to receive in writing only a summary and a consent form to sign saying that he or she has received the information summarized (Appendix 3.1, section 46.117). Most U.S. researchers provide all the required information in writing in the consent form. There is some concern that this may function as a substitute for, rather than as a supplement to, a discussion of the information, and that patients may actually be confused by the elaborate written information without much oral explanation. The Council of Europe requires as a general rule written consent (Appendix 2.2, explanation of principle 3). The British Royal College of Physicians (Appendix 4.1, section 19) believes that written consent should be used except for the most minor research procedures. Both the British and the European recommendations stress that written consent provides more than documentation; it also may make the subject think more seriously about participation and about the essential elements of the consent. The Royal College[39] also believes that oral explanations of all the required information should be supplemented by a patient information sheet (separate from the consent form) that summarizes the important information. Perhaps the best conclusion is that the optimal process of consent involves an oral explanation of items (1) through (13) followed by presenting the subject with a summary document to review and a consent form to sign. Such an approach would satisfy all of the official policies, would emphasize real communication of information (in the oral explanation) as opposed to formal documentation of it, would ensure that the potential subject receives (in the summary document) all of the required information, and would get the benefits of a written consent.

Whatever approach is adopted to the provision of written information, care must be taken to ensure that the information is written in language that is understandable by the subjects. In addition, the desire to include all the information in the written consent form has often led to so much information being included that patients do not assimilate the information and do not focus on what is crucial for them to consider. These considerations further support an emphasis on oral communication supplemented by patient information sheets and separate consent forms; those who wish to provide all of the required information in written consent forms need to think carefully about these concerns of readability and of excess information.

There are cultures in which oral understandings and agreements are standard and where attempts to obtain written consent would not be understood and/or would be viewed as insulting. Also, there are cultures in which outsiders seeking cooperation negotiate with community leaders and not with individuals. Obtaining written informed consent may be problematic in the first type of culture and obtaining individual informed consent, even orally, may be problematic in the second. The problem is partially practical; attempts to meet the usual standards may result in an inability to carry out the research. More importantly, however, such attempts may be morally problematic as they involve insensitivity to other peoples and other cultures. How, if at all, can research be carried out using subjects from such communities? These questions are discussed both in the CIOMS Guidelines and in the proposed Canadian Code. The question of written consent is easier to deal with; in certain cultures, obtaining oral consent, after providing the usual information in a culturally sensitive fashion, is clearly preferable. The harder question is that of leadership consent versus individual consent. CIOMS[40] recommends use of trusted community leaders in the consent process, but insists that such supplementary measures cannot replace individuals' understanding that they have a right to make their own decision based on the relevant information. Similarly, the 1996 draft Canadian Code emphasizes the consent of community leaders but also emphasizes that the individual members have the right to refuse to participate.[41] However, even these seemingly reasonable balancings of respect for community values and for cross-community individual rights can be criticized on the grounds that the community leaders will often include no women, so these proposals are far from gender-neutral, and that they give the community leaders an inappropriate veto over approaching individuals who may want to participate. In truth, we need studies of the success and failure of various approaches to these issues of culturally sensitive transmissions of information and culturally sensitive consent processes.

How Should Risks and Benefits Be Assessed? It is important to differentiate two different requirements about risks and benefits. The first is the requirement that the risks to research subjects be minimized. The second is the requirement that the benefits be sufficient to outweigh the minimized risks. Each of those requirements gives rise to important questions. What measures can be taken to minimize research risks? In assessing ways of minimizing research risks, to what extent should we take the costs of further measures to minimize research risks into account? In evaluating the respective benefits and risks of some proposed research, should we consider the potential benefits both to society and to the patient or should we insist that the benefits to the subject alone must outweigh the risks to the subject? Does the answer to that question depend on whether the research is therapeutic research or nontherapeutic research? Is a benefit-risk ratio satisfactory if the patient accepts it, or should the independent review panel impose its own evaluation as well?

Many possibilities exist to lessen the risks to subjects in research. Among them are the following:

1. Exclude from the study those who are put at greater risk because of co-existing medical conditions.
2. Use in the study only drugs and devices that have been adequately tested first in animal models. This result is achieved by regulation in many countries. For example, in the United States, new drugs can be tested on human subjects only after the researcher has an IND permit based, among other things, on animal data.
3. Use invasive procedures already being performed on the subjects for diagnostic or therapeutic purposes. Thus, a biopsy for research purposes may be avoided if more tissue is taken during a biopsy that is already scheduled for diagnostic purposes.
4. Experienced personnel and emergency backup procedures can be employed. Thus, in the earliest tests of angioplasty, only very experienced cardiologists were allowed to do the then-experimental procedure and backup surgery teams were ready to operate if the artery in question was perforated during the procedure.
5. A plan can be developed for monitoring ongoing results of the study to see if certain safety problems are emerging that need to be addressed. In large clinical trials, this is often done by an independent data safety and monitoring board.

How far does one have to go in minimizing risks to the subject? It is a poor balancing of values to demand that all possible measures be taken, regardless of their economic cost and of their impact on the study. But it is also a poor balancing of values to allow significant avoidable risks to subjects for modest savings of research costs or modest increases in the ease of performing the research. A balance is needed between the avoided risks and the cost of avoiding them. Unfortunately, little has been written about how this balance should be achieved.

Once the research protocol has been designed to minimize the risks, the researchers and the independent review panel must make a judgment as to whether the benefits from the research are sufficient to justify the remaining risks. If they judge the benefit/risk ratio to be unacceptable, the research protocol should not proceed. Their judgment is separate from the decision, made after the protocol is in place by individual subjects as part of the consent process, whether they want to undergo the risks so that the benefits of the research can be attained. There may be those who feel that this independent review of the risks and benefits is too paternalistic, but I cannot agree. While subjects have a right to choose in the light of their values whether or not to participate in an approved research project, researchers and independent reviewers have an obligation to not approve and conduct research when, in the light of their values, the benefits of the research are insufficient to justify its risks. Why should they approve and conduct research that they judge does more harm than good, even if there are subjects willing to participate?

The U.S. regulations (Appendix 3.1, section 46.111) and the British Royal College of Physician guidelines (Appendix 4.1, section 3) make it clear that the benefits to be considered are the benefits both to the subject and to society in general (in terms of the knowledge that may result). It is, of course, this standard that allows for nontherapeutic research that has no benefits to the patient but may be of considerable importance to the advancement of knowledge; the Royal College guidelines use this standard to justify sufficiently important nontherapeutic research even in some cases where the risks to the subjects are more than minimal. Naturally, the subjects must understand this and must nevertheless consent to be part of the research. There is less clarity about this point in the policy of the Council of Europe (especially Appendix 2.2, principle 2.1), which talks about both types of benefits but insists that the interests of the subject come first. This unclarity, which is incorporated into the International Harmonization Guidelines (Appendix 1.5), is unfortunate.

How Can Injustices and the Exploitation of the Vulnerable Be Avoided?

What classes of subjects are vulnerable to exploitation when they are enrolled in research? Are these subjects best protected by limiting their participation in research, by strengthening the informed consent process, or by imposing additional conditions on the independent review? Is there a danger that some of these classes of subjects may be unduly restricted from participating in research projects, thereby losing some of the benefits of the research? All of these questions have generated considerable discussion.

The traditional list of vulnerable subjects includes (1) children and mentally infirm adults, both of whom may be vulnerable because of their limited capacity to comprehend information about the research and to make an informed choice about whether or not to participate; (2) prisoners, other individuals who are institutionalized, and subordinates in a hierarchically structured group, all of whom may be vulnerable because their capacity to make a voluntary choice about whether or not to participate may be limited by their concern about not offending those upon whom they are dependent; (3) fetuses, who may be vulnerable because their interests and well-being may conflict with those who consented to the research impacting upon them. In recent years, a fourth type of vulnerable subject has been identified: members of less developed and less affluent communities and societies, who may be vulnerable because their lack of sophistication about modern scientific medicine and their economic status may be exploitable by researchers.

The official research policies have approached the protection of these different vulnerable groups in all of the above-mentioned ways. We shall review all of these approaches to protecting subjects in groups (1) through (3) in Chapters Five through Nine. There is, however, one general observation about all of these protections that needs to be mentioned at this point. The presupposition of most of the discussions of research involving these groups is that research is dangerous and that the members of these groups need to be protected from these dangers because their vulnerability means that they cannot easily protect themselves. There are many cases in which this presupposition is not true. These are cases in which new promising interventions are being studied and in which the only way to receive them is as a subject in a research project. In such cases, the extra protections afforded to these vulnerable subjects may actually unjustly deprive them of the benefits of being a subject. The AIDS clinical trials[42] have called attention to this type of case, but they are hardly the only example. When we discuss these populations below, we will return to the question of how to ensure that the protections do not turn into burdens.

I want to say a little about the recent discussions of the vulnerability of research subjects from less affluent and less developed societies and communities; other aspects of that issue are discussed in Chapter Three. The 1993 CIOMS Guidelines highlighted this issue. Among its suggestions[43] are the following:

1. Such research should be approved by an independent review in the sponsoring society, using its usual standards, and by an independent review in

the less advanced society, ensuring that its own ethical requirements are met. This suggestion is an example of protecting the vulnerable by imposing additional conditions on the independent review.

2. Such subjects should not be used if the research might equally be carried out in more developed communities and such subjects should be used only if the research is relevant to the health needs of the less developed community. This suggestion is an example of protecting the vulnerable by limiting their participation in research.

3. Provisions should be made, where possible, for the results of the research (especially new products) being reasonably available to members of the less developed community. This is the most controversial of the suggestions because the financing of that reasonable availability is unclear.

In short, the recent tendency is to balance protecting vulnerable subjects (including some whose vulnerability has recently been identified) with assuring their access to the benefits of research.

How Can Privacy and Confidentiality Be Protected? Can there be breaches of privacy in the attempt to enroll subjects in that the researchers need access to confidential information to determine who should be approached to be a research subject? How can those breaches be minimized? What identifying information (information that links subjects with research information) should be kept by researchers? How should this information be kept so as to minimize the risks of breaches of confidentiality? In the light of litigation, what assurances of privacy and confidentiality can be given to research subjects?

The very act of contacting potential research subjects can constitute a breach of privacy. Suppose that you are a researcher not treating HIV-positive individuals and you wish to enroll a number of such individuals as subjects in a study. It would be an inappropriate breach of privacy for clinicians to give you a list of their HIV-positive patients to contact. A number of alternatives exist: (1) Those caring for the potential subjects can enroll them in the study and give you a list of those who consent to participate. This is very protective of privacy but puts a great burden on the treating clinicians. (2) You can write a letter, describing the study and giving the potential subjects a way to contact you if they are interested in participating, which is sent to the potential subjects by the treating clinician. This is equally protective of privacy and lessens the burden on the treating clinician, but it may lessen enrollment because the burden is on the subject to contact the researcher. (3) You can write a letter describing the study and telling the subjects that they will be contacted unless they contact their clinician and ask him not to release their names to you; this letter is sent to the potential subjects by the treating clinician. After an appropriate period of time, the clinician gives you the names of all those who have not asked to have their names protected and you contact them directly. This may increase enrollment but is less protective of privacy. Clearly, none of these approaches is perfect. Researchers and independent review committees must decide on a case-by-case basis which should be adopted, depending on the importance of the relevant factors (lessening the burden on the clinicians, enrolling subjects, protecting privacy) in the particular case.

Adequate provisions should be taken by the researcher to protect the confidentiality of the research data. The standard techniques are to assign each research record a code number, to keep the information linking the number with a specific individual separate from the research record, and to limit access to that linking information. Where appropriate, the linking information can be destroyed after the study is completed or when necessary later reviews of the study data are completed. This can be done even if the rest of the data are archived for later use in meta-analyses and so forth. When the data are published, care should be taken not to present data about individuals in ways that link the presented information to identifiable individuals. Special attention needs to be paid to what research information will be shared with the subject's physician; this is very important where its inclusion will result in sensitive disclosures to third-party payers who get access to the patient's medical records.

Consent forms should contain at least some discussion of the issue of confidentiality. The more sensitive the information being collected, the more important it is that the provisions for protecting confidentiality be clarified in depth. It is important that consent forms not promise that confidentiality will be completely protected, because there is usually the possibility of the records being subpoenaed. It should be remembered that there are certain forms of research (e.g., on alcohol and on controlled substances) where it is possible in the United States to get strict confidentiality certificates, which protect the research information from subpoena, from a number of federal agencies.

All of these issues arise in epidemiological research as well, and a resolution of them will be central to our discussion of the ethics of such research in Chapter Three.

What Compensation Is Due to Injured Research Subjects? Sometimes, research is carried out in a negligent fashion, and that negligence results in serious injury to the subjects. In such cases, the subjects can use the ordinary legal processes to receive compensation. But what about injuries that are not due to negligence but result from previously recognized or previously unrecognized risks of the research? Should the subjects be compensated, recognizing that they were injured in the course of socially valuable and needed research, or should they bear those costs as part of what they agreed to when they agreed to be in the research? Does it make a difference whether the research was therapeutic research or nontherapeutic research?

The official policies are in sharp disagreement on this point. The Council of Europe (Appendix 2.2, principle 14) unequivocally requires such compensation, and the British Royal College of Physicians (Appendix 4.1, sections 58–60) supports that viewpoint. The CIOMS Guidelines (Appendix 1.8, section 13) also support compensation, but hold that compensation is required even if there is no negligence only when the research is nontherapeutic.[44] Subjects/patients involved in therapeutic research protocols should be treated like those who suffer adverse reactions to regular medical therapy. The NIH regulations (Appendix 3.1, section 46.116) make no demands about compensation but simply require that the informed consent contain no language that releases or appears to release the investigator and his or her institution or the sponsor from liability for negligence. In a world in which research is increasingly cross-national, this important issue needs greater international consensus. The CIOMS approach seems most reasonable, for it confines the compensation for nonnegligent injuries to nontherapeutic research, and it is those subjects, who have no prospect of benefiting directly from the research, who have the strongest claims of justice to be compensated for nonnegligent research injuries.

Conclusion

Clearly, there are a very extensive number of national and international policies on research on human subjects. These policies arose in response both to the World War II atrocities and to later revelations about serious problems with the ethics of research involving human subjects, but continued work on refining them seems to represent a recognition of their importance independent of any particular shocking revelation. Two good examples of this are the recent discussions of how to deal with research on the treatment of acute emergencies and how to deal with cross-cultural sensitivities in the informed consent process.

There is a remarkable consensus on a large number of issues in these many policies: researchers must submit a detailed protocol for independent review and approval; the protocol must show that risks are minimized and that the research involves a favorable risk/benefit ratio; the protocol must document how prospective voluntary and informed consent will be obtained from prospective subjects; issues of protecting privacy/confidentiality and of justice in the selection of subjects must be addressed. The biggest controversy seems to be over the question of compensation for research injuries. There are also controversies about special issues that will be discussed in later chapters. Finally, there is uncertainty about the recently emerged issues of emergency research and cross-cultural research. Still, the consensus on basic policies is real. This consensus seems to be due, at least in part, to an agreement on the fundamental ethical principles governing this area: respect for persons, beneficence, and justice.

Moreover, these basic policies do not have to deal with issues of moral status, the very sort of issue that gave rise to some of the more serious disagreements among the basic policies governing animal research.

The official policies seem to comprehensively address the major ethical issues of research using human subjects and to reasonably balance the relevant values. Still, a final evaluation of them requires examining both their ultimate theoretical soundness and how they are actually implemented. Until both these tasks are completed, no final evaluation of the official policies is possible.

Chapter three

EPIDEMIOLOGICAL RESEARCH

Research on human subjects normally involves intrusions into their bodies. These may range from modest intrusions such as blood drawing to major intrusions such as surgery. The policies discussed in Chapter Two were developed to shape the conduct of this type of research. One important type of research involving humans, however, is not intrusive research on their bodies. In this type of research, one collects information from such sources as interviews, reviews of medical records, and studies on unused biological material. When used to learn about the distribution and determinants of health-related states or events, such research is central to medical epidemiology. Although other scientific disciplines use this type of research as well, our focus in this chapter will be on epidemiological research using such techniques.

Recent years have seen a growing recognition that epidemiological research raises a special set of ethical concerns. In this chapter, we will first trace the development of this recognition and the resulting formulation of international and national policies on the ethics of epidemiological research. Then we will consider the special issues discussed in these policies. Having done that, we will examine in greater depth two cases of research that have generated great controversy in recent years, anonymous studies of human immunodeficiency virus (HIV) seroprevalence and genetic studies on stored tissue. In the final section of this chapter, we will review some of the issues raised by the relatively new area of interventional epidemiology.

The Development of Ethical Concerns about Epidemiological Research

It is customary to see the origins of epidemiological investigations in the Hippocratic writings *On Epidemics* and *On Airs, Waters, and Places*. These writings recognize, for example, that malaria and yellow fever occur in swampy areas. More generally, they display a recognition of the relation between diseases and a whole variety of conditions. These observations were based on not very systematic observations. In the seventeenth century, John Graunt began the systematic collection of data about deaths (age, gender, cause of death), thereby laying the foundation for more systematic epidemiological studies. In the centuries that followed, these more systematic studies laid the foundation for an understanding of the etiology of both infectious diseases and diet-related diseases. In the post–World War II period, epidemiological studies were also extended to such illnesses as cancer (e.g., the correlation of smoking with lung cancer) and heart disease (e.g., the identification of the risk factors for heart disease).[1]

Some epidemiological studies collect the relevant data about the people without their involvement, knowledge, or consent. Thus, in Snow's classic studies[2] of the causes of cholera, which demonstrated the role of contaminated water, he used a list with the names and addresses of those who died of cholera and he investigated whether or not their water supply was from a contaminated source. By establishing that there was a much higher cholera death rate among those who used contaminated water, he established its role. The information about deaths came from the central registry without permission from, or involvement of, the deceased's family. The same is also true about the information received from the water companies about what water company supplied whom with water for consumption. Information about private individuals was supplied to Snow without the knowledge and consent of anyone. This feature is characteristic of many epidemiological studies using already existing data, and obviously raises many ethical questions about breaches of privacy in getting the data and of confidentiality in presenting the data and about lack of consent, to be discussed below.

Other epidemiological studies, using newly generated data obtained with the consent of the subjects, are very different. The Framingham Heart study,[3] started in the 1940s, enrolled subjects who submitted themselves regularly both to physical examinations and to answering a variety of questionnaires. All of this was done with the explicit consent of those studied. Such studies can also raise ethical issues about confidentiality in the presentation of the results, but they avoid the problems of lack of consent and of breach of privacy in obtaining the data because consent both to participation and to the breach of privacy is obtained.

Invasion of privacy concerns raised by the first type of epidemiological studies resulted in the mid-1970s in the first serious discussions of ethical issues related to epidemiological research. In the United States, the Privacy Act of 1974[4] laid the foundations for protecting the privacy of various records, particularly those containing information that linked the data to identifiable individuals. Such legislation had already been passed in Germany in 1970.[5] Concern was immediately expressed about how protecting privacy could be reconciled with needed epidemiological research, and various proposals were advanced, particularly by the U.S. Privacy Commission and by a group of epidemiologists (Gordis, Gold, and Seltser) in 1977.[6] Concern was also expressed about how epidemiological research would fit into the then emerging framework for regulating human subjects research, the framework outlined in the last chapter. Would everyone whose data are being studied need to consent and would all protocols for such research need to be approved by an external review board?

These specific questions were addressed to some degree in the United States in 1981 by the HHS regulations about human subjects research (Appendix 3.1, section 46.101 b2 and b4). Epidemiological research of the first type (involving already existing data, documents, records, and specimens) are exempt from the regulations and therefore do not require either external review or informed consent. The only exception to this is private information that is recorded in a manner that allows for the identification of subjects, thereby raising concerns about adequate protection of confidentiality. Similarly, epidemiological research of the second type that employs only surveys and interviews is exempt unless it either involves minors or involves private linkable information that, if disclosed, could place the subjects at risk of legal liability or could be damaging to them. Presumably, the fact that the subject must consent by responding to the survey/interview justifies the broader exemption for the second type of research. However, guidelines from other countries questioned the legitimacy of these exemptions. In its 1985 *Report on Ethics in Epidemiological Research*, incorporated into its 1992 Statement (Appendix 4.12, supplementary note 6), the Australian National Health and Medical Research Council required review and approval of all epidemiological research protocols by a research ethics committee and required consent of the subjects even for research using already existing records unless requiring that consent would make a valid study scientifically impossible or unless requiring it would produce excessive anxiety in the subject. The approval of all protocols by research ethics committees, when they exist, was also supported by the European Union in 1991.[7]

While the subject-related concerns began to be raised in the 1970s, there also began to emerge at the same time the concept that there were broader ethical issues about epidemiological research that needed to be addressed by epidemiologists. Susser, Stein, and Kline surveyed some of these issues in a landmark article in 1978.[8] Among the issues they identified were questions related to the choice of research topics, the design of studies, and special questions raised by the new field of interventional epidemiology. C. S. Soskolne, in a 1985 proposal to the American College of Epidemiology to create a committee on ethics guidelines,[9] identified additional issues related to the role of epidemiologists as expert witnesses and as supporters of advocacy programs for public health measures, related to conflict of interests, and related to conflicting obligations to various stakeholders in the results of that research in the industrial setting. In other settings, Soskolne also suggested that epidemiologists, following the lead of the statisticians, should consider issues relating to obligations to society, to funders and employers, and to colleagues as well as the more familiar issues of obligations to the subjects. These suggestions led several professional groups to develop such guidelines. Among them were the International Epidemiological Association (1990),[10] the Industrial Epidemiology Forum (1991),[11] and the Chemical Manufacturers Association's Epidemiology Task Force (1991).[12] The most elaborate of these were the guidelines from the Industrial Epidemiology Forum, which addressed the four categories of obligations: obligations to the subject (consent, privacy and confidentiality, and protecting welfare); obligations to society (avoiding partiality and conflicts of interest, due diligence, maintaining public confidence); obligations to funders and employers (protecting privileged information, specifying obligations); obligations to colleagues (confronting unprofessional behavior, appropriately reporting methods and results).

Two major developments in the 1990s further shaped the development of ethical reflection on epidemiological research. The first was the development of *International Guidelines for Ethical Review of Epidemiological Studies* by CIOMS in 1991 (Appendix 1.7). In addition to the traditional subject-related issues of consent, privacy, and confidentiality, it devotes extensive attention to such issues as releasing of study results, respecting social mores by being sensitive to different cultures, and evaluating research done by researchers from one country in other host countries. It also explicitly incorporates the distinction that has become very important in this area, and which will be discussed below, between avoiding causing harm and avoiding wronging. The second development was a return to concerns about privacy violations when epidemiological researchers accessed already existing data without permission of the subjects. The primary focus of this discussion was a European Union Directive on the processing of personal data first proposed in 1991 but not finally issued until 1995.[13] It was widely claimed that the original version would have undercut the possibility of most research on already existing data, and major changes were made in the final 1995 version.

This brief history reveals a growing recognition that many ethical questions are raised by epidemiological research. Some of them relate to the protection of the subjects: What forms of epidemiological research require review by an IRB or by a research ethics committee? What forms of epidemiological research require consent by the research subject? Under what conditions should already existing data be made available to epidemiologists for research purposes? What measures should be taken to protect the confidentiality of that data? Others raise broader concerns: To whom should the results of epidemiological research in general, and industrially sponsored epidemiological research in particular, be released so as to avoid inappropriate conflicts of interests? What is the role of epidemiologists in public health advocacy? What are the special obligations of epidemiologists in international and cross-cultural studies? In the next section, we will see what guidelines have emerged in response to all of these questions.

The Ethics of Epidemiological Research

Independent Review of Epidemiological Research. As noted above, the early national policies differed on this point. The 1981 HHS regulations allowed for much epidemiological research to proceed without IRB review and approval so long as the data did not involve identifying information, whereas the 1985 Australian guidelines did require review and approval of all epidemiological research protocols by research ethics committees. For a period of time, the trend was clearly in the direction of requiring that review. The NIH's Office of Protection from Research Risks notes that many IRBs do review such protocols to ensure that issues of privacy and confidentiality are adequately addressed.[14] The 1991 Industrial Epidemiology Forum's Guidelines[15] also call for review of protocols, emphasizing that there is also a need to review the question of whether or not individual consent is possible and appropriate. The 1991 CIOMS Guidelines (Appendix 1.7, section 33) also call for such review in all cases except, quite appropriately, when the study is investigating the outbreak of an acute communicable disease. The Guidelines also clarify that this requirement applies only to research protocols and not to internal institutional evaluations of their programs.

In a series of articles published in the 1980s, Kenneth Rothman[16] lamented the difficulties that this independent review can pose for epidemiological research. Some of the issues he raised, about invasions of privacy and about individual consent, will be discussed below. But two deserve attention in this context. First, many epidemiological studies utilizing data from existing records examine the records in a large number of institutions to secure enough data. Does this require separate approval of the IRBs or the Research Ethics Committees in each of those institutions? This is often required, and Rothman documents how time consuming and costly that process can be. In one study involving food additives and cancer, the investigator spent a year getting separate approval from 66 hospitals. It might be more appropriate, at least in the case of researchers using data from existing records, that they only be required to secure a review and approval in their own institution and to document that approval to the independent review committees in all other institutions in which the study is conducted. While this means reliance on the standards in the home institution of the investigator, which may differ from the standards in the institutions in which some of the research will be conducted, such reliance may be appropriate when the risks are small and the burdens on the investigators are very great. Second, many independent reviewers of epidemiological studies involving already existing data forget that, at least in the United States, the protocols for these studies are eligible for expedited review, lessening the burdens both on the investigators and the IRBs. There seems to be no reason why the burdens of a full review need to be imposed, unless there are special concerns about consent, privacy, or confidentiality raised by the particular protocol.

Whether or not Rothman's arguments can be met, there now seems to be a reexamination of the requirement of independent review for all protocols. The British Royal College of Physicians allows research on existing records without review by a research ethics committee as long as the guardian of the existing records agrees and there is adequate protection of confidentiality.[17] The 1997 proposed Canadian Code, like the U.S. regulations, do not require independent review when the existing records contain only non-identifying information.[18] So the question of independent review of epidemiological research is far from settled, although most agree that it is required when the records to be studied contain identifying information.

Individual Consent in Epidemiological Research. There seems to be a general consensus about the need to obtain consent from individuals enrolled in epidemiological research that creates new data by surveying/interviewing these individuals or testing them in a variety of ways. There may be some disagreement about how formal the consent process needs to be in interview/survey research. There is also considerable disagreement about whether parents of adolescents need to be notified of, and formally consent to, survey/interview research involving their children, especially in sensitive areas such as sexual behavior and drug use, or whether the consent of the adolescents should be adequate. In the United States, as noted above, survey research involving minors is not exempt from IRB review that needs to consider these consent issues. These questions were also debated in connection with the Family Privacy Protection Act of 1996.[19]

The more controversial question, which has received more attention, is whether individual consent must be obtained to utilize information in already existing records about those individuals, and it is that question that will be the focus of our attention in the remainder of this discussion. The main argument against imposing that requirement for research involving already existing data is the practical difficulties that would result. It is not just a question of the number of individuals who must be contacted; far more important are the difficulties that would be encountered in trying to find these individuals with whom the researcher has no other relation. Naturally, the force of this argument will vary depending on the study in question. An epidemiological study using existing data from subjects who are still hospitalized will have less difficulty in meeting a requirement of individual informed consent than one using existing data from the general population. This argument from practicality is often reinforced by the observation that as long as confidentiality is protected, there is no risk of harm to the individual subject. Given that this is so, why should individual consent be required?

The CIOMS guidelines, respecting these reflections, allow for an independent review board to exempt particular research protocols from the requirement of informed consent in those cases in which the burden of such a requirement would be great, the protections for confidentiality are adequate, and the research is of sufficient importance (Appendix 1.7, section 2). This is, in fact, one of the reasons why CIOMS feels that such protocols must be independently reviewed on a case-by-case basis; given their inherent biases, the researchers are not the appropriate people to make that balancing decision. Moreover, CIOMS emphasizes the desirability of obtaining, where appropriate, consent for the conduct of the study from community representatives.

There are those who would object that this balancing approach is still too burdensome. Why should the burden of obtaining informed consent be imposed, even if doing so is practically feasible, given that the independent review has concluded that the risk of harm has been minimized because confidentiality is adequately protected? This was one of the issues raised by Rothman. Probably the best response to that question invokes the distinction between risks of harms and risks of wrongs. The use of already existing data without the consent of the individual wrongs that individual by invading his or her privacy and by treating him or her solely as a means to an end, even if confidentiality safeguards ensure that the individual is not actually harmed. This wronging is avoided if consent is obtained, and that is why it is best to obtain it where possible. There will be cases in which obtaining consent may not be practical but in which the public interest in having the research conducted may outweigh the wrongs to the subjects. In such cases, the job of the independent review is to determine whether these three conditions (confidentiality is safeguarded, consent is impractical, and the research is of sufficient importance) are satisfied and to approve the research if they are. In other words, the independent review addresses the question of whether the relevant values would have been appropriately balanced if the research is allowed to proceed without individual consent. Also, as the 1997 proposed Canadian Code indicates, it addresses the question of alternatives (e.g., consultation with a representative group) to obtaining individual consent.[20]

Invasions of Privacy in Epidemiological Research Using Already Existing Data. This last observation leads us directly to the debate about epidemiological research and the protection of privacy. As computerized databases contain a continually increasing amount of private information about individuals, information that can be synthesized by merging databases, they become ever more useful for epidemiological research. At the same time, there is a growing concern about the potential for invasions of privacy by those who can access these databases and a growing demand for the protection of privacy by limiting such access unless consent of the data subjects is obtained. This very legitimate demand directly conflicts with the need of epidemiologists to do studies employing the data in such databases. It is just these studies that would be the hardest to conduct if individual consent was required. Should such research involving invasions of privacy be allowed, after independent review has ensured that it is of sufficient importance, that individual consent is not practical, and that confidentiality is adequately protected, on the grounds that the benefits outweigh the wrongs? Or should we protect privacy by not allowing for such research?

It is just this question that was much debated in Europe in the early 1990s. The main focus was on a proposed Directive from the European Union on the processing of personal data. The earliest versions emphasized protecting privacy, and there was a great concern that this would make epidemiological research impossible in Europe. In the final version of the Directive, issued in late 1995,[21] the balancing approach is adopted, with the following major provisions:

1. In general, processing of data for statistical or scientific purposes is acceptable, provided that there are appropriate safeguards of confidentiality.
2. Data should not be kept in a form that permits identification of the subjects for longer than is necessary for the purposes for which it is collected; however, an exception is made for scientific and statistical use if there are appropriate safeguards.
3. Data may be processed without consent of the data subject if it is sufficiently in the public interest to allow that processing (presumably, much processing for the purpose of epidemiological research is sufficiently required by the public interest).
4. Although data about racial or ethnic origin and about health or sex life cannot be processed without the consent of the data subject, it may be for preventive medical purposes or for other reasons of substantial public interest.
5. Data subjects must be notified when data about them is being disclosed to third parties; however, they need not be if the disclosure is for statistical or scientific research and disclosure would be impossible or would involve disproportionate effort.

These provisions taken together allow for such research without consent when the three conditions of protection of confidentiality, impracticality of consent, and sufficient public importance are satisfied. These exceptions have been incorporated, with various subtle nuances, into 1994 statutes passed in France and Germany,[22] although there is concern about what is happening in other European countries.[23]

A similar balancing approach has been incorporated into the proposed U.S. 1995 Confidentiality of Medical Records Bill.[24] It contains a provision allowing for the disclosure of medical records for purposes of health research providing that an IRB determines that the disclosure is necessary and is of sufficient importance to outweigh the invasion of privacy and providing that there are appropriate safeguards. It is of interest to note that there is no mention of an IRB determination that obtaining individual consent is not practical, and that is a weakness of this statute.

In short, then, the balancing approach seems to have won general acceptance, although there remain a variety of subtle differences about the requirements for allowing the invasion of privacy required in epidemiological research on already existing records. One of these requirements is that confidentiality be adequately protected. We turn next to a discussion of what that means.

Protecting the Confidentiality of the Data. As early as 1977, Gordis, Gold, and Seltser[25] made several crucial suggestions about how the confidentiality of this private data should be maintained. Among those suggestions were the following:

1. Personal identifying information should be correlated with a study number. All study data forms and computerized records should employ only the study number. The records correlating the study number with the personal identifying information should be stored securely elsewhere.
2. Once the study is completed, the records with the identifying information should be destroyed. If it cannot because of possible follow-up studies, mechanisms for continuing secure storage should be carefully developed.
3. Everyone involved in the study must be cautioned about the importance of confidentiality and confidential information should be released only to those who need to use it.

These measures have now become standard.

Another safeguard of confidentiality, mentioned in several of the professional guidelines,[26] is that confidentiality should be protected in the final report/publication of the research by ensuring that individual subjects cannot be identified from the data presented. This is usually accomplished by presenting only aggregate data, although more individualized data may be presented if that is of interest so long as that presentation does not result in the data subject being identifiable. In my consultative activities with NASA in connection with its plan to develop an electronic database of information obtained from the medical records of astronauts, I was involved in a situation in which the number of subjects was so small that there was not an effective technique for protecting confidentiality in the report of the data. By checking the data against the list of astronauts on given missions, it was almost always possible to identify the data subjects. It was therefore agreed by all involved that the data subjects would have to be informed about the lack of true confidentiality, that any data about them that they did not want to be public would not be included in the reported database, and that objecting to the inclusion of data would in no way prejudice being chosen to serve on a mission. In this way, the right to confidentiality was protected because the subjects consented to the breach of confidentiality even when confidentiality itself could not be protected.

Before turning to the broader questions, let us summarize what we have learned about the protection of subjects in epidemiological research. Epidemiological research protocols, even when using only already existing but identifying data, should be independently reviewed by an IRB or a Research Ethics Committee/Board to ensure that the benefits of the research outweigh any losses from invasions of privacy, to determine whether individual consent of data subjects (or some alternative to it) is feasible/desirable, and to check on the adequacy of the measures to protect against harms from breaches of confidentiality. Unless there is controversy on one of these points, expedited review may well be appropriate. Consideration should be given to a single institution review of a multi-institutional protocol. Informed consent should usually be obtained from subjects when new data are being created with their cooperation because obtaining it will usually be feasible. It might also be obtained when feasible in research involving already existing data. It is permissible to do the research when this is not feasible as long as the independent review concurs that the research is sufficiently worthwhile and that appropriate safeguards are in place. The most important of these safeguards is the protection of confidentiality both in the handling of the data and in its publication.

Communicating the Results of Epidemiological Research. Two very different questions have been raised under this heading. One relates to communicating the results to the individual subjects. The other relates to communicating the results to the public given barriers that may be imposed by sponsors. These questions are not unique to epidemiological research, but they seem to be of particular importance in that setting.

The CIOMS guidelines (Appendix 1.7, section 13) emphasize the importance of communicating to subjects findings from the study that are relevant to their health. Getting that information is one of the benefits to the individuals that (one would hope) outweighs the risks of harms or wrongs to them posed by epidemiological studies. Providing that information may sometimes be impossible because of the unlinking of very sensitive data from identifiers to further protect confidentiality (e.g., in anonymous HIV screening programs). When providing that information to individuals is not possible either because of unlinking or because of logistic reasons and/or when it is insufficient for public health purposes, the information should be conveyed to public health authorities. These guidelines, supported in the professional standards, seem very reasonable. We will return to their application to the case of HIV anonymous seroprevalence studies below.

Much epidemiological research is sponsored by those with an interest in certain results being attained, and a concern has been raised that this funding may lead to conflict-of-interest problems in the public communication of study results. Not surprisingly, this topic has attracted considerable attention in the codes of the professional groups, as well as in the CIOMS guidelines. A number of major points have been made:

1. In addition to avoiding fraud, epidemiologists should avoid the distortions resulting from manipulating data, withholding part of the evidence, or withholding some findings entirely at the request of the funders of the research.
2. Although epidemiologists may use funder-provided privileged information, including information protected as trade secrets, in their research, final reports must contain enough information about methods as well as findings so that the results can be critically assessed.
3. No funding should be accepted whose receipt is contingent upon reaching certain conclusions.
4. All of these points should be carefully specified in the contracts between epidemiologists and the sponsors of their research.

Epidemiologists and Public Health Advocacy. Epidemiological findings have important public health implications. A classic example of this is the epidemiological finding associating smoking with lung cancer and other health problems. In many cases, the epidemiologists who discover these findings turn their efforts to public advocacy for measures designed to minimize the health problems (e.g., advocating bans on advertising cigarettes). In doing so, they speak not merely as public citizens but as scientists with a particular expertise. Is this type of advocacy an appropriate professional role or is it a mixing of roles that challenges the objectivity of epidemiology as a science? This question has been discussed in some of the professional codes and public guidelines.

Although none of the guidelines opposes this advocacy role, their discussion of that role shows differing attitudes toward it. The most cautionary discussion is contained in the guidelines from the International Epidemiological Association,[27] which cautions that "It is difficult to be an impartial advocate. To steer a true course between scientific impartiality and advocacy of actions to enhance, protect or restore health can be a difficult challenge." A somewhat more positive, but still cautionary, approach is found in the CIOMS guidelines (Appendix 1.7, section 31), which state that: "Investigators may discover health hazards that demand correction, and become advocates of means to protect and restore health. In this event, their advocacy must be seen to rely on objective, scientific data."

I would suggest that this discussion would be helped by distinguishing several different questions: Are epidemiologists who discover health hazards obliged to report those discoveries in professional publications? Our earlier discussion about communicating the results of epidemiological studies emphasized the importance of that obligation as part of the professional role of the epidemiologist. Are those epidemiologists then obliged to enter into an advocacy role for measures to deal with those hazards? I would suggest that this is not a professional obligation, but that epidemiologists have the same personal obligation as other informed citizens to play some role in the discussion of these health measures. This obligation does not, however, demand advocacy on any particular issue. If epidemiologists become an advocate on a particular issue, are there special limits on their advocacy? Here, I would suggest that in their role as advocates, epidemiologists have a special obligation to advocate in a responsible, scientifically objective fashion, in part to not discredit the objective findings of epidemiological research by irresponsible advocacy. On this point, the various guidelines are quite properly in agreement. I would also suggest that, for the very same reason, they should indicate what is reporting of objective scientific findings and what is advocacy.

Cross-Cultural Epidemiological Research. As noted in Chapter Two, the CIOMS guidelines on human research devote considerable attention to ethical issues raised by cross-cultural research. This is not surprising in the light of the international nature of CIOMS. At least three such issues are discussed in the CIOMS guidelines on epidemiological research. All three grow out of the concern that cross-cultural studies, conducted by first-world researchers on third-world subjects, not become a new form of imperialism in which first-world values and research agendas are imposed on third-world cultures in ways that are detrimental from the third-world perspective.

The first is the issue of whether obtaining individual informed consent and respecting personal confidentiality is an expression of first-world individualism that makes no sense in cultures where group cohesiveness and conformity to communal decisions are more crucial values. On this issue, CIOMS calls for respecting "the cultural expectations of the societies in which epidemiological studies are undertaken, unless this implies a violation of a transcending moral rule" (Appendix 1.7, section 25). In practice, this means that "a leader may express agreement on behalf of a community, but an individual's refusal of personal participation is binding" (section 5). As we saw in Chapter Two, CIOMS, in its 1993 general guidelines on human subjects research, strengthened that commitment to transcending cross-cultural moral rules by insisting that third-world subjects must be told everything that would be told to research subjects in a first-world country and that their right to individually refuse to participate must be clearly explained. Sensitivity to local cultural expectations, while important, is clearly seen by CIOMS as secondary to following transcending moral rules.

A similar prioritization is found in connection with a second issue in cross-cultural studies. This is the question of the appropriateness of epidemiological studies of the health hazards posed by traditional communal practices, ranging all the way from special diets to such practices as female circumcision. Once more, while agreeing that communities have a right of respect for cultural values, CIOMS concludes that "studies expected to result in health benefits are usually considered ethically acceptable and not harmful" (Appendix 1.7, section 24).

The third issue relates to the ethics of using third-world subjects in studies to advance research agendas of first-world countries. CIOMS suggests (Appendix 1.7, sections 16–17) that there should be compensating benefits to the third-world subjects. Among the benefits mentioned are the provision of research-related health care while the research is being conducted and the training of local health care workers so that there be a lasting benefit to the community of the study subjects from participating in the research. These provisions parallel CIOMS's requirement, discussed in Chapter Two, that the results of medical research be made reasonably available to the community of the third-world subjects. It remains to be seen whether these suggestions will become standard practice in cross-cultural epidemiological research.

Two Controversial Cases

In this section, we examine two special cases that have generated considerable controversy. The first has to do with genetic research on archived tissue and blood samples. The second has to do with studies of the prevalence of HIV infection. As we shall see, these two controversies involve many of the issues we have already discussed.

Genetic Research on Stored Tissue Samples. In the summer of 1994, the NIH convened a meeting to discuss genetic research on stored tissue samples. The results of that meeting, and of the follow-up deliberations, were published in the end of 1995.[28] It created sufficient controversy, particularly among the pathologists, that a new set of discussions began in 1996 and continued in 1997 as part of the mission on the newly created U.S. National Bioethics Advisory Commission (NBAC).[29] Similar deliberations were conducted in Great Britain by the Royal College of Physicians and in Canada by the research councils as they developed their 1997 proposed Code. All of these discussions revolved around the related issues of review by IRBs, consent, protection of privacy and confidentiality, and informing the sources of the material of relevant results.

Several types of research activities were differentiated in these discussions, and each raises different issues. The first is research using already obtained material that has already been stripped of identifiers, even if some information (demographic or clinical) about the source has been retained. The second is research using such already obtained material that has not yet been, but would be, stripped of identifiers. The third is research using already obtained material where it is proposed that the material not be stripped of identifiers. The final is obtaining new material for use in future research.

Two obvious points about the first type of research. First, if the already existing material is truly anonymous, there is no threat to confidentiality (eliminating a potential harm) but no potential of informing the sources of relevant results (eliminating a potential benefit). Second, if the already existing material is truly anonymous, then consent for use in the new research cannot at this point be obtained from the sources of the material. In the light of these observations, the main question raised by such research was whether such research should receive independent review before it is conducted. The British Royal College of Physicians,[30] in keeping with its general policy about epidemiological research, did not require such review. The proposed Canadian Code[31] and the NIH report[32] supported such a review. Two purposes for that review were suggested: it provided a determination both that the research soundly addressed a significant issue that could not feasibly be conducted in a protocol using other material whose use had been consented to by the sources and that the research could not indirectly harm members of the group to which the donors belonged. Presumably, these issues are relevant to the determination that the wrong from unconsented-to use is outweighed by the gains from the research. I would suggest an additional reason for independent review. That review should examine the issue of true anonymity, of whether or not the existence of the remaining information accompanying the sample is compatible with the assurance that the source cannot be identified. It is just this type of review to ensure that confidentiality has been adequately protected that is one of the reasons for the view, noted above, that all epidemiological protocols should be independently reviewed.

More complex issues are raised by the second type of research. In such cases, an alternative to conducting the research without consent after making the material anonymous would be to contact the sources and obtain consent for the use of the material with adequate protections of confidentiality. The Royal College of Physicians does not require obtaining that consent.[33] In such cases, the NIH group suggested that the independent review assess the merits of both options, taking into account such questions as the difficulty of recontacting sources (the more difficult to recontact, the more reasonable to strip the identifiers) and the availability and usefulness of medical interventions that could be offered to some sources after the results of the testing are known (the more available and useful the interventions, the less reasonable to strip the identifiers).[34] This type of balancing seems quite compatible with the more general balancing approach that has been adopted for epidemiological ethics. It has been claimed by some,[35] particularly in the community of pathologists, that the proposal of the NIH group would require always obtaining consent before using stored samples whose source could be identified, and that such a requirement would be excessively burdensome. This objection seems to be based on a misreading of the actual proposal, which allows for stripping identifiers as an alternative to obtaining consent when an independent balancing judgment supports not obtaining consent. The proposed Canadian Code is open to that objection, for it does mandate obtaining the consent.[36]

Where the researchers propose to not strip identifiers, or where tissue is now being collected for other purposes but may be used at a later date for future research, the NIH group recommended that consent for use of the material in research must be obtained unless very stringent requirements are met. One mentioned in the report is obtaining a certificate of confidentiality from the assistant secretary of health to protect the information from being compulsorily released in legal proceedings. In seeking consent, the NIH group recommended that potential sources be offered the option of not allowing the tissue to be used in research, of allowing the tissue to be used in linked research (after a realistic picture has been presented about the possible risks from breaches of confidentiality and the possible benefits from being recontacted with new findings) or of allowing the tissue to be used only in anonymous unlinked research. The sources should also be told of the extent, if any, to which they will share in the profits from commercial products. Finally, some members of the NIH group thought that they should be offered choices about the types of research in which the material could be used and the types of researchers that might use the material.[37] This set of consent recommendations has also been opposed by many both on the grounds that the complicated consent proposal is too complex for use and on the grounds that it may compromise the statistical validity of the epidemiological data obtained. These objections support the less demanding requirements of the proposed Canadian Code[38] about the information to be provided (how the tissue will be taken and preserved, what it might be used for, and how confidentiality will be protected), without the need to seek consent for use of the tissue in different types of research.

I would make two observations about these consent requirements, evaluating them in the light of broader consent requirements in epidemiological research. The first relates to the requirement of obtaining consent in all cases of linked research using already existing tissue samples. As we have seen above, such a consent requirement is not imposed in all cases of linked epidemiological research on already existing personal data in databases. Where obtaining consent would be too burdensome and where confidentiality is being adequately protected, the emerging international consensus seems to be that the research may proceed if it is of sufficient importance. Why should the same standard not apply to linked research using already existing tissue samples? The second relates to the requirement of obtaining consent for possible future research uses when collecting new tissue. Here, analogously to the case of interview research where new data is being created, there seems to be no reason why consent should not be obtained. But it remains an open issue as to whether the NIH or the Canadian approach is preferable.

In short, I would make the following suggestions about genetic research using stored tissue samples. All such research protocols should be independently reviewed. In the case of samples that have already been stripped of identifiers, the review should determine that the samples truly are anonymous and that the research is sufficiently beneficial. In the case of samples that have not yet been stripped of identifiers, the advantages and disadvantages of stripping the identifiers versus doing linked research with adequate protection of confidentiality should be carefully balanced. When it is decided to do linked research, obtaining consent is usually appropriate, but that requirement may sometimes be waived because of the burden it imposes. Consent should almost always be obtained when collecting new material that may later be used in research because obtaining it is almost always realistically possible. The precise information to be provided and the choices to be offered require more careful research in the light of both theoretical demands and practical limitations.

Unlinked Anonymous HIV Seroprevalence Studies. Once HIV was identified as the cause of AIDS and once adequate tests for HIV infection became available, epidemiologists recognized both a need and an opportunity to determine the prevalence of HIV infection. Because AIDS develops only after many years of infection with HIV, studies of the prevalence of HIV are needed if we are to be able to predict the number of future cases of AIDS, especially in different demographic groups, and to plan for the provision of care for those with AIDS. Such studies conducted repeatedly over time are also needed to quantify the success or failure of public health prevention efforts. The existence of a reliable test of HIV infection using blood samples provided the opportunity to conduct these needed studies.

From the beginning, there were strong reasons to be concerned that studies of prevalence of HIV infection using only those who volunteered to be tested would underestimate the true prevalence; many of those in high-risk groups might refuse to consent to being tested for understandable reasons. What emerged instead in the United States was a program run by the CDC of unlinked anonymous screening. This program has become a source of some controversy, especially in Europe,[39] and a review of that controversy teaches us a lot about epidemiological ethics.

The CDC program involves testing done at sentinel institutions throughout the country. It involves testing of blood samples that have been drawn for other purposes and that would otherwise be discarded. Some demographic information is kept about the sources, but identifying information is destroyed so that the testing is of anonymous samples. As a result, the sources whose blood tests positive cannot be notified and counseled, but there are no resulting threats to confidentiality.

If one examines this program from the perspective of the general standards for epidemiological research, it seems quite acceptable. The testing is being performed on already existing blood samples drawn for other purposes, and it strips the records connected with the blood samples of identifiers. We have just seen, in our discussion of genetic research on stored samples, that this type of approach may be an acceptable alternative to retaining the linking information and getting consent. In the case of HIV seroprevalence studies, what makes it acceptable is the greater reliability of the data from such a study plus the protection of privacy resulting from anonymity of the sources.

This type of approach was also supported by a Canadian Working Group in a 1988 report (Appendix 4.11), appealing to the general principles governing epidemiological research. It made a number of additional points that deserve careful attention.

The first point is that the legitimacy of this program presupposes the universal availability, separate from the anonymous testing program, of voluntary HIV testing based upon informed consent, pretest and post-test counseling, and protection of confidentiality. This seems correct. Part of the balancing required in deciding whether an anonymous program is acceptable is a consideration of the harms to those who cannot be informed of the results. In this case, the harm of not being notified of the test results, and of not being counseled about available care and about changes in behavior to limit the further spread of HIV, is lessened if those who want it can get that information and that counseling in independent programs. The sentinel institutions in the CDC program might want to ensure that such voluntary testing programs are readily available to all patients in those institutions and that the patients are notified of the existence of these separate voluntary programs.

A second major point made by the Canadian report is that such anonymous testing programs should be accompanied by public education about their existence and by the existence of a mechanism whereby individuals, at their own initiative, can contact the researchers to request that their leftover serum not be included. A similar provision was also incorporated into the British testing program, which was finally approved in 1989 after three years of considerable controversy.[40] This type of "opt-out" provision has some theoretical attraction, but its extensive use, especially by those in high-risk groups, would result in a severe limitation on the validity of the prevalence data. It remains to be seen what will be the implications of its adoption.

The Committee of Ministers of the Council of Europe addressed these questions in 1989 as part of general recommendations on HIV-related issues.[41] It accepts the legitimacy of unlinked studies done without consent, as long as this is consonant with local law, and emphasizes the importance of the ready availability of voluntary confidential testing and counseling in the settings in which such unlinked studies are carried out.

As noted above, this type of anonymous testing has drawn opposition. Some critics challenge its scientific importance. Others worry about whether the unlinking of identifiers can really be sufficient to ensure anonymity. Still others are worried about the legitimacy of denying the results of the testing to the sources of the material. These objections can usually be met in well-designed programs. But the fundamental issue for some of these critics is that such programs conscript people into research efforts that they may not want to be part of. This is, of course, an appeal to losses resulting from unconsented-to invasions of privacy and from being used without permission. For these critics, such losses outweigh any social gains. The adoption of their position would in truth require that all epidemiological research be based on informed consent. As we have seen in this chapter, the alternative is to see these losses as serious moral considerations, but ones that can be outweighed in at least some cases by the need for the research and by the design of the research to prevent harms and to protect confidentiality. On this general balancing approach, which has won wide acceptance, the anonymous HIV seroprevalence testing program is morally justified.

Interventional Epidemiology

Epidemiologists primarily study the distribution and determinants of health-related states or events. It is vital to apply the results of these studies to the control of health problems. Some of these applications are tested in classical clinical trials testing interventions directed toward individuals. Others are tested in trials testing interventions directed toward communities. These interventions usually involve efforts designed to change lifestyle factors that have been shown in observational epidemiological studies to contribute to such diseases as cardiovascular disease and lung cancer. Trials of these community-directed interventions constitute the research effort of interventional epidemiology. In 1995, the *American Journal of Epidemiology* published a major symposium[42] on methodological issues raised by such trials. In this final section, we will examine the related ethical issues.

To help identify the issues, we will use as an example the COMMIT Study.[43] This study, funded by the National Cancer Institute, tested comprehensive community-wide strategies designed to inform citizens about the importance of not smoking and to alert smokers to the various opportunities for smoking cessation. Eleven matched pairs of communities were involved. One community in each pair was randomly assigned to receive these educational interventions and the other was assigned to the control group. The primary end point was the smoking quit rate among a cohort of heavy smokers followed in each community; secondary end points included the quit rate among a cohort of lighter smokers and the prevalence of adult cigarette smoking in each community. End point cohort members were contacted annually to assess smoking status, but they were not told of their status as cohort members, presumably to avoid any biasing effects of that information. For similar reasons, those surveyed in community-wide surveys of smoking prevalence were not told of the link between the survey and local COMMIT activities. The study showed no significant difference in quit rates among heavy smokers and in overall smoking prevalence; there was a statistically significant but modest (3%) additional quit rate among the lighter smokers in the intervention communities. This result suggests that different strategies, or the same strategies focused on specific more susceptible groups, will be required if community interventions are to make a difference to smoking behavior.

There are at least two types of ethical questions raised by this sort of study. The first has to do with the consent of communities to being randomized and to receiving the intervention. Do communities need to consent to being involved in such studies? If they do, who consents for them? If they do, do all twenty-two communities need to consent to being randomized or do only the eleven who were interventional communities need to consent to the intervention? The second has to do with the consent of the individuals surveyed, especially the members of the end point cohorts. Is it sufficient that they consent to being questioned annually about their smoking habits, or do they need to be informed, in order for that consent to be an informed consent, that they are part of the end point cohort of a community intervention study?

The COMMIT intervention was delivered through a community organization approach. Before randomization, there was some informal community involvement. After randomization, a community planning group, consisting of key community representatives, was formed in each of the eleven intervention communities; each played a major role in designing the implementation of the intervention in its community. Does the existence of these planning groups, as opposed to the more informal prerandomization community involvement, constitute adequate community consent? It is difficult to accept this suggestion. After all, these groups were formed only after randomization occurred and only in the communities that were randomized to receive the intervention. So their existence is irrelevant to the participation of the control group communities as a control group for the study and is irrelevant to the consent of any community to be randomized into the study. At most, their existence represents community consent to continue in the study, and it only does so if they could be envisaged as possibly withdrawing their community as opposed to just insisting on modifications in the intervention. The role of these groups is really better understood as facilitating access to the community groups necessary for the interventions to be possible. This is a valuable role, and the COMMIT study was wise to create such groups, but the relevance of these groups to community consent is at best modest. The CIOMS Guidelines on epidemiological research (Appendix 1.7, section 6) talk of a more significant role of community representatives in designing and assessing the study and require obtaining consent from community leaders chosen according to community traditions (section 5). Naturally, many questions remain both about whom to choose and about community consent for the control group communities. The question of community-based consent for such interventional studies clearly needs then further investigation; studies such as COMMIT should lead to this needed investigation.

The nondisclosure of some information to the members of the end point cohort groups reflects a more common and quite reasonable practice. The acceptability of this practice is explicitly stated in the CIOMS Guidelines: ''For certain epidemiological studies non-disclosure is permissible, even essential, so as to not influence the spontaneous conduct under investigation, and to avoid obtaining responses that the respondent might give in order to please the questioner. Selective disclosure may be benign and ethically permissible, provided that it does not induce subjects to do what they would not otherwise consent to do.'' (Appendix 1.7, section 9) As there is little reason to believe that the members of the end point cohort groups who answered the annual questions about smoking would have refused to do so if they knew they were members of that group, this last condition is satisfied.

Conclusion

The origin of official ethical policies for epidemiological research is not primarily connected to concerns about problematic cases, although the Tuskegee study certainly had an impact. Instead, these policies were prompted to some degree by general concerns about issues of privacy in a computerized society and to some degree by the desire of professional leaders to produce greater professionalism through the development of professional ethical standards.

In the development of these policies, new ethical concerns and new ethical methods were identified. Some of the new ethical concerns relate to potential wrongs. It is not enough to ensure that subjects in epidemiological research cannot be harmed because the confidentiality of data is protected. One must also consider the wrongs of unconsented-to invasions of privacy and of being used in research without consent. Others of the new ethical concerns relate to communities. We must be respectful of community values and of the agreement of communities as well as of individual values and individual consent. The new ethical methods relate to the idea of balancing. The new concerns about wrongs and about community involvement were not taken as absolute moral constraints but as values to be balanced against other values. If the research is of sufficient public importance, if obtaining consent is sufficiently burdensome, and if confidentiality is adequately protected, the research may proceed even if these wrongs occur. The new concerns about community values/consent do not displace either the need to respect universal moral standards or the need to obtain individual consent.

While neither of these achievements were reached easily, they do now seem to have won considerable support in the newest official policies. Nevertheless, the debates over research using stored tissue samples and over the program of unlinked anonymous HIV seroprevalence show that the full implications of these achievements have not yet been fully understood. Ethical reflection that involves recognizing new values and then responsibly balancing them against competing values involves many subtle reflections that are successfully completed only over a period of time. My own recommendations on many of the issues in the chapter (especially about stored tissue research, about anonymous HIV seroprevalence research, and about community intervention research) are my attempt to contribute to the balancing involved in the elaboration of the new consensus.

Chapter four

GENETIC RESEARCH

In 1953, the structure of DNA was identified by Crick and Watson. This sparked a revolution in biology. By the early 1970s, scientists learned how to isolate genetic material from one species and to attach it to genetic material from another species, thereby creating the technology of genetic engineering. Later in that decade, scientists began to identify the specific genetic foundations of various diseases, thereby laying the foundation for a program of gene therapy. By the early 1980s, scientists began to envision the possibility of mapping all of the human genes, thereby laying the foundation for the Human Genome Project. Much of the research required to carry out these programs required considerable investments, and the investors hoped that patents on the resulting discoveries would be the basis of the economic return on their investment. This served as the source of the interest in patenting the results of biotechnology.

Each of these topics (genetic engineering, gene therapy, the genome project, and patenting the results of biotechnology) has given rise to extensive ethical controversies. Nevertheless, on most of these topics, a fair amount of consensus has emerged in the official policies, even while there are remaining areas of controversy. In this chapter, we will look at each of these topics separately. We will examine the ethical issues associated with each of them, see the extent to which they have been resolved, and identify the remaining areas of controversy. We will see in the official policies an emerging pattern of greater acceptance of genetic research and greater willingness to treat the ethical issues raised by genetic research in a fashion analogous to how those issues are treated in other areas of research. It is this emerging pattern that is to a considerable extent responsible for the emerging consensus.

Genetic Engineering

In June of 1973, as the techniques of genetic engineering were first becoming available, a Gordon Conference was held on nucleic acids. At that conference, there was a discussion of the ethical issues related to the new technology.[1] Central to that discussion were concerns about possible hazards to those working in the laboratories and to the general public. This discussion led to a remarkable set of events.

A letter was sent from the participants to the National Academy of Sciences, with a copy published in *Science*, calling for the creation of a committee to look at these issues.[2] That committee was created and it called in 1974 for a moratorium on certain types of research and caution in the conduct of other types of research until standards could be developed. It organized a February 1975 meeting at the Asimolar Conference Center in California. That international meeting called for an ending to the moratorium subsequent to the adoption of provisions for physical and biological containment measures that were graduated according to the risk of the experiment. This led to the adoption of the first NIH Guidelines in 1976 by a newly created NIH Committee, the Recombinant DNA Advisory Committee (RAC).[3] Similar guidelines were adopted in Great Britain by the Genetic Manipulation Advisory Group (GMAG)[4] and in other countries. These guidelines, modified many times in the years to follow, were the foundations of the guidelines currently in place that will be described below.

Two very different evaluations of these events are possible. The first sees them as a responsible proactive attempt by the scientific community to identify the crucial ethical concerns about genetic engineering, concerns about the risks and benefits of these new techniques, and to deal with these concerns by a thoughtful program of risk minimization. The second sees them as a social failure to deal with the harder ethical issues raised by genetic engineering by allowing the scientific community to focus attention only on manageable questions of risk minimization. Let us look briefly at this latter evaluation and the broader issues about which it is concerned before we focus in on the current regulatory schemes.

What are the broader issues that have been identified as possible ethical concerns about genetic engineering? One often cited document that seems to embody a broader perspective is the 1982 Recommendation of the Parliamentary Assembly of the Council of Europe on Genetic Engineering.[5] It does distinguish between health and safety issues and broader ethical issues. But the broader issues turn out to be about the limits of gene therapy, about the uses of genetic information concerning humans, and about the patenting and commercialization of biotechnology. These are all legitimate issues; they will in fact be the central issues of the remaining sections of this chapter. But none of them are direct challenges to the ethics of genetic engineering itself. Perhaps the most important of the direct ethical challenges to genetic engineering itself are the claim that genetic engineering involves arrogantly interfering with nature by creating new life forms and by crossing the species barrier and the claim that genetic technology could be misused for purposes of biological warfare. In David Baltimore's opening address at Asimolar, these issues were explicitly excluded from the agenda, and the critics of the post-Asimolar developments see this as evidence of the failure.[6] These challenges, while rhetorically persuasive to some, have not been effective because they have not been formulated in a way that adequately differentiates genetic engineering from many other technological developments undertaken to improve the quality of human life, all of which interfere with nature and have the potential for misuse. In short, then, I would suggest that the post-Asimolar focusing on safety issues may reflect a failure of the critics to adequately demonstrate that there really are broader concerns about genetic engineering itself, rather than legitimate broader concerns about gene therapy and/or about the use of genetic information, (which will be discussed in the later sections of this chapter).

We turn then to the regulatory issues about safety. There are a number of general points about genetic engineering and safety that should be kept in mind. First, there are at least three sets of safety issues that have been addressed. These are the contained use of potentially dangerous genetically modified organisms, the protection of workers from risks related to exposure to genetically modified organisms at work, and the deliberate release into the environment of genetically modified organisms. In addition, the products of genetic engineering must pass the usual regulatory standards for foods, drugs, and so on before they can be sold in the marketplace. Second, regulatory systems can either have special regulations governing safety issues related to organisms produced by genetic engineering or they can cover them by relevant general safety regulations. Third, regulations can incorporate standards that are very stringent, emphasizing safety, or they can incorporate less stringent standards, taking some safety risks in order to increase the potential benefits obtained from genetic engineering. Finally, regulatory schemes need to be regularly updated in light of greater experience with, and knowledge of the risks of, genetic engineering.

The regulations governing genetic engineering in the European Union illustrate all of these points. There are three directives issued in 1990 covering the three safety issues mentioned above. Two, the regulations on contained use and on deliberate release into the environment, deal exclusively with genetically modified organisms; the third, on worker safety, is a general directive relating to exposure to biological agents. In 1994, the two directives on genetically modified organisms were made less stringent, partly in response to experience and partly in response to a recognition that excessive stringency can interfere with valuable scientific and technological developments.[7]

Although we will not be reviewing all the details of any of the regulatory schemes, a brief review of the major provisions of the European regulations on containment and on release are in order. We will also contrast them with the U.S. regulations.

The European regulations on containment distinguish two types of genetically modified microorganisms: the safer type I GMOs and the more risky type II GMOs. Under the 1994 revisions, a GMO is classified as type I if it is unlikely to cause disease or adverse effects in the environment because the recipient organism is unlikely to do so and because the vector and the insert do not endow it with a phenotype likely to do so. The regulations also distinguish type A teaching or research operations from type B industrial or commercial operations; the former is our concern. Type A operations using type I GMOs need to do a risk assessment, need to keep exposure to the lowest practical level by maintaining control measures and equipment, and need to formulate and regularly review local codes of practice. After an initial notification of operation to the local regulatory agency, no further submissions to any agency are required, although records must be kept. Stricter regulations (governing such topics as closure of the system, exhaust gases, sample collection, and effluent treatment) are imposed on type II GMOs. In addition, regulatory authorities must be informed of each research project involving type II GMOs, and they have 60 days to object before the research can commence. It is this last provision that is most burdensome on researchers, keeping in mind that the 60-day period can be extended if the regulatory authority asks for further information. This is why the adoption in 1994 of a broad definition of a type I GMO was so important.

The regulations governing release of GMOs into the environment are more demanding, even if this is done for research and not for general marketing. Regardless of the type of GMO, all such research must be approved by the regulatory authority. Researchers must submit extensive technical information and a detailed risk analysis and the research cannot proceed without approval from the regulatory agency. The 1994 modifications simplify things by allowing for a single application and approval for a series of related experiments. Nevertheless, more might be done if GMOs were classified according to risk and less stringent requirements were imposed on the release of less risky GMOs. The regulations also allow for individual countries to require that the public be notified and allowed to comment before approval is given. This requirement has been imposed in the United Kingdom.[8] It remains to be seen whether this provides for further useful input and offers an appropriate role for those most directly affected or whether this just adds an additional barrier to research.

Comparing these European regulations with the U.S. regulations is complicated by the lack of a single comprehensive regulatory scheme in the United States. The closest the United States comes to this is a 1986 Coordination Framework for Regulation of Biotechnology,[9] which sets out the responsibility of various federal agencies for the control of biotechnology and the basic principles adopted by those agencies. In terms of regulations on research in contained environments, the most crucial regulations are the NIH's Guidelines for Research Involving Recombinant DNA Molecules, the latest version of which was promulgated in June of 1994.[10] In terms of regulations on research involving the release of GMOs into the environment, the most important of the regulations are from the Department of Agriculture, the latest version of which was adopted in 1993, with further liberalizations developed in 1995.[11]

The NIH regulations incorporate a number of major elements. There are various levels of review required for such experiments. Depending on the level of concern for danger, experiments must be approved either by an institutional biosafety committee or by such a committee and the NIH. In reviewing protocols, a major emphasis is on the appropriate level of containment, where that involves standard lab practices, special physical barriers, and highly specific biological barriers. Four biosafety levels are recognized, with level 1 requiring the least stringent containment measures and level 4 requiring the most stringent containment measures. The regulations carefully describe the containment measures normally expected at each of the biosafety levels. Strictly speaking, the regulations apply only to research conducted at institutions receiving NIH funding for recombinant DNA research. Voluntary compliance by others is encouraged, and special measures have been adopted to protect crucial trade secrets.

The Department of Agriculture regulations govern field testing of genetically engineered crops. Originally, no such research could be conducted until approved by the agency. There were extensive precautions taken to prevent the escape of pollen, plants, or plant parts. Finally, the agency had to do an environmental assessment; this last requirement often gave rise to litigation by those opposed to such testing. Since 1993, applicants can just notify the agency, and not wait for approval, for field testing of genetically engineered corn, soybeans, cotton, potatoes, tomatoes, and tobacco, as extensive experience has shown the safety of such field testing. Since 1993, approximately 90% of all testing has been performed under this notification system, and the 1995 proposals would extend it to many more species.

These U.S. regulations, like the European regulations, still involve special regulatory schemes for genetically modified organisms, as opposed to covering them by relevant general safety regulations. However, in limiting the procedural requirements (by relying in more cases on institutional approval and on mere notification), they have been updated to reflect the good safety profile from initial experience. The U.S. regulations on containment are certainly more detailed and demanding than the European regulations, but they are increasingly less demanding on the issue of introducing genetically modified plants into the environment.

Some of the critics of these modifications[12] have suggested that they are due more to the commercial concerns of biotechnology firms and to the research concerns of the scientific community than to a real appreciation of the risks associated with genetic engineering. It is hard to be persuaded by this criticism in the light of the failure of the critics to specify any actual harms caused by laboratory genetic research or by research involving the introduction of genetically modified plants into the environment.

With the development of techniques of genetic engineering, a variety of ethical concerns were expressed. Some of these, raising very broad ethical concerns about genetic engineering itself, have not been articulated in an adequate enough fashion to have an impact on the official policies governing research on genetic engineering. Others, having to do with safety concerns, have been extensively addressed in these policies. They have become less demanding as experience has lessened some of these safety concerns. Eventually, they may simply be incorporated into general safety regulations. For now, however, those doing research using the techniques of genetic engineering need to be aware of the specific regulations in their own country.

Gene Therapy

In the early years of genetic engineering, the main applied focus was on the genetic modification of organisms for the production of pharmaceuticals and on the genetic modification of plants to improve food production. As the techniques of genetic engineering were better understood, and as better vectors for transferring genes into target cells were developed, researchers began to consider the possibilities of treating genetic disorders through use of these new techniques. The thought was that one could treat incurable illnesses due to single defective genes by using the right vector to introduce the normal genes either into the cells in the affected tissue or into other targeted cells (e.g., bone marrow) that can alter the disease process.

As these ideas were being considered, an experiment using these techniques was conducted in 1980 at UCLA on two patients, one from Israel and one from Italy, without the appropriate approval of an IRB.[13] This approval was, of course, required by all of the regulations covering human research discussed in Chapter Two. This incident, combined with general concerns both about the safety of gene therapy and about the limits on gene therapy, led to an extensive public discussion of, and a set of international policies for, gene therapy. Those discussions and the resulting policies are the focus of this section. But before turning to them, we need to keep in mind a few points about the development of gene therapy.

The first approved gene therapy experiment[14] was a protocol for treating children with adenosine deaminase (ADA) deficiency. Such patients lack a gene that expresses the enzyme ADA essential to the immune system, and children with this deficiency usually die of infections. The children enrolled in it have been doing well, but it is hard to know whether this is due to the gene therapy or to their also receiving a synthetic form of the enzyme, polyethyleneglycol (PEG)-ADA. Researchers are reluctant to take the patients off that additional treatment because it is clearly effective. Other experiments to treat genetic ill-nesses have gone less well. For example, attempts to treat cystic fibrosis through gene therapy using adenoviruses as vectors either don't result in enough ex-pression of the corrected gene or result in acute inflammations. Surprisingly, the majority of the gene therapy experiments approved by June of 1995 were for treating nongenetic diseases such as cancer or AIDS by using inserted genes to stimulate processes that might fight the diseases in question. Few positive results have been published. Nevertheless, there has been enough enthusiasm for these techniques that emergency approvals were granted for their use in desperate cases in 1993. Despite this enthusiasm and the resulting extensive private in-vestment in biotechnology firms working on gene therapy, there developed a feeling by early 1995 that much more basic research might be required before gene therapy would succeed. This led the NIH to create in 1995 a panel to develop a plan for a more rational approach to research in this area. In short, then, the initial excitement about gene therapy has turned to a cautious optimism tempered by a recognition that much more basic research may be required.[15]

During this period (1980–95), there was also much discussion of a number of fundamental ethical issues. Although there was near unanimity in the accep-tance of research on at least some forms of gene therapy, at least three issues emerged as deserving careful attention: What process and standards of review should be used for gene therapy protocols? What limits, if any, should be placed on the conditions eligible for treatment by gene therapy? Should gene therapy be confined to somatic cells or can it also be applied to germ cells? We shall examine each of these questions separately.

All gene therapy protocols are research studies involving human subjects. They must, therefore, be approved by an IRB or a research ethics committee/board using the standards discussed in Chapter Two before they can be imple-mented. In addition, as they involve new biological products used therapeuti-cally, national drug regulatory agencies, as will be explained in Chapter Eight, must be notified and must agree (or, at least, not object) before clinical trials can commence. Despite these standard layers of approval, it was initially quite common to require an additional level of approval for human gene therapy protocols. This is a continuation of the trend, noticed in the previous section, to begin by treating genetic research as a special case requiring special control.

In the United States, the requirement of additional review was imposed by the NIH and that additional review has been provided by its RAC. It issued in 1985 an extremely important set of standards, the "Points to Consider" docu-ment,[16] which will be analyzed below. In 1988, the European Medical Research

Councils called for additional review and monitoring at the national level for gene therapy protocols (Appendix 2.6, section on Regulation). In 1992, the U.K. Clothier Committee on the Ethics of Gene Therapy concurred with this recommendation; this led to the establishment of the Gene Therapy Advisory Committee, which provides the additional level of review. It has issued a guidance,[17] which provides a standard for review, also analyzed below. Similar groups have emerged in other countries. Australia is a bit of an exception. It has a national Genetic Manipulation Advisory Committee, which monitors research and is available for consultation, but its approval is not required for gene therapy protocols under the policies of the National Health and Medical Research Council (Appendix 4.12, Supplementary Note 7).

A number of reasons have been put forward for requiring these additional levels of review. One is the desire to allay public fears about unregulated gene research. Another is to ensure that these protocols, which are often very technically complex, are reviewed by those who have the requisite technical expertise. Finally, there is the fear that purely local review may not address larger issues that are special to gene therapy.

A reaction to this trend has begun to emerge. There is an increasing sense that extra layers of review are not required and that institutional review and national drug regulatory agency review should be adequate, especially in those countries in which drug regulatory agencies carefully scrutinize research protocols using new agents before clinical trials can commence. In the United States, this reaction led to the decision in 1994–95 to confine RAC review to protocols that involve new target diseases or vectors, that involve uncertain health or environmental risks, or that require public review for some other reason. In November of 1996, after much public discussion, the Director of the NIH went one step further and decided that the RAC would no longer review individual protocols. Review of individual gene therapy protocols would be done locally by IRBs and nationally by the FDA. Discussion of larger policy issues would be initiated by the Office of Recombinant DNA Activities at the NIH. Although the RAC will continue to exist, it remains to be seen what will be its role.[18]

The U.S. guidelines are incorporated into the RAC's "Points to Consider"[19] and in the FDA's "Points to Consider."[20] Both sets of guidelines call for the submission of basic science and preclinical data related to safety and efficacy. The RAC guidelines address patient selection, confidentiality, and consent; the FDA guidelines address manufacturing process and quality control. These differences reflect the differences in mission of these groups. The RAC guidelines reflect the usual ethical standards for research and special standards in the area of gene therapy about assuring accurate public information in a fashion consistent with preserving confidentiality and about assuring full communication among investigators in a fashion consistent with protecting patents and trade secrets. The same is true for the Guidance from the U.K. Gene Therapy Advisory Committee.[21] The differences between the standards in these different countries reflect underlying differences on how they approach human subjects research. For example, the U.K. emphasis, noted in Chapter Two, of encouraging subjects to consult their own physician is reemphasized in the British gene therapy guidance, and is viewed as essential for pediatric protocols.[22] The limited number of special issues in these different guidelines supports the view that extra levels of review may not be necessary.

One large issue that has attracted much attention, even if not emphasized in the U.S. and U.K. guidelines, is possible limits on the conditions to be treated by gene therapy. Two limits have been proposed in many of the official policies on gene therapy: gene therapy should not be done for the sake of enhancements and gene therapy should not involve germ line therapy.

The motivation for the first of these limits is found in the unfortunate connection between genetics and the eugenics movement in the first part of the twentieth century.[23] The eugenics movement was devoted to using genetic knowledge to "improve the human condition" by encouraging the breeding of "socially desirable people" and by preventing the procreation of "undesirables." This movement came to be dominated by a variety of prejudicial stereotypes, leading to discrimination against various groups and, at its most extreme, to racial purges and holocausts. It also encouraged the practice of compulsory sterilization, as well as other infringements on individual rights. In the post–World War II period, this type of thinking fell out of favor, although it has reemerged in a variety of settings. With the development of genetic engineering and of gene therapy, concerns were expressed that these new techniques could be used as part of a revised eugenics program. Many of the official policies for gene therapy attempted, therefore, to prohibit the eugenics use of gene therapy.

In general, the Europeans have supported this first limitation. The European Medical Research Councils, in a 1988 statement (Appendix 2.6, section on Scope of Gene Therapy), said that: "gene therapy for the enhancement of general human characteristics such as physical appearance or intelligence . . . raises profound ethical problems and should not be contemplated." A similar limitation is found in the Council of Europe's 1996 Convention on Human Rights and Biomedicine (Appendix 2.3, Article 13). The 1993 Guidelines from the Health Sciences Council of Japan goes even further, limiting gene therapy research to research on treating conditions that are fatal (Appendix 4.13, Article 4). Some of the official policies are less absolute. The British Clothier Committee (Appendix 4.6, section 8.7) simply said that "In the current state of knowledge any attempt to change human traits not associated with disease would not be acceptable," suggesting that it might be after further knowledge is gained.

This limitation requires, of course, the ability to differentiate acceptable treatment of diseases or dispositions to diseases from unacceptable mere "improvements'' or ''enhancements.'' Many cases of each type are easy to classify; genetic modifications to treat cystic fibrosis are acceptable on this approach whereas genetic modifications to change eye color are not. However, there are others that might be more problematic to classify. Consider, for example, dispositions to antisocial behavior. If genes favoring such dispositions were discovered, would their replacement be an appropriate use of gene therapy? Moreover, cosmetic enhancements by other medical techniques (e.g., cosmetic surgery) are commonly allowed; why should genetic interventions to produce these enhancements be banned? As long as no coercion or violation of human rights is involved, as was the case in the eugenics movement, what is wrong with genetic enhancements?[24]

When the prospects for genetic enhancement become more realistic while the safety profile of gene therapy becomes more established, and when the distinctions come under greater pressure, these limitations may not be maintainable. In March of 1997, the United States RAC called for a public conference to discuss genetic enhancement.[25] Perhaps we may see the emergence of a disagreement in official policies over genetic enhancements.

A second limit found in many official policies restricts gene therapy to somatic cells only. The European Medical Research Councils in 1988 proclaimed that ''germ line gene therapy should not be contemplated'' (Appendix 2.6, section on Distinction between Somatic and Germline Gene Therapy). Similarly, the 1996 Council of Europe Convention allows for genetic interventions ''only if its aim is not to introduce any modification in the genome of any descendants'' (Appendix 2.3, Article 13).

At first glance, this ban seems very problematic. Treating genetically based diseases by modifying only somatic cells results in the need to treat the same disease in each succeeding generation as the defective genes are passed on from one generation to another. Why not solve the problem definitively by modifying the germ cells so that the defect is not passed from one generation to another?

Some of the considerations that are offered in support of the ban are only cautionary observations. Germ cell genetic therapy is an intervention that involves considerable scientific uncertainties about long-term benefits and risks that need to be resolved. These types of cautionary observations do not support the complete ban in question. They support instead a cautionary approach that would hold off on experiments to test germ line therapy until the risks and benefits are better understood, through both basic research and research using animal models. Such a cautionary approach has been adopted by the RAC in the United States, which has stipulated that it will not at this time consider protocols for germ line gene therapy, suggesting that it might at later times when the needed scientific information was available.

What are the arguments of those who would ban germ line therapy entirely? The following are often mentioned:

1. Experimentation to test germ line therapy would be experimentation on future generations that could not give their consent. We are not entitled to perform this type of experimentation.
2. Future generations have a right to inherit a genetic endowment that has not been intentionally modified. The advocates of this right have described it as the right to the integrity of genetic patrimony. Germ line therapy violates this right.
3. Experimentation on germ line therapy opens up still further opportunities for the use of genetics in discriminatory eugenic programs.

Those who support experimentation to develop germ line therapy would argue that progenitors can consent to therapeutic experimentation that indirectly affects their descendants much as parents can consent to therapeutic experimentation on their children, that there is no right to inherit a genetic endowment that produces serious diseases, and that germ line therapy is no more necessarily connected to inappropriate eugenics than somatic cell therapy.[26] These responses seem adequate, and all that seems to be justified is a cautionary approach to germ line therapy.

As one reviews the development of the ethical issues surrounding research on the development of gene therapy, a familiar theme reappears. It is the theme of greater liberalization in official policies after greater familiarity with the technology. The clearest example of this is that there is less of a felt need for further levels of review of individual protocols as more gene therapy protocols have been carried out, despite the limited success of the early protocols. Moreover, as possibilities for further protocols are being explored, there may develop a greater level of comfort with the idea that we will eventually move into well-defined areas of germ line therapy and of appropriate enhancements. Alternatively, this may become an area in which official policies disagree.

The Human Genome Project

By the mid-1980s, the advances in genetic engineering combined with the promise of gene therapy led to the suggestion that an organized effort should be made to sequence the entire human genome and to map the entire complement of human genes. In a five-year period (1985–1990), that concept grew from a vision into a formal plan, supported in the United States with considerable public funds as a joint project of the NIH and the DOE and coordinated with similar efforts elsewhere. For the first time, biological research had a big science project comparable to some of the big science projects in the physical sciences.[27]

There are many fascinating issues of science policy raised by this development. Among them: Are the benefits of this type of big science sufficient to justify the potential loss of funding to smaller projects in a time of limited research budgets? Is it possible to coordinate the efforts of researchers in many laboratories in many countries to ensure that all areas of the human genome are sequenced and mapped without expensive and needless duplication of efforts? How can one facilitate the sharing of information among all of these researchers without depriving anyone of appropriate credit and reward? These issues are not unique to the Human Genome Project, but they arose with particular urgency in that project because of the necessity for considerable collaboration and sharing of information. It should also be noted that many of these policy issues raise questions about appropriate rules for intellectual property rights in the results of the genome project; those questions will be discussed in the next section of this chapter.

There is, however, another aspect of the history of the genome project both in the United States and elsewhere that must be mentioned because it relates directly to the rest of this section and to the central concerns of this chapter. By the late 1980s, the U.S. effort contained as a significant component a program devoted to studying the ethical, legal, and social implications of the Human Genome Project. This was called the ELSI program. Funding for this activity was set at a definite percentage of the federal budget for the genome project, making the ethics of the Human Genome Project the best-funded area of bioethical research. Similar funding became part of the funding of human genome projects in other countries. These seemed to be a clear recognition that the ethical issues associated with the Human Genome Project could not be neglected.

What were these issues? It is fair to say that they were primarily issues related to the use of the results of this research, rather than challenges to the ethical validity of the research itself. Among the issues that have attracted considerable attention are voluntary choices as the basis for genetic testing, proper criteria for universal screening programs, privacy and confidentiality of information obtained from genetic tests, and nondiscrimination against those genetically disposed to various illnesses in insurance and employment. Although a full treatment of each of these issues lies beyond the scope of this book, researchers in this area need to be familiar with at least the basic concerns about each of these issues and the fundamental policies that have emerged.

The theme that voluntary choices must be the basis for genetic testing has been reiterated in many of the international declarations on the Human Genome Project. The Declaration of Inuyama (1991), from the Council for International Organizations of Medical Sciences,[28] declared that "Voluntarism should be the guiding principle in the provision of genetic services." The World Medical Association Declaration on the Human Genome Project clarified what voluntarism implied when it declared that "One should respect the will of persons screened and their right to decide about their participation and about the use of the information obtained'' (Appendix 1.4, section on recommendations). Most recently, the principle has been reaffirmed in a draft of a declaration on human rights and the genome to be presented for UNESCO's adoption in the fall of 1997.[29]

This emphasis on voluntarism in genetic testing has been particularly important for testing programs related to Huntington's disease, where it is well documented that many who are at risk don't want to know whether they will develop this disease. After the detection of the gene defect in 1993, which made it possible to test individuals directly without necessarily testing other family members, the guidelines from the International Huntington Foundation and the World Federation of Neurology[30] reaffirmed the principle that ''The decision to take the test is solely the choice of the individual concerned.'' It went on to affirm that with the exception of prenatal testing, ''The test is available only to individuals who have reached the age of majority.'' It explained that this would enable the child to make his or her own decision upon reaching the age of maturity so as to preserve children's right to decide whether they want to know. In doing this, of course, it explained why the standard principle that parents can make decisions about what forms of medical interventions will be provided to their children does not apply to this case.

The principle of voluntarism in genetic testing, as normally formulated, relates to well-validated genetic tests and insists that individuals have the right to decide whether or not to be tested. But there is a possible extension of that principle to genetic tests still in the process of being validated through research protocols. Should individuals have the right to receive that genetic testing outside of research protocols if they so wish (the extended principle of voluntarism) or may society decide to limit these genetic tests to those who are enrolled in research protocols relating to the validation of the tests? This question has created great controversy as new genetic tests emerged for susceptibility to Alzheimer's disease (APOE4 gene test)[31] and for breast cancer (BRCA1 mutation gene test).[32] Individuals desiring such testing outside of research protocols and commercial labs willing to provide it came into controversy with professional groups wanting to limit the testing to individuals in research protocols. One side argued that the principle of personal autonomy that lies behind voluntarism justifies extending voluntarism to such cases. Commercial firms began to make such tests available.[33] The other side argued that with important scientific questions about the validity of the test as a predictive test unanswered, with the implications of a positive finding for preventive treatment nonexistent (in the case of Alzheimer's disease) or questionable (in the case of breast cancer), and with the damaging psychosocial implications of a positive finding uncertain, it would be wrong to offer the test except in research protocols designed to answer these questions.

These controversies about the use of newly emerging genetic tests will no doubt continue to arise as the genome project continues to provide new information about genetic susceptibility to diseases.

A universal screening program would be one that made a validated genetic test either for disease susceptibility or for carrier status available to all relevant individuals in the society who wished to be tested. What criteria should be employed in deciding whether a universal screening program should be developed? This issue has proved particularly contentious in the area of cystic fibrosis carrier screening. Most children with cystic fibrosis are born into families without a family history of cystic fibrosis. Therefore, identifying all the families at risk would require a universal screening program. The genetic defect for cystic fibrosis was identified in 1989. The American Society for Human Genetics (in 1989) and a workshop convened by the NIH (in 1990) concluded that carrier screening was not justified because of the inadequate sensitivity of the tests then available and because of a lack of pilot program data.[34] As the sensitivity improved, such pilot programs began both in the United States and in the United Kingdom. A 1997 summary[35] reported that interest in being screened was very variable, with the greatest interest being shown by those who would be screened for free as part of routine prenatal care. It also reported considerable uncertainty about the meaning of the results. Task forces were working in 1997 to develop guidelines in the light of these findings, with the greatest support being for screening programs offered to people planning to become pregnant so that they could make reproductive decisions.[36] In the meantime, one 1994 study estimated that a universal screening program would not be cost effective to the health care payer because the screening costs would be greater than the medical costs saved due to terminated pregnancies. The authors concluded that the justification would have to be from the perspective of the expectant parents.[37] It remains to be seen whether universal cystic fibrosis screening for those willing to be screened will emerge as the standard of practice. Cystic fibrosis screening is the original test case for universal genetic screening, much as Huntington's disease is the original test case for the voluntarist approach to genetic testing.

Three very important policies have been articulated on genetic screening: a 1993 report from the U.K.'s Nuffield Council on Bioethics,[38] a 1994 Council of Europe policy,[39] and 1997 recommendations from a U.S. ELSI Task Force on Genetic Testing.[40] Each attempts to identify the criteria for a legitimate voluntary screening program with adequate protections of confidentiality, and there is considerable overlap in their criteria, with some subtle disagreements. Among the criteria mentioned are:

1. The program should involve tests that are highly sensitive and specific and that have a high positive predictive value.
2. There must be available therapy or other interventions that are more useful

if applied before symptomatic disease appears or the knowledge gained must be otherwise valuable to the individuals being screened.

3. The program can be justified economically in comparison to other ways in which health funds could be used.

4. The program must be based on lab work whose high quality can be assured.

5. The program must involve adequate counseling before the screening to ensure informed consent and adequate counseling about the meaning of the results afterwards.

One of the results of the genome project will be the ability to better identify individuals that are more likely to develop various expensive diseases. There is the possibility that such information could be used by insurance companies to deny health or life insurance coverage to such individuals and by employers to deny them employment. These concerns are not just theoretical. A 1983 study by the Office of Technology Assessment of the U.S. Congress showed that a considerable number of large companies had engaged in refusals to hire based upon genetic testing in the period 1970–82.[41] With the emergence of far greater abilities to test, the potential for denials of insurance or employment will only increase.

Various attitudes toward this potential are possible. Some view this potential as a legitimate opportunity for insurance companies and employers to respond to real differences among people in a legitimate fashion. Why should those who are at less risk have to share the costs of insuring those who are at greater risk? Why should companies have to bear the costs of hiring workers who are more likely to be sick? On this account, genetic testing is no different from the traditional testing done by insurance companies before policies are written and by employers before workers are hired; properly validated genetic testing can be mandated and its findings can be taken into consideration. Others, at the opposite end of the spectrum, view this potential as the beginning of a pattern of discrimination against those who are genetically predisposed to various illnesses. The goal of insurance is to spread risks among large populations and that only happens when everyone has equal access to insurance regardless of genetic heritage. Similarly, equal opportunity for employment mandates that genetic heritage not become the basis for discrimination in employment. Even properly validated genetic testing should never be mandated for insurance or employment purposes, and those who are voluntarily tested should have total control over who receives the results. Naturally, various in-between positions are also possible.

It is fair to say that at both the international and the national level, the second attitude has prevailed in the official policies that have been developed in the early 1990s. Thus, the World Medical Association concluded in 1992 that ''The disclosure of information to a third party or the accessibility to personal genetic data should be allowed only with the patient's informed consent'' (Appendix 1.4, section on recommendations). The Council of Europe was even more explicit when it said in 1992 (Appendix 2.5, Principles 6 and 7) that ''Insurers should not have the right to require genetic testing or to enquire about results of previously performed tests, as a pre-condition for the conclusion or modification of an insurance contract'' and that employment should not be dependent on undergoing genetic testing unless that can be justified ''by reasons of direct protection of the person concerned or of a third party and be directly related to the specific conditions of the activity.'' This last exception raises many questions that will, no doubt, need to be resolved in the next few years.

Two 1993 reports, one from the United States and one from Great Britain, reinforce this trend. The U.S. report is from an ELSI Task Force on Genetic Information and Insurance.[42] Given the serious problems about access to health care faced by those in the United States who lack health insurance, its focus was on health insurance. Among its conclusions about a fundamentally reformed health care system were that in it genetic information should not be used to deny health care coverage to anyone and the cost of health care coverage should not be affected by genetic information about the covered individual. In the interim, it recommended that ''health insurers should consider a moratorium on the use of genetic tests in underwriting.'' In Great Britain, with its system of universal health care coverage under the National Health Service, the health insurance issue was less central. Instead, a report from the Nuffield Council on Bioethics focused on life insurance and on employment.[43] It recommended that insurance companies should not require genetic tests as a prerequisite for obtaining life insurance, with the exception of policies with a high monetary value or policies written on individuals whose genetic problem is revealed through traditional family histories. Following the Council of Europe, it allowed for genetically based refusals of employment only when there is a direct threat to the health of the employee or others, but it added the important proviso that ''the condition is one for which the dangers cannot be eliminated or significantly reduced by reasonable measures taken by the employer to modify or respond to the environmental risks.'' Finally, in 1995, the United States EEOC (Equal Employment Opportunity Commission) ruled[44] that employers that discriminate against individuals on the basis of genetic information violate the general laws against discrimination in employment, and the U.S. Congress passed a bill[45] banning discrimination in insurance based on genetic susceptibility to disease.

These issues are far from completely resolved. It is of interest to note that the American Council of Life Insurance, which had a representative on the 1993 ELSI Task Force, opposed the report in that it ''directly conflicts with ACLI policy'' and that the Health Insurance Association of America, which also had a representative, concluded that ''the association's policy should be one of neutrality.''[46] Both in the United States and in the United Kingdom, life insurance associations attempted in 1995–96 to develop alternative approaches, emphasizing their view that a ban on genetic testing for insurance underwriting would enable those at risk to take unfair advantage of the system. A full response to their opposition may require a total rethinking of the role of testing in both insurance and employment, a rethinking that has already begun in many countries.

To summarize, the human genome issue has raised many important ethical questions about the use of the resulting information. The emerging consensus in the official policies seems to be that the principle of voluntarism should guide the decision as to who will be tested, that universal screening programs, even if voluntary, should be introduced only after stringent criteria are met, and that those who genetically are at higher risk for developing diseases should be protected against discrimination both in employment and in insurance. Many, but not all, of the aspects of this consensus represent the application of traditional bioethical standards to the use of genetic information.

Patenting the Results of Genetic Research

The growth of scientific research has been greatly encouraged by providing researchers and/or investors with patents governing the useful results of their research. In the area of genetic research, however, this patenting has given rise to many ethical concerns. In the final section of this chapter, we will focus on the special ethical issues related to the patenting of the results of genetic research.

Three major events in the United States, with parallels elsewhere, provoked an intensive discussion of the patenting of the results of genetic research. The first was the decision by the United States Supreme Court in *Diamond v. Chakrabaty* (1980) that human-made living microorganisms were patentable as new and useful compositions of matter. The European Patent Convention of 1973 has also been interpreted to allow for the patenting of such microorganisms. The second was the decision of the U.S. Patent Office in 1987 that nonnaturally occurring nonhuman animals would be patentable; on the basis of this decision, Harvard University received a patent for a mouse, the Harvard Oncomouse, which was genetically altered to be very susceptible to developing cancer, thereby making it an excellent model for scientific research.[47] This decision was also adopted by the Appeals Board of the European Patent Office in 1990, reversing an earlier refusal to allow the patent, and was implemented in 1991–92 by the European Patent Office.[48] The third were 1992 filings by commercial interests, by the NIH, and by the British Medical Research Council for patents on expressed sequence tags for human genes, with the claim covering the tag, the entire sequence, and the protein product.[49] Each of these events provoked considerable controversy, and the result of this accumulated controversy is a widespread feeling that there are major ethical difficulties with the patenting of the results of genetic engineering.

Why this controversy over patenting the results of genetic research given that patents are regularly issued for other results of scientific research? Some of the controversy was really about other regulatory issues, with the opponents of patenting using that opposition to indirectly raise the regulatory issues. As discussed in Chapter One, there was a recognition that the regulations in some countries (e.g., the United States) protecting transgenic animals from inappropriate suffering were inadequate. As discussed earlier in this chapter, there were also concerns about safety and environmental impact. All these concerns, however, were best dealt with by the proper regulatory mechanisms we have described, not by limiting genetic research through banning patents on its results.

Some of the controversy was really an attempt by those who opposed genetic engineering (because it interfered with the integrity of nature or because it posed a threat of misuse for biological warfare) to stop genetic engineering by banning the patents needed to support research. We have already discussed those issues earlier in this chapter and suggested that they have never been properly developed into compelling concerns.

The rest of the controversy really was about the patents themselves. It raised moral questions about what can legitimately be patented and extent of discovery questions about what research discoveries justify the issuing of a patent so as to promote rather than to hinder research. Let us examine each of these questions separately.

The patenting of genetically modified microorganisms and animals already raised questions about whether living entities should be ownable through patents. But in the light of the fact that living things are owned in other ways, it was unclear why they could not be patented. In the minds of many, however, human genes are different. A number of considerations have been offered to explain why. One is that much as we don't allow human beings—as opposed to other living things—to be owned, because that is incompatible with human dignity, we should also not allow for the ownership of human genes. Another is that the human genome consists of naturally occurring genes that are part of our common heritage. No one should be able to make that common heritage into their private property through a patent.

In addition to this fundamental moral question about the patentability of human genes, there was also the question of what needed to be discovered before the rewarding of a patent was appropriate. This issue was raised by the NIH and the British Medical Research Council 1992 filings. Those filings were based on expressed sequence tags, and contained no information about the function of the gene or about the use of the results. Those filings were followed by, and were intended to preempt, commercial filings of a similar nature. By 1994, the U.S. Patent Office had rejected these filings, claiming that their utility is not clear, but it made clear in October of 1996 that other such filings might be accepted, keeping in mind the utility of the sequences as probes.[50] What is needed to justify the issuing of a patent?

The moral issue and the extent of discovery issue were mixed together in a proposed European Union Directive.[51] Exclusion from patentability on moral grounds is more common in European patent law than in U.S. patent law. Not surprisingly, therefore, the 1992 proposed European Union Directive on the Legal Protection of Biotechnological Inventions expressed the first concern. While allowing for the patentability of biological material, it prohibited the patenting "of the human body or parts of the human body per se." The explanatory memorandum accompanying the Directive made it clear that this ban covers the patenting of human genes only as a part of the human body. But it also suggested that the ban applies only when the function of the gene and the protein for which it codes is unknown, suggesting that the drafters were also concerned about the extent of discovery issue. In any case, the Directive was rejected in 1995, but a version was reconsidered in 1997. Developments in the summer of 1997 make it likely that a compromise Directive, allowing for some patenting of human genes, will be adopted.[52]

A compromise approach has recently emerged. This approach would not allow for the patenting of the genes, but it would allow for the patenting of uses of the genes (or of the sequences), presupposing of course that it was the use and not just the gene or the sequence that had been discovered. This approach directly addresses the extent of discovery issue and its relation to promoting research. On the one hand, this approach would provide the needed encouragement for research, for it is the patentable uses that bring in the desired revenues and that need to be protected by intellectual property rights. On the other hand, this approach would not hinder research on uses because the sequence had already been patented. Moreover, it indirectly satisfies those concerned about the moral issue of patenting human genes because the human genes themselves would remain part of the common heritage of humanity, which could not be patented by anyone.

This compromise position was proposed by the U.S. National Center for Human Genome Research in April of 1996 (Appendix 3.10), following an international scientific conference that supported it. According to this policy, all researchers supported by the Center must quickly release to public databases all human genomic DNA sequences and must not patent such sequences until they can demonstrate the use.

The patenting of the results of genetic research is still highly controversial. The opponents of such patenting marshalled a group of U.S. religious leaders to issue in early 1995 a general opposition to patenting both transgenic animals and human genes.[53] As noted above, the European Directive on these matters was defeated in the European Parliament, in part by those generally opposed to patenting life. Within the research community, where patenting has found greater acceptance, there is still considerable debate about what must have been achieved before a patent should be issued. But there seems to be a growing international official acceptance of the patenting of genetically modified micro-organisms and transgenic animals and of the patenting of specific uses of human gene sequences, although perhaps not of the human genes themselves. This compromise has yet to be fully realized in international intellectual property law. The development of an international agreement supporting such a compro-mise seems highly desirable.

Conclusion

The quantity of official policies on issues related to genetic research is very great. Moreover, the origin of these official policies on genetic research is truly unique. It represents the clearest case of extensive official policies developed to prevent the development of problems, rather than policies designed in response to problematic cases. The policies adopted after Asimolar are one example, but there are others. We had, for example, policies limiting gene therapy before the first gene therapy protocols reported their first limited successes. This represents to me a major accomplishment. Preventive ethics is preferable to curative ethics in the same way that preventive medicine is preferable to curative medicine.

The trend in all of these policies is clear. They begin with special limitations and procedures, but rely more on standard policies and procedures as time goes along. Thus, the very strict safety regulations were modified as experience with genetic engineering accumulated and special national reviews for gene therapy protocols have increasingly come under challenge. It is increasingly clear that the standard principles of autonomy, confidentiality, and nondiscrimination should apply to genetic testing, to the release of genetic information, and to the use of genetic information in employment and insurance decisions. Of particular interest is the growing willingness to apply the standard policies of intellectual property law to patents resulting from genetic research.

From the very beginning of the development of these policies, critics have argued that this trend toward the normalization of the policies governing genetic research is mistaken. From their perspective, this trend has failed to take into account the truly unique issues raised by genetic research. We have confronted this objection several times in the chapter, and our judgment about it has always been the same: the critics have failed to support their case by an adequate articulation of their concerns and/or an adequate defense of them.

There is much that remains to be done: further decisions need to be made about safety regulations for research involving genetic engineering; the limits of gene therapy remain to be defined; adequate protections of autonomy, confidentiality, and nondiscrimination need to be built into national laws; final decisions need to be made about the issue of patents. But the right questions have certainly been asked, and the trend toward normalization in the answers given seems appropriate.

Chapter five

REPRODUCTIVE AND FETAL RESEARCH

In recent years, great interest has developed in doing research involving fetuses. At least three forms of research have emerged. First, there is therapeutic and nontherapeutic research using fetuses in utero as subjects. Second, there is research employing tissue from aborted fetuses. Finally, with the emergence of in vitro fertilization, there is research on zygotes to study the early stages of development and to improve the techniques of technologically assisted reproduction.

This great interest has been accompanied by considerable ethical concern. This is not surprising. As a result of the general debate on abortion, the citizens of most developed countries are divided on such questions as the moral status of the fetus at various stages of development and the permissibility of abortion under various circumstances. Similarly, as a result of the general debate about the claims of feminism, the citizens of most developed countries are divided on such questions as the authority of pregnant women over decision making that has an impact on fetuses and the legitimacy of technologically assisted reproduction. These differing views influence the official policies governing reproductive and fetal research. As one result, the development of such policies has been a very contentious process; there probably are more governmental and professional reports on the development of these policies than on any other issue in research ethics. As another result, the development of these policies has often been based on the formulation of a moral compromise designed to secure acceptance of the research policy by adherents of as many of the differing views on abortion and on feminism as possible. We will be looking at the nature of the compromises involved, and the success in developing the compromises, throughout this chapter.

In this chapter, we will separately examine each of these types of research.

We will identify the major ethical issues that have been raised about each and analyze what the policies have to say about these issues.

One preliminary terminological point. The use of language to differentiate the various stages of development from conception until birth varies considerably. Moreover, the terms employed often seem to be chosen for their emotional connotations, with different sides choosing different terms. When we want to differentiate the various stages of development, we shall employ the term *zygote* to refer to the product of conception for the first two weeks following conception (until the primitive streak appears), the term *embryo* to refer to it for the next six weeks following conception (until organogenesis is completed), and the term *fetus* to refer to it from then until birth. We do so without making any judgment that these stages, whatever their medical significance, are morally different in any significant way.

One preliminary substantive point. There has also been in recent years a significant discussion about the involvement of women as subjects in research, about the use of women of childbearing potential as research subjects, and about the use of pregnant women as research subjects. The second and third of these issues are related to our concerns in this chapter, especially to those discussed in the first section on research on fetuses in utero. Because of their importance, however, they will be discussed separately in Chapter Nine.

Research on Fetuses in Utero

All official policies treat research on fetuses in utero as human subjects research governed by the policies for human subjects research discussed in Chapter Two. Independent review of the research protocol is required, the requirements on risks and benefits must be met, and informed consent must be obtained.

It is clearly understood by all that at least some therapeutic research on fetuses in utero must be allowed. How else can we discover and validate new methods for treating fetal health problems? ACTG 076, the trial that showed that the use of AZT lessened maternal-fetal HIV transmission, is an excellent example of why such research is required.[1] Moreover, some basic research on fetuses in utero may also be necessary as the foundation for the later development of new forms of treatment. However, additional requirements on research employing fetuses in utero have been imposed, requirements that are responses to special aspects of this type of research.

Because fetuses in utero and pregnant women are linked to each other, research on one may affect the other. Such research may have a differential impact on the pregnant woman and the fetus, with one benefiting while the other does not. At the extreme, the research that is beneficial to the one may actually be harmful to the other. The fundamental presupposition of all of the official national policies is that the independent review process for human subjects research must consider the interests and rights of both parties in reviewing research protocols on fetuses in utero. Some have also imposed additional requirements on the acceptable level of risk to the fetuses.

This is the major way in which those policies accord some moral standing to the fetus. This stands in opposition, of course, to any view that fetuses have no moral standing and that their interests and rights do not need to be considered at all. It does not presuppose, however, any commitment to the view that their moral standing is that of full personhood, equivalent to the moral standing of the pregnant woman. All that the policies presuppose is that fetuses have some moral standing so that some concern must be devoted to their interests and rights. The assumption of this presupposition constitutes our first example of the moral compromises adopted in the development of fetal research policies.

The U.S. regulations from the DHHS (Appendix 3.1, section 46.208) provide a good example of this compromise. Recognizing its importance, they allow for therapeutic research on fetuses in utero. In such therapeutic research, the fetus must be placed at risk "only to the minimum extent necessary," although if necessary, that could still be a quite substantial risk. They also require that appropriate studies on animals have been completed first. The regulations also allow for nontherapeutic research on fetuses in utero after the completion of appropriate studies on animals. In such nontherapeutic research, however, the risk to the fetus must be "minimal." This is less strict than the 1986 policy of the Council of Europe, which seems to ban all nontherapeutic research on fetuses, no matter how minimal the risk.[2] But the U.S. standard is stricter than the U.S. requirements on nontherapeutic research for pediatric subjects, discussed in Chapter Six, which allow for at least some nontherapeutic research that imposes somewhat greater risks, and the Council of Europe standard is stricter than the European policies that allow nontherapeutic research on children if the risks are no greater than minimal. The justification for these stricter requirements on nontherapeutic research involving fetuses than on nontherapeutic research involving children is unclear. The Council of Europe policy was in the process of being reexamined in 1997 as part of the follow-up to the 1996 European Convention.[3] It remains to be seen whether this stricter European standard will be modified.

Because fetal consent is meaningless, the only party whose consent can be sought is the pregnant woman. There is some potential for conflicts of interest in that maternal consent may not reflect fetal interests. There is also the possibility that pressure may be put on pregnant women to consent to fetal research that is not in the interests of the pregnant woman. This has led at least some of the official policies to impose additional requirements on the informed consent process for research on fetuses in utero.

The U.S. regulations also illustrate these additional requirements on the informed consent process. The process of selecting subjects and obtaining their consent must, where appropriate, be monitored. Moreover, the consent of the father as well as of the pregnant woman must be obtained, unless the research is therapeutic research related to maternal health needs or unless his identity is not known or he is not reasonably available or the pregnancy is the result of rape (Appendix 3.1, section 46.208). In all these ways, the normal informed consent process is modified.

Other official policies represent important variations on this theme of additional consent. The British Royal College of Physicians does require that fathers ''normally be consulted'' in all cases of research in pregnant patients, including therefore research on fetuses in utero.[4] On the other hand, the proposed Canadian Code treats maternal consent as necessary and sufficient.[5] Of special interest is the discussion of these problems in the CIOMS Guidelines.[6] It is concerned with ensuring input from the women in those societies in which female self-determination is not fully recognized. It recommends a number of culturally sensitive techniques, such as using other women from the culture in question to probe the subject's willingness to participate in research.

This basic approach has recently come under criticism by those who feel that it is insufficiently sensitive to the substantive and decisional rights of the pregnant women involved. Substantively, it is claimed, pregnant women are deprived of the benefits from participating in research on better therapies out of a fear for fetal harm. Procedurally, it is claimed, pregnant women are deprived of the authority to make decisions for themselves and their fetuses.

The substantive issue is really related to the issues of research on pregnant women and women of childbearing potential and will be discussed in Chapter Nine. In the United States, the procedural issue arises only in cases where the woman's health needs are not at stake; it is only in such cases that the father's consent is required. In the United Kingdom, the Royal College suggests getting the father's consent in all cases. Because no evidence has been offered to show that the above-discussed potential problems have actually occurred, these requirements have not been justified. It should also be noted that these extra consent requirements are not imposed on pediatric therapeutic research and minimally risky nontherapeutic research. It seems best then to adopt the Canadian view that maternal consent is sufficient.

To conclude, then, official policies allow therapeutic research on fetuses in utero as long as the risks are minimized and earlier animal testing has been done. They differ over allowing nontherapeutic research on fetuses in utero even if the risks are minimal and earlier animal testing has been done. Where these requirements on nontherapeutic research are stricter than the requirements on nontherapeutic research on children, they should be liberalized. Various countries also impose a standard of obtaining the consent of the fetus's father in at least some cases; that additional requirement should be abolished.

Research Using Fetal Tissue

Although the ethical issues surrounding research on fetuses in utero are related to the moral status of the fetus portion of the abortion debate, such research does not directly involve abortions. This made it relatively easier to develop official policies based upon moral compromises that have won widespread support, even if some of their provisions need to be modified. The research to which we now turn, using fetal tissue, does more directly involve abortions because the fetal tissue is usually obtained from aborted fetuses. Developing official policies based on moral compromises has been more difficult in this area. Not surprisingly, therefore, the attempt to develop such policies has become very controversial, even playing a role in the 1992 presidential election in the United States. In this section, we will first trace the development of this issue, then note the compromise-based consensus that has emerged in official policies, and finally assess the objections and alternatives to that consensus. We shall see that despite the controversies, the compromise-based consensus has rightfully won widespread acceptance in official policies.

Research using fetal tissue is not new. Fetal kidney tissue was used in the research that led to the culturing of the polio virus and the development of the polio vaccine. It continues to be used in research in virology. It is also used in screening products for toxicities and carcinogenicity, in studying fetal development, and in creating animal models for human diseases. This research continued quietly through all of the debate on fetal tissue research. That debate was provoked by the emergence in the 1980s of suggestions that transplanting fetal tissue might be helpful in the treatment of such diseases as diabetes and neurodegenerative diseases (e.g., Parkinson's, Huntington's). These suggestions needed to be tested in research protocols, and it is those protocols that provoked the controversy.

Why use fetal tissue rather than tissue from adults? Four reasons are usually given[7]:

1. Fetal cells develop rapidly, hastening the desired effects.
2. Fetal cells are less antigenic, minimizing rejection problems.
3. Fetal cells are more resistant to damage both in vitro and after transplantation.
4. There is a large supply of such cells available from elective abortions, and a much smaller supply available from spontaneous abortions and ectopic pregnancies.

It is this last advantage that gives rise, at the same time, to a series of concerns about fetal tissue research, concerns felt primarily by those who have significant moral hesitations about, or opposition to, abortions: Would the taking of this tissue for research purposes actually involve the illicit killing of still alive embryos or fetuses? Even if not, would that practice encourage, or at least involve complicity with, morally inappropriate abortions? Is it appropriate that the pregnant woman be allowed to consent to the tissue donation, given that she has consented to the termination of the life of the embryo/fetus, and if she cannot, who can?

A significant number of official policies and professional guidelines have emerged in response both to the promise of fetal tissue transplantation and the moral concerns about it. All attempt to base a research policy on a moral compromise. In sketching the consensus that emerged in those responses, we will be employing the following major responses: (1) the 1989 Polkinghorne report, whose recommendations were adopted as a code of practice for the United Kingdom (Appendix 4.5); (2) 1986[8] and 1989 (Appendix 2.4) recommendations of the Parliamentary Assembly of the Council of Europe, which have been followed in 1994 guidelines issued by NECTAR (Network of European CNS Transplantation and Restoration)[9]; (3) interim U.S. regulations issued in February of 1993, the laws on fetal tissue transplantation contained in the U.S. National Institutes of Health Reauthorization Act of 1993 (Appendix 3.11), and earlier H.H.S. regulations dating back to 1981 (Appendix 3.1); (4)a 1993 report of the Canadian Royal Commission on New Reproductive Technologies,[10] which contains an important discussion of the uses of fetal tissue, and the 1997 draft Canadian Code.[11]

Some controversy developed in connection with each of these responses, but the greatest controversy arose in connection with the U.S. response. In 1987, following a promising report about fetal neural tissue transplants into patients with Parkinson's disease, the NIH began considering running an intramural research protocol on fetal neural tissue transplants. That was postponed until a 1988 report of an advisory committee approved such protocols using material from induced abortions as long as certain guidelines were in place. Despite that recommendation, HHS officials in the Bush administration imposed a ban on federal funding for fetal tissue transplantation research. Such research could be done in the United States only with private funds. Congress in 1992 attempted to overturn that ban, but a presidential veto stopped that. Just prior to his veto, President Bush established through presidential order a fetal tissue bank using tissue only from spontaneous abortions and ectopic pregnancies. In 1993, President Clinton lifted the ban on fetal tissue transplantation research using tissue from induced abortions, and interim guidelines for such research were issued.[12] That permissive stance was incorporated in 1993 into the NIH Reauthorization Act (Appendix 3.11, section 111), which also abolished the Bush fetal tissue bank. The provisions of that act superseded the interim guidelines. Those centers involved in the tissue bank program reported in early 1995[13] that usable fetal tissue was recoverable in less than 1% of spontaneous abortions and ectopic pregnancies. In the meantime, in 1994–95, the first federally funded research projects under the 1993 act, fetal tissue transplantation projects at the University of Colorado and at Mount Sinai Medical Center, began.[14] Despite renewed Congressional discussions in 1996, to be discussed below, about the related issue of research on preimplantation zygotes, the permissive position on fetal tissue research now seems to be firmly established.

What consensus is embodied in these various official policies? The following are the crucial principles:

1. As a form of respect for embryo/fetal life, even if that life is not accorded the same respect as the life of a newborn, research involving tissue donation should be performed only after death of the embryo/fetus has occurred. When the material is obtained from an induced abortion in the first trimester employing standard vacuum aspiration techniques, as is often the case in Parkinson's disease fetal transplantation research, this is not an issue, because intact embryos/fetuses are not recovered. It becomes an issue when other techniques are used later in pregnancy. This principle stands in distinction to an earlier British report, the Peel Report,[15] which had allowed such research on the pre-viable embryo/fetus, and to earlier NIH regulations that had also allowed some research on nonviable embryos/fetuses ex utero (Appendix 3.1, section 46.209). Adopting this first principle was one of the crucial components of the moral compromise embodied in the consensus. The Polkinghorne Report defines death as absence of spontaneous circulation and respiration,[16] whereas the NIH regulations refer to the absence of spontaneous movement of voluntary muscles and of pulsations of the umbilical cord (Appendix 3.1, section 46.203). The best discussion of this issue, and the related issue of management of the embryo/fetus ex utero until death occurs, is found in the NECTAR guidelines.[17]

2. Tissue may be harvested from induced abortions as well as from spontaneous abortions and ectopic pregnancies. As is evidenced in the U.S. debate surrounding the Bush veto, this is the most controversial of the five principles.

3. The abortion decision and the tissue donation decision must be separated. This point is the other crucial component of the moral compromise embodied in the consensus. It justifies the use of tissue from induced abortions for at least some of those who have moral objections to those abortions by beginning the research only after the abortion is completed. It also helps meet their concern that a fetal tissue transplantation program encourages induced abortions. Among the many common provisions for separating the two are the following:

      a. the issue of tissue donation should only be raised subsequent to the decision to have the abortion;

      b. no financial inducements should be offered to the pregnant woman nor may she specify the use to which the tissue will be put;

      c. the timing and technique of the abortion should not be influenced by the decision to donate the tissue;

      d. separate physicians should be involved in the abortion and in the fetal tissue research.

4. The pregnant woman is the person who must consent to the tissue donation. The Polkinghorne Report[18] contains a defense of this view against two alternatives, one that says that she is ineligible because she has consented to the abortion and the other that says that her consent is insufficient and that the father of the embryo/fetus must consent as well. The NIH Reauthorization Act (Appendix 3.11, section 111) agreed that maternal consent was sufficient.

5. All protocols for such research should be approved in advance by an independent review committee such as an IRB or a Research Ethics Committee.

There are two issues that are worth special notice. First, The U.S. policy, as found in the NIH Reauthorization Act, specifically requires (Appendix 3.11, section (c3)) that potential recipients be informed of the source of the tissue, presumably to allow them to refuse the tissue if accepting it offends their conscience given its source. Some might reject this provision, arguing that the principle of separation [principle (3) above] means that the material carries with it no moral taint. The U.S. position seems more sensitive to the reality of the moral feelings of those who oppose the use of fetal tissue in transplants and who might disagree with the claim that the material carries with it no moral taint. It also seems more appropriate for a compromise policy designed to secure maximum support. I believe that it should therefore be adopted. Second, as part of its development of the principle of separation, the British created a single tissue bank that collects donated fetal tissue and makes it available to researchers. There is no such agency in the United States, but the U.S. National Advisory Board on Ethics in Reproduction (NABER), a privately funded but professionally supported group, has urged its creation.[19] In addition to helping meet the ethical principle of separation, such an approach allows for better monitoring for safety and efficacy issues. Another alternative would be a national licensing board that would review the activities of, and license, programs that supply fetal tissue for research purposes. The Canadian Royal Commission has recommended that alternative.[20]

This consensus embodied in principles (1) through (5), with the variations just noted, has won widespread support, but there are still dissenters. Some of these dissenters are found, as might be expected, among those who strongly oppose abortions, and their views have been adopted in the laws of some U.S. states that prohibit research using fetal tissue from induced abortions. Others are found in the pro-choice community; they have challenged the consensus as too restrictive. We turn now to a consideration of both of these dissenting views.

Although many issues of concern have been raised in the anti-abortion community, I want to focus on three that are deserving of special attention. They are the concerns about changed technique, about maternal consent, and about complicity.

One of the requirements in the consensus is that tissue donation should not have any impact on the abortion technique used. This is an important component of the separation principle because it ensures that the research component begins only after the abortion is completed so that the abortion is not part of the research project. In fact, however, prominent investigators have reported modifications in abortion technique to ensure more and better fetal tissue. For example, the Swedish investigators of transplanting fetal neural tissue reported in *Lancet*[21] the modifications they adopted to the standard suction technique to ensure that fetal tissue will not be macerated; a similar modification was reported in *The New England Journal of Medicine* in 1992.[22] This seems to be in violation of a literal reading of the separation requirements of the consensus; even more importantly, it makes the abortion part of the research. Either these changes must not be employed or the consensus approach must be modified to allow for some changes in technique that are viewed as compatible with separation and with the research beginning only after the abortion is completed. NECTAR called attention to this issue and supported the latter approach, but it did not develop an account of acceptable changes in technique.[23]

The second of the concerns, about the pregnant woman's role as the donor of the tissue, has provoked considerable controversy, but I am unpersuaded about the need for this controversy. We need to remember that given the principle of separation, the implementation of which ensures that the question of fetal tissue donation only comes up after a decision has been made to terminate the pregnancy, the issue being considered is who is authorized to make a decision relating to the disposition of the remains of the embryo/fetus after an abortion. I would suggest modifying the consensus so that the decision about donating the fetal tissue for research is made by whatever party (the pregnant woman, she and the father, the physician performing the abortion, the institution in which it is performed) is normally authorized to make that decision when no research involving fetal tissue donation is involved.

The last of the concerns is about complicity. It argues that use of fetal issue from induced abortions requires that one stand in a relation of approbation to the induced abortion. It feels that a partnership whereby one achieves direct benefit from another's immoral behavior, even if that happens after the fact, is an immoral partnership. So, concludes this last concern, the attempt of the consensus to approve of the use of fetal tissue from induced abortions while remaining neutral on the moral licitness of the abortions fails; separation is not enough. This last concern strikes at the very heart of the attempt to fashion a research policy for the use of fetal tissue based on a moral compromise. If it is correct, the attempt fails. It is very difficult to evaluate this concern, however, as we don't have a very good theory of complicity.[24] Many of the discussants of this question appeal to the analogy of the appropriateness of using data from illicit human experiments of the type described in Chapter Two, such as the Nazi experiments that gave rise to the Nuremberg Code. The trouble with this analogy, even if one accepts the resemblance, is that its conclusion is unclear; after all, there is a continuing debate about the licitness of using such data.[25] Some see it as unacceptable complicity while others see it as obtaining some good from an already completed evil. Clearly, we need a better theory of complicity to enable us to finally settle these difficult questions that often arise when one attempts to fashion a research policy based on moral compromises. For now, however, I am unpersuaded by the complicity objection, in part because I have always supported the above argument for using the scientifically sound results (if there are any) obtained in the Nazi experiments.

From the pro-choice perspective, most of the concerns that have been expressed are about the restrictiveness of the consensus. Why, for example, shouldn't the pregnant woman be allowed to consider the good that might result from her terminating a pregnancy when she is considering termination anyway? The current consensus attempts to stop that by mandating that the issue of tissue donation not even be raised until a definite decision is made about the termination. Similarly, having made a decision to terminate the pregnancy and to donate the tissue, why shouldn't the pregnant woman be able to stipulate that the technique used be modified to maximize the usable tissue obtained? The current consensus prohibits that by mandating that the technique not be modified. Again, why shouldn't the pregnant woman, from whose body the tissue comes, be allowed to determine the beneficiary of her donation? Once more, the current consensus prohibits this specified donation. In short, from the pro-choice perspective, the implementation of the separation principle in the current consensus is an illegitimate interference with the pregnant woman's right of self-determination.

I believe that these objections, like the complicity objection of the anti-abortion community, raise a fundamental challenge to the current compromise-based consensus. The consensus, as we have seen, is an attempt to develop official policies based on moral compromise. The objectors are proposing alternatives that embody their moral beliefs and that are not part of the current social compromise. Does that mean that the compromise has not done enough justice to the pro-choice position or does that mean that the objectors are making excessive demands on the compromise? Clearly, a final resolution of these objections depends on our developing a fuller understanding of the whole idea of policies based on moral compromises. For now, however, there seems to be much merit in the argument in the 1996 version of the proposed Canadian Code[26] that the lack of a moral consensus justifies official policies that are restrictive in the ways just mentioned in order to ensure that the possibility of the use of the resulting tissue does not indirectly affect the abortion decision.

The consensus that has emerged in official policies is certainly far from perfect. The issue of abortion technique clearly needs to be readdressed and the whole question of consent to donation needs to be rethought. Moreover, a better understanding of both moral complicity and moral compromise may lead to further more fundamental modifications. However, it seems like a reasonable noncomplicitous compromise, and its widespread acceptance in official policies reflects the possibility of compromise-based official policies even in areas where there exists considerable moral debate.

Research on Preimplantation Zygotes

With the emergence of in vitro fertilization, exciting opportunities for research on newly created zygotes ex utero (hereafter called preimplantation zygotes) became available. Such research could be conducted on ''spare zygotes,'' zygotes already created in a clinical attempt to produce a pregnancy but not implanted at the time in question. These zygotes would otherwise be disposed of or would be frozen for use in future clinical attempts to produce a pregnancy. Such research could also be conducted on zygotes produced purely for research purposes by obtaining gametes from sperm and egg donors. These egg donors might be women involved in in vitro fertilization programs, other living donors willing to help the research effort, or cadaveric donors. In addition to these opportunities for research on zygotes, IVF programs allow for the opportunity of obtaining eggs to be used for research on parthenogenesis (egg development without fertilization).

What are these exciting research opportunities? What might be learned from such research efforts? The following are among the areas usually mentioned:

1. research to improve the success rates of IVF;
2. research on preimplantation genetic diagnosis;
3. research on isolating pluripotent stem cell lines for eventual differentiation and clinical use in transplantation;
4. research on nuclear transplantation to avoid disorders due to maternally inherited cytoplasmic defects;
5. basic parthenogenetic research on the role of maternal and paternal genetic material in development;
6. basic research on the fertilization and early zygote development processes.

Although much can and has been learned in each of these areas by preliminary research on preimplantation zygotes from other species, there reaches a point both in basic and clinical research where interspecies differences necessitate research on human preimplantation zygotes.

The research potential of preimplantation zygotes is great, but the ethical concerns for those who see preimplantation zygotes as entities with a moral status deserving of protection are also great. This research is usually nontherapeutic research leading in the end to the destruction of the zygote rather than to its implantation. This destruction differentiates it from therapeutic or nontherapeutic but minimally risky fetal in utero research in a way that makes developing a compromise-based official policy problematic. This research necessarily involves living entities as it cannot be conducted using tissue harvested from the already dead. This requirement for using living entities differentiates it from fetal tissue research in a way that makes developing a compromise-based official policy problematic. Not surprisingly, then, developing such official policies for this area has turned out to be very difficult.

It is possible to differentiate two radically different types of official policies that have emerged, with many other official policies incorporating components from these two very different types. One is the *permissive policy*: it allows, after appropriate review, for research on preimplantation zygotes subject to consent from the donors and subject to the restriction that they not be paid for their donation; it sets a time limit (most commonly, 14 days after fertilization) for the conduct of the research; it allows for the creating of zygotes for research purposes; it bans at least some types of this research, most commonly cross-species research and research on post-cloning transfer of zygotes. The other is *the restrictive policy*: it prohibits the creation of zygotes for research; it prohibits the use of spare zygotes for destructive research; in the official versions, it usually rests upon the view that such research on human life at any stage fails to show adequate respect to human life and fails to adequately protect vulnerable human life. It may, however, also rest on concerns about the implications of the medicalization of reproduction for the status of women.

Because countries differ in their official policies, and because there have been so many changes in, or controversies about, the official policies of some countries, a review of the official policies of the major research countries seems to be in place.

One of the clearest examples of consistent support for a permissive policy is Great Britain, which adopted such a policy in the 1990 Human Fertilisation and Embryology Act (Appendix 4.4), an act based on the 1984 Warnock Report.[27] The British have created a special agency, the Human Fertilisation and Embryology Authority, that must license each act of reproductive research. The British Act also requires that consent be contained from the gamete and/or the zygote donors that their donation will be used for research and prohibits payments to secure that consent. The time limit for research is 14 days after "the gametes are mixed." This is based on the appearance of the primitive streak at this point in time rather than on its being the end of the period of implantation. After the primitive streak appears, the zygote cannot divide into two or more embryos, so this time marks, as the Warnock Report noted, "the beginning of individual development of the embryo."[28] The British do allow for the creation of zygotes for research purposes. Finally, the British impose a number of restrictions on the type of research that can be approved. Research cannot be approved if it involves trans-species placement of embryos, nuclear transplantation, or genetic alteration of any cell while it forms part of the embryo. In addition, embryos used in research cannot be used in treatment.

One of the clearest examples of consistent support for a restrictive policy is found in Germany. After a series of reports in the 1980s, the German parliament passed in late 1990 the Embryo Protection Law (Appendix 4.7). It prohibits artificial fertilization for any other purpose than bringing about a pregnancy, so the creation of zygotes for research purposes is banned. It also prohibits attempts to fertilize more eggs than will be transferred in one cycle, so there are no spare preimplantation zygotes on which to experiment. Finally, it directly prohibits research by prohibiting the extracorporeal development of a human embryo for purposes other than pregnancy.

The French developments are particularly interesting, because France moved from almost adopting a permissive policy to adopting a restrictive policy. In the 1980s, the National Ethics Committee and the Conseil d'Etat had devoted considerable attention to the issue of assisted reproduction, and had recommended a moderately permissive policy, prohibiting the creation of zygotes for research but allowing for research on spare zygotes up to 7 days (emphasizing the normal time for implantation rather than the normal time for the formation of the primitive streak).[29] Legislation incorporating these proposals was introduced. The government then changed, and a far more restrictive law was passed in July of 1994. The full text of the statute[30] is as follows:

> The in vitro conception of human embryos for the purpose of study, research, or experimentation shall be prohibited. All experimentation on embryos shall be prohibited. As an exceptional measure, the man and the woman making up a couple may agree to studies being carried out on their embryos. This decision shall be expressed in writing. Such studies must have a medical objective and may not be harmful to the embryo.

The opening clause represents a ban on creating zygotes for research that had been part of the original legislation. The rest represents a general ban on preimplantation research, with the last clause allowing for very limited exceptions to that ban, exceptions that do not cover destructive research. In May of 1997, the

National Ethics Committee proposed a limited extension to allow research on embryonic stem cells derived from conserved surplus embryos whose parents have decided to terminate that conservation.[31] It remains to be seen whether the new legislature will accept this suggestion.

These differences on preimplantation research have had a considerable impact on discussions in the Council of Europe. When the Council of Europe attempted to develop a general bioethics convention, the article dealing with research on embryos in vitro attracted great controversy. It originally banned creation of zygotes for research, but allowed research on spare zygotes up to 14 days if that was allowed under national law. That was too permissive for many states. In February of 1995, the whole of the article was dropped except for the ban on creating zygotes for research, but that ban was unacceptable to Great Britain. As a compromise, the final version (Appendix 2.3, Article 18) kept the ban on creating zygotes for research, but ambiguously recognized the legitimacy of some research by saying "Where the law allows research on embryos in vitro, it shall ensure adequate protection of the embryo."

These European differences and changes are paralleled by developments in Australia, Canada, and the United States. We turn then to those developments.

Australia formulated what is, I believe, the earliest officially adopted permissive policy. It is found in a 1982 statement of the Australian National Health and Medical Research Council (Appendix 4.12), supplemented by the Victoria Infertility (Medical Procedures) Act of 1984.[32] It is not surprising that the Australians would take a leadership role in this area of research ethics, given the importance of their in vitro fertilization research effort.

Several themes that became prominent in permissive policies are found in this Australian material. There are time limitations on the research; it is permitted only until the time at which implantation would normally occur if the zygote were in vivo. This is defined as between 7 and 14 days after fertilization. There are limits on the types of research permitted; the NHMRC statement prohibits, for example, cloning experiments. Unlike the British permissive policy, The Victoria Act, with one special exception (research prior to the time of syngamy), prohibits creating zygotes for research purposes. Finally, there is a special review process for this type of research; the Victoria Act created a special Standing Review and Advisory Committee that had to approve research proposals. Employing these restrictions, the Committee, chaired by Louis Waller, approved in 1985 experiments involving the chromosomal testing of zygotes frozen and then thawed with the restriction that they be conducted only on spare zygotes.[33]

The Victoria Act made it clear, in defining the mission of that Advisory Committee, that it was to attempt to satisfy both the principle that "childless couples should be assisted in fulfilling their desire to have children" and the principle that "human life shall be preserved and protected at all times."[34]

The former principle supports the research effort whereas the latter supports the restrictions. The Australians saw their modified permissive policy as a compromise-based policy.

The compromise was not to last. In May of 1995, the state of Victoria repealed its 1984 act and replaced it with an act that bans destructive research even on surplus zygotes.[35] That language seems to allow for research only if it is followed by an attempt at implantation. This sharp reversal in Australian policy testifies to the difficulty of creating a compromise-based official policy that will remain acceptable over time.

Recent developments in Canada involve a 1993 report of the Canadian Royal Commission on New Reproductive Technologies,[36] the two drafts of the Canadian Code,[37] and 1996 proposed legislation.[38] Although they do not involve quite as dramatic a reversal as the Australian changes, the important changes in those few years testify once more to the difficulties in creating a compromise-based official policy in this area.

The 1993 report contains a very fine presentation and defense of a permissive policy. Several points deserve special mention:

1. It presents the clearest statement of the compromise nature of the 14-day limit:

   > It also recognizes the legitimate value of medical knowledge and the need to find a morally acceptable compromise in a pluralistic society in which there are various views about the relative importance of different stages of embryo development. People disagree about issues such as the role of potentiality, the importance of individuation, or the value of medical knowledge, and the 14-day limit is a prudent and legitimate compromise among these differing views and interests.[39]

2. It accepts the need for zygotes created for research purposes, in the light of the fact that freezing spare zygotes for later implantation has limited the numbers available for research. At the same time, it is concerned that obtaining eggs for creating such zygotes not be done in a way that excessively burdens the donors. It therefore prohibits the use of invasive procedures specifically to retrieve eggs for purposes of creating zygotes for research. These eggs must be retrieved during procedures already being performed.[40]

3. It prohibits research that involves altering genetically human zygotes, cloning by nuclear substitution, transferring zygotes across species, or creating animal/human hybrids.

4. It accepts at this time the British restriction on transferring the zygote experimented on to a woman's body in order to produce a successful pregnancy. It recognizes, however, that this may become legitimate in

clinical trials of techniques that might be therapeutic or might increase the chance of a successful pregnancy. It allows for that eventuality, requiring only a special review of such protocols. In this respect, it embodies the feminist perspective that women not be denied the benefits from the research in which they participate.

This report was not the final word in Canada. In July of 1995, an interim moratorium on research was adopted, pending the formal adoption of an official policy. In 1996, the draft Canadian Code modified the recommendations of the 1993 report by extending the time limit to 17 days for research into implantation failures and clarified that the ban on implanting a zygote after research did not extend to research involving the testing for genetic disorders of one cell separated from the rest of the zygote.[41] The 1997 draft dropped the extension of the time limit to 17 days and incorporated an explicit ban on creating zygotes for research.[42]

Finally, in June of 1996, the government introduced the Human Reproductive and Genetic Technologies Act.[43] This Act, which is a compromise between the permissive and restrictive policies, is one of the first to specifically appeal to feminist concerns about exploitation of women, as well as to concerns about threats to human dignity, in limiting such research. The major change from the 1993 Report is a prohibition on creating preimplantation zygotes for research purposes. Given the increasing unavailability of spare zygotes for research, that prohibition may severely limit research on preimplantation zygotes in Canada. Very few official policies, with the British policy being the most notable example, are now fully permissive policies, allowing for the creation of zygotes for research.

The U.S. history is even more complex. Until 1993, HHS regulations (Appendix 3.1, section 46.204) prohibited the federal funding of IVF research unless it was approved by an Ethics Advisory Board. That Board was abolished in 1980. As a result, preimplantation zygote research in the U.S. was confined to privately funded research, which was not limited by any official national policies. That requirement for approval of federally funded research was abolished by the 1993 NIH Revitalization Act, the same act that lifted the ban on fetal tissue transplantation research. The director of the NIH created an advisory panel to develop guidelines for federally funded research in this area. In 1995, this panel developed a set of recommendations (Appendix 3.9) that represent the fullest and in some ways the most liberal version of a permissive policy, although its proponents saw it as a proposal for a compromise-based official policy. The compromise is, once more, on the moral status of the preimplantation zygote. The combination of the basic permissibility of the research and the limitations on it are meant to reflect a pluralistic evaluation of the status of the preimplantation zygote, seeing it as deserving of respect but not of the same respect due to infants. It is this lesser respect that allows for the permissibility of destructive research.

One of the areas in which the panel moved beyond the standard version of the permissive position was on the question of the time limit on research. It recognized two cases in which such research should be allowed beyond the 14-day limit, and one in which it might be allowed after further study. It allowed for research beyond the 14-day limit on the reliable identification of the appearance of the primitive streak and on the development of cell lines from pluripotential stem cells, noting in the latter case that there would not be an embryo continuing to develop as an organized integrated whole. It also allowed for the possibility, after further study, of research on preimplantation embryos until the beginning of the closure of the neural tube (days 17–21) so as to allow for a better understanding of early defects in the development of the nervous system.

On the question of zygotes created for research purposes, the NIH panel rejected one of the usual reasons for allowing such zygote creation while accepting it for other reasons. It rejected as a reason for zygote creation the scarcity of spare zygotes remaining from infertility procedures, a scarcity resulting in part from successful programs for freezing spare zygotes for later implantation. It allowed for zygote creation for research purposes when "the research by its very nature cannot otherwise be validly conducted" or when it is necessary "for the validity of a study that is potentially of outstanding scientific and therapeutic value" (Appendix 3.9, section on Fertilization of Oocytes Expressly for Research Purposes). Examples of the former are studies on prefertilization oocyte freezing and/or maturation; examples of the latter are studies on the possible harmful effects of new drugs to induce ovulation. It also allowed for the possibility, after further study, of creating zygotes for research on developing embryonic stem cell lines.

In discussing the types of research that might be allowed, the NIH panel supported parthenogenetic research and research on nuclear transplantation, as long as both involve no transfer to establish a pregnancy. It rejected, however, research on cross-species fertilization or chimera development, as well as research on preimplantation gender selection, a topic that had not been extensively addressed by other groups, although it is banned in the 1996 proposed Canadian legislation. The NIH panel raised the question for further study of whether research on nuclear transplantation with transfer to circumvent inherited cytoplasmic defects and research on cloning by separation or splitting without transfer might be allowed.

The immediate reaction to the NIH report was not positive. President Clinton rejected any creation of zygotes for research purposes. Congress temporarily banned all federal funding for preimplantation zygote research unless similar research would be allowed on fetuses in utero (therapeutic research or nontherapeutic research of minimal risk), and that ban was extended in June of 1996. This ban led to the suspension of research funding for Mark Hughes, a distinguished geneticist who was doing research on preimplantation genetic diagnosis.[44] It remains to be seen what will become official U.S. policy for federally funded research on preimplantation zygotes, keeping in mind that there is no offical federal policy governing privately funded research.

There is one 1997 development that deserves special notice. The NIH report, in agreement with the other reports and official policies we have discussed, opposed research on human cloning followed by transfer. One of the only groups that supported such research was the U.S. National Advisory Board on Ethics in Reproduction (NABER), a privately funded but professionally supported group that had allowed for such research in certain circumstances subject to the limitation of creating no more than four clones.[45] In the light of successful 1997 research on mammalian cloning, many official groups, including the U.S. National Bioethics Advisory Commission, were asked to reexamine the issue of cloning research.

Two groups associated with the European Union, the Advisers on the Ethical Implications of Biotechnology to the European Commission[46] and the European Parliament,[47] were opposed in principle to human cloning, the former because of "considerations of instrumentalization and eugenics" and the latter because "each individual has a right to his or her own genetic identity." The U.S. National Bioethics Advisory Commission was less firm in its rejection of human cloning. It recognized both safety concerns and ethical concerns, and called for a moratorium accompanied by continued research on safety issues related to the technology and by continued reflection on the ethical issues.[48]

I suggested at the beginning of this section that the development of a compromise-based official policy on preimplantation zygote research would be far more difficult than the development of such policies on the other issues discussed in this chapter. The basis for such a compromise-based policy, a compromise on the status of the preimplantation zygote, would be hard to develop. That has turned out to be correct. Official policies range from a permissive policy in Great Britain to a restrictive policy in much of Europe and in parts of Australia. The emerging Canadian policy is in-between these two extremes, and it is unclear what the official policy in the United States will be. Researchers in different parts of the world are likely to face different policies, and changing policies, in the years to come.

Conclusion

As in the case of genetic research, the official policies on reproductive and fetal research did not originate as responses to questionable cases of earlier research. They represent, instead, an attempt to regulate the research contemporaneous with the actual development of the research.

There is a feature of these official policies on reproductive and fetal research that makes them unique. They were all developed with an awareness that there was a need to find compromises among the varying positions on such divisive questions as the moral status of fetuses and the decisional authority of pregnant women. In other words, they are compromise-based research policies. This makes the official policies discussed in this chapter quite different from the ones discussed in other chapters, where the policies were usually based on a consensus about the relevant fundamental moral values to guide the policies.

We have seen that the ability to develop internationally convergent compromise-based official policies varied from one area to another. It was easiest for research on fetuses in utero, more difficult for research using fetal tissue, and most difficult for research on preimplantation zygotes.

Some have drawn the conclusion that the efforts in question were mistaken.[49] Given the difficulties we have seen, they suggest that it would be best to develop official policies based on a single coherent view of such issues as the status of fetuses and the decisional authority of pregnant women. This suggestion is theoretically attractive, for its adoption might well result in policies that could be given a theoretically satisfying justification. Its adoption is also likely, however, to result in even greater controversy over official policies in these areas. It needs to be remembered that the development of official policies based on moral compromises has at least resulted in widely accepted useful official policies in two of our three areas. Would that have happened without the compromises incorporated into those policies?

I would draw a different conclusion. The real problem is that we lack any good understanding either of the value of moral compromises in shaping official policies or of the standards for a good moral compromise. Too often, the fashioning of a compromise-based official policy is viewed as a political necessity and the terms of the compromise are dictated by the counting of votes. We need, instead, a positive understanding that the adoption of moral compromises as the basis for official policies is the morally appropriate way of respecting differing views in a pluralistic society. We need, in addition, a positive theory about how such compromises should be shaped in a pluralistic society. I would conclude, then, that the development of better official research policies in this area awaits the development of a positive social theory of moral compromises as the basis for official policies, in general, and for official research policies in particular.

There is one other conclusion that I would draw. The need for a positive theory of appropriate moral compromises is particularly important when the fundamental issue is about the moral status of the entities in question. The two areas of research ethics examined so far in which there are the most significant differences in principle in official policies are research on animals and research on preimplantation zygotes. The differences between human priority policies on animal research and balancing policies on animal research reflect at least in part differences on the moral status of animals. Similarly, the differences between permissive and restrictive policies on preimplantation zygote research reflect, at least in part, differences on the moral status of preimplantation zygotes. Unfortunately, it is precisely about issues of moral status that we have the least understanding of proper moral compromises as the basis for official policies. So further progress in developing better official policies in these areas is particularly dependent upon the development of a better theoretical understanding of moral compromises on issues of moral status as the basis for official policies.

Chapter six

RESEARCH INVOLVING VULNERABLE SUBJECTS

When we examined the ethical questions raised by research on human subjects in Chapter Two, we noted a special set of concerns raised by research involving members of certain vulnerable classes of human subjects. On the one hand, we want to provide them with special protection from abuse and exploitation. On the other hand, we recognize that there may be a social need for research on these subjects and that they may personally benefit from participation, and we need to make sure that the special protections are not excessively onerous. How can these competing demands be met? This chapter will explore this issue in reference to three classes of vulnerable subjects: children, mentally infirm adults, and prisoners. We will see, at least in connection with the first two classes, a growing recognition of the need to support research involving such subjects.

Research Involving Children

The early history of experimentation on children, going back to Jenner's work on smallpox, involved testing vaccines by exposing the vaccinated children to the disease in question. By the end of the nineteenth century, such vaccine experiments, and others on issues of nutrition, were often conducted on institutionalized children on the grounds that their conditions of living could be standardized, making the study more scientifically valid. Some of this experimentation, such as Joseph Goldberger's 1916 demonstration in orphanages in Mississippi that improved diet decreased the incidence of pellagra, was clearly beneficial to the subjects. Others, such as the many late nineteenth and early twentieth century experimental infections of children with gonorrheal cultures and Alfred Hess's research, which involved modifying diets to induce diseases such as scurvy and rickets, were clearly less benign, even when they yielded valuable information. By 1941, when William Black submitted an article describing applying herpes simplex virus to a twelve-month-old baby "offered as a volunteer," the article was rejected on ethical grounds by the *Journal of Experimental Medicine* but was published by the *Journal of Pediatrics*. So the very beginning of scientific research on children was clouded by ethical concerns, some about the very licitness of pediatric research and some about its legitimacy in the special case of institutionalized patients.[1]

In the post–World War II period, further incidents provoked further ethical concerns. Some of the worst of the experiments carried on under the Nazi regime involved children and were condemned at Nuremberg. But as we noted in Chapter Two, it was easy for physicians to dismiss those revelations as abuses of a horrendous regime and to not see them as part of a continuum of illicit research that extended to much research that had taken place in democratic societies. For that reason, Beecher's 1966 article in *The New England Journal of Medicine*,[2] which documented many questionable cases of post–World War II research in the United States, was more influential. Four of the twenty-two studies involved children. The most widely known example was the Willowbrook study, in which institutionalized children were deliberately infected with hepatitis to study the natural history of the disease and to lay the groundwork for vaccine research. The parents consented, but many questions were raised about that consent. Two of the others seem even more objectionable. In one, fifty patients of a children's center were treated with Tri-A to demonstrate the extent of hepatic dysfunction produced by this drug; several, with marked dysfunction, were re-treated after hepatic function returned to normal and once more developed abnormal liver function. In the other, described by Beecher as a "bizarre study," twenty-six normal newborns were exposed to extensive x-rays to study ureteral reflux.

These revelations about abusive pediatric research led to the development of official policies for the ethical conduct of research in children. Some of this occurred before World War II. In 1900, in response to a case in which four children were inoculated with syphilis serum to serve as a control group for a vaccination study, a Prussian ministry issued regulations prohibiting non-therapeutic research on children and on incompetent adults. Thirty years later, that prohibition was relaxed in that such non-therapeutic research was allowed only if it did not in any way endanger the child and only if consent was obtained from the child's legal representative.[3] In the post–World War II period, similar themes emerged. For example, from the first 1964 version of the World Medical Association's Declaration of Helsinki (Appendix 1.2), there has been much emphasis on obtaining the consent of the parents before research on children is performed.

The basic framework that has emerged resembles the general framework for research on human subjects described in Chapter Two. Researchers must submit their research protocols for approval by an independent committee before the research can be conducted. That committee should not approve the protocol unless adequate measures have been taken to obtain voluntary informed consent. Moreover, that committee should not approve the protocol unless risks have been minimized and there is a favorable risk-benefit ratio. There are, however, two major differences. One is that consent must usually be obtained from the parents because the child is judged to have insufficient capacity to comprehend the information about the research and to make an informed choice as to whether or not to participate. A second major difference is that there is a need to place additional limits on the risks to which pediatric patients/subjects can be exposed, especially in research that is not directly beneficial to them. This brief description leaves several crucial questions open:

1. Until what age is someone considered a child for the sake of requiring these special protections?
2. Does the pediatric patient/subject need to consent as well?
3. Can nontherapeutic research on children be justified by benefits to other patients from the knowledge obtained from the research, and if so, at what risk to the child?
4. Are there special groups of pediatric patients/subjects who should be treated differently?

Many official policies have appeared that respond to these questions. The Declaration of Helsinki (Appendix 1.2), the CIOMS Guidelines (Appendix 1.8), and the 1996 International Harmonization Guidelines (Appendix 1.5) provide international guidance. In the United States, official policy is set by HHS regulations issued in 1983 (Appendix 3.1); they are usefully supplemented by 1995 Guidelines from the American Academy of Pediatrics.[4] In Canada, a 1993 report was issued by the National Council on Bioethics in Human Research,[5] and this report was the foundation for the relevant sections in the proposed Code.[6] A similar report was issued in Australia in 1992 by the National Health and Medical Research Council (Appendix 4.12). For Europe in general, the 1990 Guidelines of the Council of Europe (Appendix 2.2) developed an approach to pediatric research that was incorporated into the 1996 Bioethics Convention (Appendix 2.3). In the United Kingdom, the British Pediatric Association issued guidelines in 1980 (revised in 1992),[7] and additional guidance is found in the 1991 report of the Royal College of Physicians on research involving patients (Appendix 4.1), the 1991 report of the Medical Research Council on research involving children (Appendix 4.2), and the 1996 Royal College of Physicians Guidelines on the Practice of Ethics Committees.[8] The French 1988 statute on research also addresses pediatric research (Appendix 4.8).

The most recent of these policies, particularly those coming from the community of pediatricians, emphasize the value of research on children, even while advocating special protections for them. Thus, the British pediatricians[9] begin their guidelines with the claim: "Research involving children is important for the benefit of all children and should be supported, encouraged and conducted in an ethical manner." The American Academy of Pediatrics,[10] writing about pediatric research on drugs, makes the stronger claim that justice requires pediatric research: "There is a moral imperative to formally study drugs in children so that they can enjoy equal access to existing as well as new therapeutic agents." Following their lead, the NIH has announced[11] that it will require all grant applicants proposing to do relevant research to either include children as subjects or justify their exclusion. We shall see whether or not this more recent emphasis on encouraging research on children, as well as the more traditional emphasis on protecting them in the research process, appropriately shapes the official policies we will now examine.

While these official policies are in agreement about the basic framework outlined above, they disagree about how issues (1) through (4) should be resolved, and their respective views will be the main focus of the rest of this section.

The Age Limit for Special Protection. The 1983 HHS regulations governing research on children do not specify an age (such as 18) after which the special regulations do not apply and after which, for example, the consent of the subjects is sufficient. Instead, they specify that a subject is a child if he or she has "not attained the legal age for consent to treatments or procedures involved in the research, under the applicable law of the jurisdiction in which the research will be conducted" (Appendix 3.1, section 46.402). What this means is that the researcher, and the independent committee reviewing the research protocol, must determine whether or not the subjects could have legally consented on their own in the jurisdiction in question to the treatment in question if it were being used for purely therapeutic purposes. If he or she could have, then the special regulations governing pediatric research do not apply; if he or she could not have, then the special regulations do apply. The answer to this question may, of course, vary from one jurisdiction to another, and this may become a source of confusion, especially for multicenter trials taking place in different legal jurisdictions.

Why did the HHS regulations not specify a specific age? Why did they require researchers and independent review committees to examine what are often very complicated legal questions? The answer to these questions is to be found in the tremendous differences among the states about the authority of older adolescents (especially those between 16 and 18) in health care decision making. The traditional view was that everybody below a certain age was a minor who had no authority to make health care decisions; now, the different states in the United States allow some adolescents (emancipated minors, mature minors, perhaps all older minors) to make at least some health care decisions (reproductive, treatment of venereal diseases, psychiatric treatment) for themselves.[12] In recognition of this variability in giving authority to older adolescents in the health care setting, HHS accepted the same variability about consent in the research setting.

This recognition of legal ambiguities seems to have shaped the response to this issue in other policies. Many of the official policies simply refer to the protections applying to all those who are legally recognized as minors. Others are more respectful of the rights to independence of older minors. The British Pediatric Association,[13] for example, affirms the view that when children have sufficient understanding and intelligence to understand what is proposed, it is their consent, not the consent of the parents, that is crucial. The Medical Research Council, somewhat more cautiously, says that the research ethics committee, in dealing with this question as it approves protocols involving older children, should "consider carefully the maturity and independence of the children to be approached and the likely expectations of their parents. For example, an LREC may agree that it would be inappropriate to approach the parents of children who are living independently of them" (Appendix 4.2, section 6.1.3). The Royal College of Physicians is even more cautious: "Even if an investigator believes that a child is capable of giving consent, the approval of a parent or guardian should be obtained before any research procedure is comtemplated on a child under the age of 16 years. It may also be desirable to obtain parental consent in some older children." (Appendix 4.1, section 22) For medicolegal reasons, it now recommends obtaining parental consent for all nontherapeutic research on patients under the age of 18.[14]

The policy that most affirms the right to independence of the pediatric subject is found in the 1993 Canadian report.[15] It specifies the age of 14 as the approximate age of maturity, and it makes it clear that although parental involvement is encouraged, the consent of the subject over the age of 14 is sufficient at least for therapeutic research. It is of interest to note that no age for maturity is explicitly incorporated into the proposed code.[16]

There has been little published about how these different policies actually operate; we do not know, therefore, whether the theoretical differences have an impact on what research is actually done, what is the actual role of parents under these different policies, and what are the wishes of older children about parental involvement. It is, therefore, difficult to form any firm convictions about which policy is actually best, whatever their respective theoretical merits.

The Assent of the Pediatric Subject. We have seen that one of the special protections provided to pediatric patient/subjects who are not sufficiently mature to consent on their own to participate in research is the requirement that their parents consent to their participation in the research. This does not mean, however, that such minors have no role to play in the consent process. The major international and national guidelines are in agreement that, at least in many cases, pediatric patient/subjects must also agree to participate in the research before it can be performed. To quote the Declaration of Helsinki: "Whenever the minor child is in fact able to give a consent, the minor's consent must be obtained in addition to the consent of the minor's legal guardian." (Appendix 1.2, section I.11) Similar provisions about obtaining pediatric consent (which has come to be called the child's assent) are built into the HHS regulations in the United States (Appendix 3.1, section 46.408) and the various British guidelines (Appendix 4.1, section 21 and Appendix 4.2, section 6.1.4). A nice explanation of why this additional requirement is imposed is found in the Explanatory Memorandum accompanying the 1990 Council of Europe Guidelines:

> Owing to the fact that the research concerns the person himself, the experts considered that it was necessary to take account of the view of the incapacitated person [their term which covers immature minors as well as incompetent adults] when he is able to express such views. No medical research may be carried out on that person if he refuses to undergo medical research, regardless of whether consent has already been given by his legal representative(s).(Appendix 2.2, section 36)

Imposing this additional requirement has raised several crucial questions. At what age is pediatric assent required as well? Are there cases in which the research can be performed with parental consent despite the minor's refusal to participate or with the minor's assent despite parental refusal? The various policies have answered these questions differently.

Obviously, pediatric assent cannot be required if the patient/subject is very young. At what age, then, should the process of obtaining assent begin? Some have attempted to answer this question by specifying an age. The 1995 report from the American Academy of Pediatrics, following its 1980 report, suggested an intellectual age of seven years.[17] The age of seven was also adopted in the 1993 Canadian report.[18] The British Pediatric Association, following that approach, required getting assent from school-aged children.[19] The HHS regulations (Appendix 3.1, section 46.408) adopted the alternative approach of allowing local IRBs to determine when the pediatric patients are capable of assenting, taking into account their age, maturity, and psychological state; assent is required for all subject/patients whom the IRB judges to be capable of assenting. Such an approach has the advantage of allowing for greater flexibility and variability, properly reflecting both differences among children of the same age and differences among research projects. On the other hand, it poses a problem for multicenter research (because different IRBs may disagree) and it also allows for lax IRBs to excessively weaken the requirement of pediatric assent. At the author's own institution, assent must be obtained from all pediatric patient/subjects who are twelve and older and need not be obtained from patient/ subjects who are younger than seven years. Assent from children ages seven to eleven is obtained where appropriate in light of the nature of the research and of the maturity of the patient/subjects. This policy is an attempt to avoid both excessive flexibility and excessive rigidity about assent and to take into account developmental facts about the increasing intellectual capacities of adolescents to meet the requirements for adult competency.

Whatever approach is adopted, appropriate attention must be paid to how assent is obtained. Asking the pediatric patient/subject to countersign the parental consent form in front of the parent is questionable, in part because of doubts about the minor's ability to comprehend the meaning of a form written for adults and in part because of questions about the voluntariness of the assent in those circumstances. Age-appropriate assent forms are far more meaningful, and discussing the issue with the minor alone is important, especially if there are reasons to believe that the minor is not in agreement with his or her parents.

A related and very difficult question is whether pediatric research is ever permissible on minors who are old enough to assent and who have not assented. The U.S. regulations (Appendix 3.1, section 46.408) explicitly allow for such research in those cases in which "the research holds out a prospect of direct benefit that is important to the health or well-being of the children and is available only in the context of the research." An example often given is new chemotherapy protocols for pediatric cancer patients who have failed all conventional treatments. However, the NIH's Office for Protection from Research Risks has issued an important clarification in connection with this exception:[20]

> ... IRBs should be sensitive to the fact that parents may wish to try anything, even when the likelihood of success is marginal and the probability of extreme discomfort is high. In general, if the child is a mature adolescent and death is imminent, the child's wishes should be respected.

The French law on research (Appendix 4.8, Article 209-10) absolutely opposes this permission to override the refusal by the minor to participate: "The consent of the minor or major under guardianship must also be sought when he/she is apt to express his/her will. The refusal or revocation of consent of such person may not be overridden." Adopting a somewhat intermediate but less well-defined position, the 1993 Canadian report[21] says that "dissent from a child with a reasonable understanding of the nature of the interventions proposed be given serious consideration"; the proposed 1997 Code[22] stipulates that exceptions to this rule should occur only when "there are sufficient compensating benefits for the participants that can only be provided through research participation," bringing the Canadian position close to the U.S regulations.

It is worth noting that all of this discussion is directed to the case in which the parents consent to the experimental therapy while the minor refuses to assent. Much less has been written about the case in which the dying minor wants to participate in one more research protocol in the hope of deferring death but the parents refuse their consent.

My own view about both of these cases is that it is more important to focus on getting the minor and his or her parents to talk to each other and to come to a joint agreement about participation in a research protocol than it is to judge whose decision should win out if they cannot. Colleagues who have followed this approach have reported that it usually works and that it is far more satisfactory than the more legalistic alternative.

Imposing Risks on Pediatric Subjects. Research protocols often impose risks on the subjects. When the subject is an adult, those risks are justified by a combination of the subject's consent and the benefits to the subject and/or to society. Is that same approach appropriate in the case of pediatric subjects? Can the risks of the research using them as subjects be justified by consent and by benefits to society, or should such research be confined to cases where there are sufficient benefits from participation to the minors themselves? These questions have been extensively debated for many years, and have been dealt with in different ways in the different official policies.

There are those who have argued that parents do not have the right to consent to research involving their children that puts their children at risk unless there are sufficient compensating benefits to the children themselves. This approach would obviously not allow for nontherapeutic research involving any risks, however small, on children. Others have suggested that if the risks are sufficiently small, parents can consent to the research even if it holds out no promise of direct benefit to the minor subjects. This approach would obviously allow for more nontherapeutic research on children.[23] The various official policies have adopted the second approach, but they disagree on the permissible level of risks.

The United States HHS regulations (Appendix 3.1, sections 46.404–7), which are the most permissive, have identified different risk levels for different types of pediatric research:

1. No greater than minimal risk (e.g., urinalyses, small blood samples, EEGs)—research is permitted as long as adequate provisions are made for parental consent and for pediatric assent.
2. Greater than minimal risk (e.g., biopsies, spinal taps, and many drugs) but presenting the prospect of direct benefit to the subjects— research is permitted as long as the anticipated direct benefits justify the risks, no better alternative is available, and adequate provisions are made for parental consent and for pediatric assent.

3. Greater than minimal risk and no prospect of direct benefit to the subjects but likely to yield generalizable knowledge—research is permitted as long as the risk is only a minor increase over minimal risk, the information is of vital importance to understanding or ameliorating the subject's condition, the intervention presents experiences that are reasonably commensurate with the subject's actual situation, and adequate provisions are made for consent from (usually) both parents and for pediatric assent.

4. Other research—requires approval of the Secretary of HHS after consultation with a panel of experts who agree that it is ethically sound.

In my experience, most approved pediatric research in the United States falls under the first two categories, although some approvals are certainly given for the third category of research.

Less permissive positions have been adopted in other official policies. The Council of Europe (Appendix 2.3, Article 17.2) allows for nontherapeutic research on children only when the risks are no more than minimal, thereby not allowing for the third category of research permissible under the HHS regulations. Even more stringent on this issue are the guidelines from the British pediatricians.[24] They classify as minimal risks only such interventions as urine samples and analysis of blood drawn for other purposes, treating injections and venipuncture as low-risk procedures (a category analogous to the HHS's category of minor increase over minimal risk), which are not allowed in nontherapeutic research on children. Their justification for doing so is the fear that children have of these procedures and of the brief pain or tenderness accompanying them.

It seemed to many that a similarly strict approach was adopted by the Canadian Medical Research Council in 1987. Clarifying this issue was one of the major purposes of the 1993 Canadian report.[25] Its standards accept such procedures as injections and venipuncture in nontherapeutic research as long as the benefits to children in general from the knowledge gained are sufficient, but it did not go as far as the NIH regulations in permitting nontherapeutic research with more than minimal risks. The 1996 International Harmonization Guidelines (Appendix 1.5, section 4.8.14) seems to come closest to the HHS position in that it allows for such nontherapeutic research when the risks are low (as opposed to minimal).

There are two related aspects of these policies that are troubling. The first is that most (with the exception of the HHS regulations and the International Harmonization Guidelines) do not do justice to the needs for research on children, although they all talk about its importance. They are just too restrictive on nontherapeutic research, especially on older children. This leads to the second point. All of these policies treat all minors alike. This seems wrong. As minors get older, their assent should become of greater significance and this should allow them, with parental consent, to assent to participate in nontherapeutic research whose risks are more than minimal, with the risk level approaching that for which adults can volunteer as the minors get closer to full maturity. Although it is difficult to formulate a precise rule that incorporates this approach, a rule that allowed independent review committees the flexibility to approve such nontherapeutic research involving older minors who assent would be appropriate, especially in policies designed to properly balance the positive value of research on children with the need to protect them in the research process.

Research Involving Special Pediatric Subjects. Many of the abuses in pediatric research that prompted the development of the official policies occurred in children who were institutionalized or who were wards of the state. They are particularly vulnerable because of a lack of parents to review the research's acceptability. This has led to the formulation of stricter protections for such pediatric subjects. Typical of such policies are the 1983 HHS regulations (Appendix 3.1, section 46.409), which focus on specifying the conditions under which such minors can be used as subjects in nontherapeutic research with more than minimal risks. In addition to the general restrictions noted above, the use of such wards is restricted to research on their status as wards or to research in which the majority of subjects are not wards and the reviewing IRB must appoint an independent advocate to protect such subjects.

More problematic is the fact that many of the states in the United States have not given to those caring for wards the authority to enroll them even in therapeutic research, even though that would clearly be allowed under NIH regulations. As a result, such wards are sometimes not enrolled in trials that offer them access to the latest and best therapies. A good example is the exclusion of HIV-infected children living in foster homes from the trials of new therapeutic agents. This has led some to advocate a rethinking of these restrictions on the participation in therapeutic research of pediatric wards of the state, particular in policies designed to balance the importance of pediatric research with the needs for special protections.[26]

Conclusions. There is a growing recognition that two values need to be balanced in policies on pediatric research. Pediatric research is of great value, both to the subject and society, and must be encouraged. At the same time, there is a need to protect pediatric subjects/patients from being abused in the research process. The current official policies have created a framework that needs to be assessed in the light of its success in balancing these two values.

According to that framework, all pediatric research protocols must be reviewed by independent review committees. In conducting their review, they must ensure that there is appropriate agreement from the parents and the minor.

In some cases, appropriate agreement may simply be the consent of the parents. In other cases, assent from the minors should be obtained as well. That requirement becomes more significant as the minors get closer to full maturity, and the minor's refusal in such cases may be binding. Special sensitivity must be shown to parental-minor disagreement in cases of research on potentially life-prolonging interventions on minors with lethal illnesses. In conducting their review, the independent review committees must also ensure that the minors are not exposed to excessive risks. The decision as to whether certain risks are excessive is particularly controversial in the case of nontherapeutic research involving anything more than the most minimal risks.

Is this framework a success? The current official policies may not have properly balanced the values of promoting pediatric research while protecting pediatric subjects. With the exception of the HHS regulations and the International Harmonization guidelines, they may be too strict on the risks allowable in nontherapeutic research. There is, moreover, a concern that institutionalized minors may be denied the benefits of participating in therapeutic research. These two areas of the current official policies should be carefully reexamined. We will return to related issues about balancing in Chapter Eight, when we discuss the relation between research and the approval of drugs and devices for use in the pediatric population.

Research Involving Mentally Infirm Adults

A second class of subjects who need special protection in the research setting are mentally infirm adults. This is a diverse class of subjects including seriously retarded adults who have never been fully competent, psychiatric patients who may alternate between competency when their illness is less severe and incompetency when their illness is more severe, and senile individuals who were once competent but are no longer and never again will be competent. As in the case of pediatric subjects, these mentally infirm adults may lack the capacity to sufficiently comprehend and process information about research to make an informed choice as to whether or not to participate, and this leads to the need for special protections.

A 1994 finding by the NIH's Office of Protection from Research Risks reminds us that this group may be vulnerable to exploitation in the research setting.[27] In a study conducted at UCLA, and eventually challenged by the NIH, a group of schizophrenic patients were taken off their medications for a period of time, resulting in regression of their disease. Questions have been raised both about the adequacy of their consent and about the risks to which they were exposed. It has been shown that similar questions arise for many other drug studies involving this type of mentally infirm adult.[28] Without making any final judgment about that particular study, it certainly illustrates the issues that need to be addressed.

It is important to remember at the same time that research on these infirmities is very important and requires the use of such infirm adults as subjects. Moreover, these adults should not be deprived of the benefits of participating in therapeutic research designed to evaluate new treatments for their concurrent medical problems. So we once more need to strike the proper balance between protecting these individuals from being exploited because of their vulnerability and ensuring that needed appropriate research involving them moves forward. We will assess the various policies in the light of their success in balancing those values.

In this section, we will examine the official policies governing mentally infirm adults as research subjects. It might seem that they should be treated very similarly to pediatric subjects. After all, in both cases, the need for the special protections are due to the same lack of sufficient cognitive capacity. Therefore, the obvious suggestions for additional protections are that the research be authorized by an appropriate combination of surrogate consent and subject assent and that there should be limits on the risks to which they can be exposed in nontherapeutic research. This is what has emerged in a variety of official policies. The Council of Europe, both in its 1990 recommendations on research on human subjects (Appendix 2.2, Principles 4 and 5) and in its 1996 bioethics convention (Appendix 2.3, Article 17), treats these two types of subjects analogously. This is also true for the 1996 International Harmonization Guidelines (Appendix 1.5, section 4.8.5).

In the United States, however, this is not true because there are no official national regulations analogous to the HHS regulations on pediatric research, despite the fact that such regulations have been recommended. How did that come about? The HHS regulations governing human research grew out of the work done in the 1970s by a National Commission. In creating that National Commission, Congress defined one of the issues to be examined as research involving the institutionalized mentally infirm. Two concerns were lumped together in this charge, a concern with the lack of competency due to mental infirmity and a concern with the possibility that the subjects might be coerced into participation because of pressures from institutional officials. The resulting recommendations, attempting to deal with both of these issues, were widely perceived in the research community as too cumbersome and bureaucratic. In the end, no special regulations were adopted for mentally infirm subjects.[29] Many have blamed either the research community or the regulatory community for this unfortunate result, but my suggestion is that the problem was primarily due to Congress's lumping two issues together. When these issues are kept separate, there is no difficulty in producing quite appropriate policies for research on mentally infirm adults, analogous to those for research on pediatric subjects, with special additional protections for the institutionalized.

Such policies would have to address a number of questions, most of which parallel the questions addressed in policies on pediatric subjects: Which mentally infirm adults require extra protection because they are sufficiently incompetent and who makes the determination that they are that incompetent? When the mentally infirm adult is incompetent to give consent to participate in the research, who shall be the surrogate decision maker? What role is there for the incompetent infirm adult in the consent process? What are the limits on the risks to which these subjects can be exposed? How should we deal with the extra problems that arise when these subjects are institutionalized and subject to pressures to consent to participate in research?

In answering these questions, it is important to consult, in addition to the usual official policies, three additional sources which provide considerable guidance. These are (1) a 1986 policy from the NIH (Appendix 3.8) governing intramural research on such subjects at the NIH's clinical center; (2) a 1989 policy from the American College of Physicians on research involving cognitively impaired subjects[30]; (3) a 1991 report of the British Medical Research Council's Working Party on Research on the Mentally Incapacitated.[31]

The Determination of Incompetence. None of these policies offers a general definition of incompetency to consent to participate in research. This is not surprising, for there is much ethical and legal ambiguity and uncertainty about that definition in many medical contexts. I have advocated a definition of competency that relates it to the capacities to receive information, to remember information, to make a decision, and to appropriately assess and use the relevant received/remembered information in making a decision.[32] Even if that account were adopted, there would still remain the question of the extent to which the mentally infirm subject must have those capacities in order to be judged competent so as to not require the extra protection provided by special policies.

Several of these policies make a number of useful substantive observations. To begin with, the question of competency must be settled independently of the determination of infirmity. There are many who are mentally infirm but who are still competent to decide about participating in research. Second, competency is a task-specific issue related to the difficulty of what is proposed. Some mentally infirm individuals might be competent to decide about participating in simpler research protocols but incompetent to decide about participating in more complex protocols. In addition, as stressed in the NIH intramural policy (Appendix 3.8), some mentally infirm individuals might be competent to decide about the choice of a surrogate decision maker even if they are incompetent to decide about participating in any protocols, Third, the clarity of the explanation of information might be relevant to the competency of some subjects to consent to participate. Better explanations will increase the comprehension range of more-infirm individuals.

In addition to these substantive points, several of the policies address the crucial procedural issue of who shall determine the subject's competency to make his or her own decision to participate in the research. This is a particularly crucial question in the light of the ambiguity and uncertainty about the definition. The British Working Party[33] felt that it cannot be the researcher, because that involves obvious conflict of interests. On the other hand, it would be excessively cumbersome on the research effort to insist on a formal judicial assessment of incompetency for every potential research subject, although such an approach has been mandated by a New York court.[34] The Working Party recommended that the determination be made by the subject's physician if the physician is not involved in the research; otherwise, it should be made by an independent party acceptable to the review committee that reviews and approves the research protocol. The NIH policy (Appendix 3.8), by contrast, seems to place the responsibility on the physician caring for the research subject, not addressing the possibility of conflict of interest if that physician is also the researcher. The Working Party's policy is preferable because it avoids that potential problem.

Choice of Surrogate Decision Maker. In the case of pediatric research, the parents are the obvious choice for surrogate decision makers. But who should have that authority in the case of mentally infirm adults? Should it be family members, and if so, who? Should it be a court-appointed guardian? Many of the official policies talk about legally authorized or acceptable representatives, without clarifying that issue. This is particularly troublesome because the law of many jurisdictions may be unclear on this point.

The NIH intramural policy is in one way very innovative on this question. In cases where the subject is still competent to choose a surrogate decision maker, even if not competent to consent to participate, the choice of surrogate decision maker is to be made by the subject (Appendix 3.8, cases 1,3,4). However, when the subject is not competent to choose a surrogate decision maker and the research risks are greater than minimal, a court-appointed guardian is required for such research even if it is therapeutic research and even if the family wishes the subject to participate (Appendix 3.8, cases 5 and 6). This requirement, especially in the case of therapeutic research, seems excessively burdensome and insufficiently appreciative of the need to balance protecting the subject against the need to not deprive the subjects of the benefits of participating in research. Nevertheless, this policy provides more guidance than the British Working Party,[35] which simply talks about the agreement of "an informed independent person acceptable to the LREC [Local Research Ethics Committee]." It is also more useful than the American College of Physicians' policy,[36] which envisages a role for the subject in appointing a surrogate decision maker only in advance while still competent. However, the American College's policy is clearer on allowing family members to consent to participation in therapeutic research without needing to seek court approval.[37]

Consent and The Role of the Subject. What about the incompetent mentally infirm individual? Does he or she have any role to play? The clearest policy is that of the British Working party, which requires that, to the extent possible, the research should be explained to the subject and that the subject does not object or appear to object to participating in the research.[38] Although the American College of Physicians did not directly impose that requirement, it did say that surrogates should withdraw agreement if the subjects become uncooperative.[39] The NIH intramural policy (Appendix 3.8, section 2) talks about the consent of the infirm subject as necessary but not sufficient.

A comparison to the consensus in official policies about assent in pediatric research suggests that these discussions are too weak in most cases but too strong in a few cases. If pediatric subjects must positively assent even if they are not competent to consent, why is it sufficient that incompetent, but aware, mentally infirm adults simply not refuse? In general, the requirement of non-refusal is too weak. On the other hand, if pediatric subjects can sometimes be compelled to participate in therapeutic research that is in their best interest, why is the same not true for mentally infirm adult subjects? In those limited cases, the requirement of non-refusal is too strong. I would suggest, therefore, that researchers using mentally infirm adult subjects provide them a role similar to pediatric subjects with the same level of competency. As noted above, this type of parallelism is appropriately adopted in many of the recent official policies. The 1997 proposed Canadian Code is particularly valuable on this point, requiring the positive assent of the mentally infirm adult but allowing for some therapeutic research in rare cases even when they object.[40]

Acceptable Levels of Risk. All of the policies agree on the levels of risk that are acceptable in therapeutic research on incompetent mentally infirm adults. Surrogates can agree to the subject's participation in therapeutic research if they judge that participation to be in the subject's best interest, even if risky. The policies disagree about nontherapeutic research. Some feel that surrogates can agree to the subject's participation in nontherapeutic research only if the risks of participation are minimal (the term used the American College of Physicians[41]) or negligible (the term used by the British Working Party).[42] But the NIH intramural policy allows for court-appointed guardians together with families to agree to the subject's participating in nontherapeutic research with more than minimal risks (Appendix 3.8, case 6). This is analogous to the third type of research (nontherapeutic research involving minor increases over minimal risks) allowed under U.S., but not under European, policies on pediatric research. Whether this is justified, as part of a policy of balancing the need to protect subjects with the need to encourage valued research, is an important unanswered question.

The American College of Physicians made two additional important observations about surrogate decision making concerning participation in therapeutic research[43]: (1) On the whole, the surrogates should focus on judging whether participation is in the subject's best interest (the best interest standard) rather than whether or not the subject would have wanted to participate (the substituted judgment standard). This is different from the usual approach to surrogate decision making in nonresearch settings. The difference is justified on the grounds that the subjects are unlikely to have thought about these issues of participation in research in advance and that substituted judgments would therefore be highly speculative. Nevertheless, if there is evidence that the subject would not have consented to participate in research, the surrogate should withhold agreement even if he or she judges that it would be in the subject's best interest to participate. (2) In those cases in which participation in the research means forgoing standard treatment, the surrogate decision maker must carefully consider whether the speculative benefits of receiving the experimental treatment outweigh the forgone benefits from the standard treatment.

Protecting the Institutionalized Subject. As noted above, when a subject is institutionalized, the issue of the voluntariness of the subject's or the surrogate's consent also arises. Both the institutionalized subject and his or her surrogate may be subjected to subtle coercion or inducement. How can they be protected without impairing the conduct of needed research that may even be beneficial to them?

The American College of Physicians' treatment of this issue is useful, although perhaps incomplete. The major observations that it made are the following[44]:

1. Institutionalized patients are very dependent on their caregivers and they or their surrogates may be coerced into agreeing to participate in research by the tacit fear, whether or not justified, that refusal might lead to a diminished quality of care. At the same time, they are very susceptible to minor positive inducements such as a change in living quarters.
2. The independent review committee should carefully examine the protocol to see whether it might involve coercion or undue influence.
3. Useful input might be received from a standing committee composed of, and chosen by, the residents of the institution.

It is of interest to note that the American College does not advocate the appointment of a consent auditor to monitor against subtle coercion of dependent individuals, one of the recommendations of the U.S. National Commission that attracted considerable controversy.[45] Does the input from the resident committee adequately deal with problems of subtle coercion? If not, under what conditions would the appointment of such auditors be helpful?

Conclusion. Research on mentally infirm adults is of great importance, and must be encouraged. At the same time, there is a need to protect such subjects from being abused in the research process. The heart of that protection is a careful review of research protocols by independent review committees. In conducting their review, they should first ensure that there are appropriate standards and mechanisms for determining whether the subjects are competent to make their own judgment about participation in research and require no special protections or whether they are incompetent and do require special protections. In the latter case, consent must be obtained from an appropriate surrogate, keeping in mind legal ambiguities and ethical concerns about whom that might be in particular cases. There may in some cases be a role for the subject in choosing the surrogate. For some of these subjects, their positive assent to participate should also be obtained; for others, the research should not be conducted against their refusal to participate. In conducting their review, the independent review committees should also ensure that surrogates should not consent to research involving excessive risks, a problem that is particularly troublesome in nontherapeutic research. Finally, when the subjects are also institutionalized, extra care may need to be paid to subtle coercions to participate. Input from the institutionalized and or independent consent-auditors are some of the mechanisms that have been suggested to deal with this extra concern.

On the whole, this type of balanced approach has been adopted in the major official policies. Their major shortcomings are that many are too demanding on the risk level for nontherapeutic research and that many are not demanding enough on the requirement of positive assent.

Research Involving Prisoners

A third group of vulnerable subjects who may need special protection in the research setting are prisoners. Traditionally, prisoners were used in phase I drug trials and drug metabolism and bioavailability studies, all of which involve risks but little if any likelihood of benefit. They were also infected with various diseases to study both the natural history of those diseases and possible vaccines. Once more, these studies involved risks but little if any likelihood of benefit. Finally, they were enrolled in various studies of rehabilitative techniques, including behavior modification and aversive conditioning studies.

Why was so much research of these types done on prisoners? After all, only the last type of research requires the use of prisoners. A number of answers can be offered. To begin with, the prisoner population is a stable population (you can count on their being there) and the environment is more controllable (especially if research subjects are placed in special cell blocks). Second, it was often easier to get prisoners to volunteer for studies involving risks but no benefits. They might volunteer to get better conditions, to earn a few dollars, or in the hope of earning earlier release from prison.

It was, of course, this second fact that gave rise to the concern about the ethics of doing research on prisoners. If the conditions in a prison (including fears of personal safety) were intolerable, but conditions were much better in a research area, were the prisoner subjects really voluntarily consenting to participate in the research or was their participation really coerced? If participation offered prisoners the best (or the only) chance to earn a little money to be used in the prison canteen, were the prisoner subjects really voluntarily consenting to participate or was their participation really coerced? If participation helped them secure earlier release, were the prisoner subjects really voluntarily consenting to participate or was their participation really coerced?

There was an additional concern raised by some commentators. One of the accepted principles of research ethics is that there should be a fair and just distribution of the benefits and burdens of research. But the suspicion was that prisoners were being used for those forms of research that were more burdensome and less beneficial. This research on prisoners might be an unfair and unjust exploitation of them even if their consent was voluntary.

As these questions were raised in the 1960s and the 1970s, a number of points quickly emerged. Research on prisoners raises different questions than research on children or mentally infirm adults; the issues are about the voluntariness of the subject's consent to participate and the fairness of using prisoners in burdensome research, not the competency of the subject to consent to participate. These issues of voluntariness and exploitation are very difficult to resolve, both practically and theoretically. The practical issue arises out of the recognition that subjects in many research projects are offered inducements to participate and they often volunteer to participate because of these inducements. How can we distinguish between legitimate inducements and inducements that are "too good to refuse"? To what extent should these judgments be modified by one's views of the conditions under which prisoners live? The theoretical issue arises out of worries as to whether offers to improve people's conditions are ever coercive or exploitative. Why shouldn't competent adults be able to accept any offers they find attractive? Nevertheless, it was thought by many to be easiest to deal with these concerns by banning or severely limiting research on prisoners. In the case of minors, we need them as research subjects if we are to find better ways to treat sick children. In the case of mentally infirm adults, we need them as research subjects if we are to find better ways to treat those infirmities. There is much less of an analogous need to use prisoners as research subjects, even if their use is very convenient.

This approach was adopted by the Council of Europe in the 1990 recommendations of its Committee of Ministers. Because of the concern about the voluntariness of consent, research on "persons deprived of liberty" cannot be carried out unless "it is expected to produce a direct and significant benefit to their health" (Appendix 2.2, Principle 7). This exception for promising therapeutic research seems appropriate; HIV-positive prisoners need access to trials of new therapies. Participation in research may be a benefit that we do not want to deny to members of vulnerable groups in the course of protecting them from abuse and exploitation.

The HHS regulations (Appendix 3.1, Subpart C) are more permissive in principle but perhaps more restrictive in practice. In addition to allowing promising therapeutic research (with special extra protections if the prisoner/subject might be assigned to a placebo control group), it allows research involving no more than minimal risk on causes or effects of incarceration and criminal behavior or on prisons as institutional structures or prisoners as incarcerated persons. These extra exceptions are justified on the grounds that the risks are minimal and prisoners are needed as research subjects. They apply primarily to social science, rather than biomedical, research. Finally, the Secretary of HHS, after an elaborate procedure, can give permission for research on health problems particularly affecting prisoners as a class. Here, the justification is that the prisoners are needed as research subjects. These extra exceptions to the ban on research on prisoners are more nuanced and appropriate.

In all cases, however, the IRB approving the research is subject under the HHS regulations to many additional requirements, and in practice this may undercut the theoretical gains in the HHS regulations. The IRB that approves the research must be substantially independent of the prison in which the research will be conducted and must contain at least one prisoner or prisoner representative. It must find that the prisoners are not receiving excessive inducements, that the risks of participation are commensurate with the risks that would be accepted by nonprisoner volunteers, that the procedures for selecting subjects are fair and immune from arbitrary intervention by prison authorities or prisoners, that each prisoner is informed that adequate measures have been taken to ensure that parole boards will not take into account their participation in research, and that adequate provisions have been made, where appropriate, for follow-up care. Although each of these provisions makes sense, their practical implications, taken together, may excessively restrict research on prisoners, even therapeutic research that might be of benefit to them.

In conclusion, although there are questions that can be raised about the foundations of the concerns about the use of prisoners as research subjects, the concerns have led to official policies that have minimized the use of prisoner subjects. To some degree, this may be acceptable because the need for their use is small. But there are grounds for concern that prisoners may be excluded from beneficial therapeutic research and that society may be losing out on some research that is needed. Some empirical studies of the impact of these regulations are probably appropriate at this point. To return to the point with which we began this chapter, we need to balance the goal of protecting the vulnerable with the goal of promoting appropriate research.

Conclusion

Official policies on research involving such vulnerable subjects as children, the mentally infirm, and prisoners originated in response to various questionable cases that suggested that such subjects needed special protection. In more recent years, however, these policies have increasingly recognized the value of research using such subjects. Participation in such research can provide valuable benefits to the subjects and important knowledge to society. We must therefore evaluate the resulting official policies in light of the balance they draw between these potentially conflicting values.

Our review of the essentially convergent official policies indicate that they have done a good job in balancing these values. There are two areas of concern. To begin with, most of the official policies on pediatric research and on research on mentally infirm adults may be too restrictive on nontherapeutic research. Such research may sometimes be justifiable even when the risks are more than minimal. Second, the institutionalized vulnerable may not have adequate access to beneficial therapeutic research. This may be due to special procedural issues (e.g., restrictive laws about institutionalized children, uncertainties about the surrogates for the mentally infirm, and special requirements for review of protocols on prisoners) rather than fundamental research policy issues, but the constraints are still there. Both of these concerns require changes, but neither undercuts the fundamentally positive achievement of the official policies in many countries in balancing the relevant important values. All of this makes the U.S. failure to develop a formal official policy on research involving mentally infirm subjects, as opposed to the NIH policy governing intramural research on such subjects, inexcusable.

Chapter seven

CLINICAL TRIALS

One of the important characteristics of research in the past few decades is the emphasis on clinical trials to validate interventions before they are widely used in the clinical setting. Whatever the theoretical scientific reasons for believing that these interventions would be beneficial, and whatever the favorable initial experience with their use, clinical trials to validate their use have become increasingly common. This is not to say that clinical trials are now used in all cases; it is to say that a variety of intellectual forces (e.g., the emergence of a science of clinical trials) and societal forces (e.g., the insistence by regulatory agencies on the use of clinical trials before drugs and devices are approved for sale) have combined to emphasize the value of such trials. It is, therefore, important that we examine the ethical issues raised by such trials.

Because such trials involve the use of human subjects, all of the discussions in Chapters Two and Six about human subjects research are relevant to clinical trials as well. In this chapter, we will not revisit those issues; instead, we will focus only on those special ethical issues raised by clinical trials. Before doing that, we will briefly review the history of clinical trials and the main characteristics of those trials; this well help us both define and deal with the ethical issues.

One preliminary observation. The extensive official policies on research to which we have referred in previous chapters will be of less use to us in this chapter. Although they have a lot to say about the general issues of human subjects research, they have much less to say about the specific issues raised by clinical trials. We will refer to the official material for guidance on some points, but we will in most cases have to rely more heavily on the proposals of scholars. We will return in the conclusion to the question of why official policies are less helpful in this area.

A Brief Introduction to Clinical Trials

Although the contemporary clinical trial is a product of the post–World War II period, there were certainly anticipations of such trials in earlier times.[1] Lind's 1747 study of treatments for scurvy, where twelve sailors aboard ship were divided into six treatment groups, laid the foundation for the widespread use of oranges and lemons to prevent scurvy. Semmelweis's study in the 1840s of handwashing before examining women in labor, which sharply reduced the incidence of mortality from puerperal fever, laid the foundation for antiseptic measures to prevent infection. In both cases, an intervention (eating citrus fruit or handwashing) was validated by being studied prospectively by comparison with a control group (those patients simultaneously getting other treatments for scurvy or those in labor who had previously been treated by physicians who had not washed their hands). But patients were not randomly assigned to the various groups and everyone was aware of who got what treatment, so there were considerable opportunities for unintended biases. In the 1920s, J. Burns Amberson and his colleagues evaluated the use of sanocrysin, a gold compound, in the treatment of pulmonary tuberculosis. In that trial, half the patients received the treatment and half received intravenous injections of distilled water; neither the patients nor most of the professionals knew which patient got which treatment, so the trial was nearly a double-blinded controlled trial. Also, the decision as to who got what was determined by the flip of a coin, so the trial was a randomized trial, even if the method of randomization was somewhat primitive. All of these features were brought together in a more sophisticated fashion in a 1948 study of use of streptomycin to treat pulmonary tuberculosis, a study headed by Sir Bradford Hill.[2] It was also notable for its attention to ethical issues, including a decision to not blind the patients and the treating physicians to who got what treatment by using placebo injections; this was done to avoid unethically subjecting the control group in the trial to unnecessary intramuscular injections four times a day for four months.

This very brief historical survey has already introduced many of the important features of the modern clinical trial. Although no official list of crucial features exists, I think that most would agree upon the following as being essential:

First, it is a prospective trial of a well-defined intervention. A clinical trial must be distinguished from a retrospective case review study, in which the subjects in both groups have already received or not received the intervention in question, and the study examines differences in outcomes. By its very nature, the subjects in such a retrospective review cannot be randomly assigned to the treatment or control groups and neither they nor the treating clinicians are blinded to which group they are in. Prospective clinical trials assign patients *in advance* to the two groups and can therefore have both of these desirable features. This is not to say that retrospective studies are of no value. They are often the source of hypotheses for prospective clinical trials. For reasons that will emerge below, they are sometimes the only studies that can be done. They are the major source of information as to how well interventions validated in clinical trials work in clinical practice. Contemporary medical outcomes research is a sophisticated form of retrospective review and it is attracting considerable attention. It is only to say that the evidence from a retrospective study cannot be as conclusive as the evidence from a well-designed prospective trial, because certain sources of possible bias cannot be excluded from retrospective reviews.

Second, it studies a population carefully defined by inclusion and exclusion rules. A clinical trial is designed to answer the question as to whether a certain intervention does or does not make certain differences. In general, that answer will depend on the population in which the intervention is used. Therefore, the trial must specify what population is being studied. This is done by specifying inclusion criteria and exclusion criteria. In general, the inclusion criteria are supposed to reflect the patient population for which there are scientific reasons to believe that the intervention will work. If there are several such populations, and if there are reasons for thinking that the results might differ in those populations, it may be best to define a series of substudies that separately examine the effectiveness of the intervention in each of the populations, thereby preserving a certain homogeneity in the study population. In general, the exclusion criteria are supposed to keep out of the study those populations for which there are scientific reasons to be concerned about the safety of the intervention, although they can also be used to better define the group for which efficacy is anticipated. Finally, it should be noted that there is a trade-off between using broad inclusion and modest exclusion criteria (thereby making it easier to find subjects to enroll in the study but weakening the science and the safety protection) and using very precise inclusion and extensive exclusion criteria (thereby improving the science and the safety protection but making it harder to find subjects to enroll in the study).

Third, it involves a control group as well as an intervention group. Clinical trials must involve a control group to compare with the intervention group, but they differ on the type of control group employed. The control group may be a concurrent group receiving a placebo instead of the intervention (a concurrent placebo-controlled trial), it may be a concurrent group receiving a standard intervention to which the new intervention is being compared (a concurrent active-controlled trial), it may be a concurrent group receiving the same drug intervention at a different dosage (a concurrent dosage-controlled trial), or it may be an earlier group that had not received the intervention in question (a historically controlled trial). The first three types of trials can all be run as randomized trials, where patients are randomly assigned to one or the other of the groups, but the fourth cannot, and this means that certain forms of biases cannot be eliminated from such trials. Also, because other factors might have changed between the earlier time and the time of the trial, differences between the intervention group and the historical group cannot necessarily be attributed to the intervention. For these two reasons, concurrent controlled trials must in general be preferred to historically controlled trials. The comparative advantages of the three types of concurrently controlled randomized trials, and the reasons for sometimes using historically controlled trials, will be discussed below in our examination of the ethical issues.

Fourth, it assigns subjects to these groups randomly. Randomization is crucial to clinical trials for a number of reasons. To begin with, it minimizes the possibility of unconscious biases leading to more favorable subjects being assigned to one group rather than the other, invalidating the study's comparison of the two groups. Also, randomization tends to produce two groups that are comparable to each other in important baseline characteristics. For these two reasons, as well as for reasons of statistical methodology, randomization to treatment and control groups is seen as vital to clinical trials; as explained above, the inability to randomize is one of the major weaknesses of retrospective studies and of historically controlled studies.

Fifth, it blinds both the subjects and the treating professionals to the assignment of individual patients to the control or the treatment group. Such trials are called double-blinded trials. If only the subjects are blinded to the assignment, the trials are called single-blinded trials. Blinding the subjects helps prevent excessive dropout, especially from the control group. It also helps avoid subjects being influenced by their knowledge of their assignment to seek different concomitant treatments or to assess subjective outcomes differently. Blinding the investigators helps prevent their offering different concurrent treatments to the different groups and helps prevent their knowledge of the assignment influencing their clinical assessment of the outcomes. It is sometimes very difficult and/or inappropriate to blind either the subjects or the clinicians. As noted above, in the classic 1948 study of streptomycin, blinding would have required injecting the control group with a placebo four times a day for four months, and this was judged to be inappropriate. When blinding cannot be employed, it is important to minimize the above-described potential biases by using outcomes that are very objective and by defining as carefully as possible the conditions under which concurrent treatments can be used. This is often not easy to do, so while blinding is not as essential to a good clinical trial as randomization, it certainly should be carried out where possible.

Sixth, it is of an adequate size to determine whether well-defined end points are found more often in one group than in the other. A clinical trial is meant to test hypotheses about the differences that an intervention makes in a population. The differences may range from better relief of pain to increasing survival. Some investigators, rather than defining the possible differences to be studied in advance, indiscriminately collect data and then see what differences exist between the control group and the intervention group. This is not valid; the more "fishing" you do for differences, the more likely you are to find differences that occurred just by chance. We have already indicated the importance of defining the intervention and the population in advance. It is equally important to specify what differences are being looked at; these are the defined end points of the trial. It is also very important to make sure that your trial looks at enough patients. If it does not, you may not see a difference that the intervention really makes. In the past, many negative results were announced that were mistaken; not enough patients had been looked at. Today, good clinical trials are planned with the help of statistical calculations to enroll enough patients so to have adequate power to detect real differences. The calculations vary depending upon the end points being studied, so this is another reason why the end points must be specified in advance.

Finally, it has been approved as ethical in advance by an independent review process, and it is carefully monitored during the trial by an independent data board that is authorized to stop the trial if conclusive positive data about efficacy or negative data about safety emerge. We have already discussed in Chapter Two the role of independent review of the trial before it commences as a crucial mechanism for ensuring that the trial is ethical. The only additional point that needs to be added to that discussion here relates to the fact that many of these trials are run as multicenter trials. The Royal College of Physicians[3] allows for a central review by one Research Ethics Committee, with the others considering only local issues; the 1997 proposed Canadian code[4] insists that each local Research Ethics Board must do a full review of the protocol. We do need to add some additional remarks about the monitoring of the trial while it is being conducted. During the time the trial is being run, data about safety or efficacy may become available from other trials, and this may make the trial unnecessary (because efficacy has been established) or inappropriate (because excessive risks have been established). There is also the need to periodically review in a planned fashion the data emerging in the trial to decide whether the preliminary data settles the issues in question. To ensure that these questions are adequately reviewed by a group that has no vested interest in the continuation of the trial, it has become customary to have these questions assessed by an independent Data and Safety Monitoring Board (DSMB).

It has often been observed that there are far more clinical trials evaluating new drugs or new devices than clinical trials evaluating new surgical techniques. Part of this is due to the·existence of regulatory review mechanisms for new drugs and devices but not for new techniques; these mechanisms, and their influence on clinical trials, will be discussed in Chapter Eight. But this difference is also due in part to the greater difficulty in conducting clinical trials of new surgical techniques with the above seven features. Most crucially, people may be unwilling to be randomized in a trial where the treatment arm involves invasive surgery. Moreover, blinding is difficult in such trials. Finally, having a concurrent control group may be problematic when the new surgical intervention offers a treatment for a previously devastating or lethal condition. We will return to these issues below, and we will examine the prospects for ethically acceptable trials of new surgical techniques.

With this understanding of the major features of clinical trials, we can now turn to the major ethical issues raised by such trials.

The Major Ethical Issues

Commencing a Clinical Trial. There is a limited period of time during which an intervention can be tested in a prospective concurrently controlled clinical trial. On the one hand, it would be inappropriate to subject a complete treatment group to the risks of the intervention until its details have been worked out and until there is adequate reason to believe that it might be sufficiently beneficial, and it would also be inappropriate to spend the resources on such a trial until those conditions are satisfied. On the other hand, it would be inappropriate to deny to a control group the benefits of the intervention once the sufficiency of those benefits of the intervention have been adequately established.

An excellent example that illustrates the difficulties in defining this limited period is the introduction of ECMO (extracorporeal membrane oxygenation) in the management of neonatal respiratory insufficiency. In the late 1970s, this technique was introduced in the neonatal population. While the details of its use were being worked out in the management of the first patients, the early reports involving those patients showed such a significant improvement over historical controls that there was great unwillingness to run a concurrent controlled trial, even though the use of historical controls was questionable because of the many other dramatic improvements in the management of these patients. ECMO increasingly became a standard therapeutic intervention, even though its use had not been validated in a classical clinical trial.[5] Finally, in 1993, the community of British neonatologists ran a randomized concurrent active-controlled trial, with the understanding that ECMO could be used only in the context of such a trial; it was stopped in 1995 when the data showed a clear advantage to those receiving ECMO as opposed to conventional treatment.[6]

Some might suggest that a concurrently controlled trial should have been started with the very first neonate to receive ECMO, but I believe that this suggestion misses the point about the need to adequately develop the intervention and to find some evidence suggesting its effectiveness before running a clinical trial. But then the question remains as to when there is too much evidence to conduct the trial. By the end of 1992, the International ECMO Registry had showed an 81% survival rate in 7,647 gravely ill infants, with only 17%

suffering severe neurological damage, but these data were not from randomized trials.[7] Was 1993 too late to run such a trial?

Many have viewed our question as being about the conflict between a clinician's obligation to do the best for the individual patient (leading to using the therapeutic approach best supported by the preliminary evidence) and the researcher's obligation to gather sufficient evidence to guide future practice (leading to enrolling the subjects into the clinical trial). Such analysts have placed much emphasis on decisions about clinical trials being made by independent monitoring boards who don't have that obligation to the individual patient. I believe that this approach misses the issue. Would it have been any easier for an independent board to have authorized the commencement of a concurrently controlled trial of ECMO once the early data about improved survival was in? The heart of the problem is defining the window of opportunity for an ethically legitimate clinical trial, when there is some but not conclusive evidence for the benefits of the proposed intervention, not on defining who makes the decision.

Some have suggested that the informed consent process can take care of this problem. As long as the potential subjects are informed about the preliminary data but are still willing to be enrolled in a concurrently controlled trial, running such a controlled trial is morally acceptable. Thus, the British ECMO trial made a great effort to inform the parents and to receive their consent before any neonate was randomized into the trial, although there were several problems with their efforts.[8] However, this suggestion misses the point, already discussed in Chapter Two, that even the best informed consent process is only one of the conditions required for legitimate human subjects research. If there is enough evidence supporting the use of the intervention, then enrolling subjects in a concurrently controlled trial of the intervention would not have a favorable risk-benefit ratio because of the losses to those in the control group and would be illegitimate despite the consent of the subjects. Any justification of a clinical trial, while referring to the consent of those enrolled, must also refer to the evidence being suggestive but insufficient, and that requires defining the window of opportunity.

Charles Fried, in 1974,[9] introduced the term "equipoise" to define that state of uncertainty that must exist in order for a concurrently controlled trial to be justified. As he used that term, it seemed to mean that the available evidence must offer no reason for preferring one of the treatments arms in the trial over the others. But if that were truly the situation, we would not have any reason to start the trial; as noted above, clinical trials begin with evidence suggesting that the intervention is more efficacious and are designed to see whether or not that suggestion holds up. So that type of complete equipoise cannot be a presupposition of ethically legitimate clinical trials. Benjamin Freedman, in a much discussed 1987 article,[10] suggested instead that the equipoise required for a legitimate clinical trial is a clinical equipoise, a remaining disagreement in the expert clinical community, despite the available evidence, about the merits of the intervention to be tested. When experts still disagree despite the evidence, there is enough evidence to justify starting the trial but not enough evidence to make running the trial inappropriate. This type of disagreement apparently existed in the British neonatology community and provided the impetus for the trial.

This condition for the legitimacy of initiating a clinical trial is ambiguous because it leaves the degree of remaining disagreement unclear. It has, however, acquired a wide following, and it is incorporated into the 1993 *Institutional Review Board Guidebook* of the NIH's Office of Protection from Research Risks,[11] one of the few official documents to discuss these issues. Nevertheless, this approach is excessively dependent on the sociological fact of continuing disagreement in the clinical community. That disagreement may reflect the fact that the evidence is suggestive but not sufficient, in which case the trial is legitimate. But it may just reflect a conservatism toward accepting change in some segments of the clinical community, and why should that be enough to justify running the trial?

A more reasonable approach was first suggested by Paul Meier.[12] According to that approach, the prospective subject is viewed as someone with a legitimate sense of self-interest but also with a certain sense of community altruism, leading to a desire to help settle important clinical questions. If the evidence of the benefits of the intervention is so great that such a person would not, out of self-interested concerns, volunteer to be in the trial, then the evidence is sufficient to make the trial morally unacceptable. If, on the other hand, such a person would volunteer out of a sense of altruism, despite his or her legitimate self-interested concerns, then that indicates that the evidence on behalf of the intervention is at best suggestive. In thinking about the legitimacy of initiating a clinical trial, one should try to imagine oneself as such a person and ask whether or not one would be willing to volunteer to be in the trial.

Obviously, much more thought needs to be devoted to this issue, but certain conclusions are clear:

1. It is a mistake to suggest that the very first person receiving a new intervention should do so in the context of a concurrently controlled randomized clinical trial.
2. At the same time, it is clearly desirable to begin such trials as soon as possible, before there is enough evidence to make a clinical trial unacceptable, even if the evidence is not conclusive.
3. There is no simple definition of the window of opportunity for running a concurrently controlled clinical trial once suggestive evidence has emerged, but several formulas (Friedman's, Meier's) are available to guide us in thinking about this difficult issue.

4. In the light of the extra conditions discussed in Chapter Six for legitimate pediatric research, these formulas may require modification as one applies them to trials involving children such as the British ECMO trial.

5. In cases in which running such a trial would be unethical, we may have to rely upon the evidence derived from comparing those receiving the intervention with the members of a historical control group, even if such evidence faces some of the issues raised above. We will return to this point in our discussion of control groups.

Defining the Study Population/Recruiting Subjects. Participation in a clinical trial can bring to individual subjects benefits (from receiving a beneficial new intervention or from better monitoring and care because one is in the trial) as well as burdens (from receiving a harmful new intervention or from having to undergo burdensome testing procedures). Moreover, when individuals from a particular group are included as research subjects in a trial, information from that trial may be more beneficial to other members of that group as future subjects. One of the fundamental principles of ethical research on human subjects identified in Chapter Two is that the burdens and benefits of research should be distributed equitably. But there are grounds for concern as to whether this principle is being respected in clinical trials, whether one looks at it from the perspective of individual subjects or from the perspective of the groups to which they belong.

Some of these concerns, related to the underinvolvement of children and mentally infirm adults in clinical trials, have already been discussed in Chapter Six. Other concerns grow out of the underrepresentation of women and of members of various minority groups in clinical trials, either because they are excluded directly or indirectly by the inclusion and exclusion criteria or because the mechanisms for enrolling patients fail to enroll them. Because of the importance of these issues, we will devote much of Chapter Nine to a consideration of them.

The Selection of the Control Group. Although the control group for a clinical trial can be a historical control group, the use of a concurrent control group is obviously scientifically preferable. This allows for randomization and for blinding and avoids the problem of ascertaining whether observed differences are due to the intervention being tested or to other changes that took place between the earlier period and the period in which the intervention was tested. Nevertheless, there are occasions in which the use of a concurrent control group would be unethical and only historical controls are acceptable.

· A very clear example was the trials of new surgical techniques (transplantation, the Norwood Palliative Procedure) for treating neonates born without a functioning left side of the heart (hypoplastic left heart syndrome).[13] Until these techniques were developed, there were no therapeutic options and all the children died relatively quickly; in fact, it was common to just keep them comfortable and to do nothing to prolong their dying. After some initial successes, these new techniques were tested in a series of patients, and the results were compared with the earlier results of uniform mortality; this was, in effect, a historically controlled trial of these techniques. It would have been unethical to randomize neonates into a trial of either of these promising techniques against nothing, so a concurrent trial was inappropriate. Moreover, the usual problems with historically controlled trials were less present. Nothing else had changed, the outcome difference was very objective (survival versus death) so there was less room for the influence of biases due to a lack of blinding, and so forth. It is important to note that there was and still is room for a randomized concurrently controlled trial of the two techniques to see which is preferable. Even in the case of new surgical techniques for treating previously lethal conditions, some randomized clinical trials may be ethically appropriate.

Obviously, not all cases are so clear. As the ECMO case illustrates, there are many cases in which it is debatable whether a concurrently controlled trial is still ethical despite initial promising results. This is particularly true when the scientific problems of using a historical control group, due to other changes in treatment, are far greater. Those are the cases in which the choice of a historical versus a concurrent control group is far more troubling ethically.

Similarly troubling problems arise in the choice of which type of concurrent control group to use. For example, when a new drug is being tested for the treatment of a condition, often there are many other drugs available and approved for treating that condition. The question being tested is whether the new drug is as good as, or is better than, the already approved drugs. Should one test the new drug against the already approved drugs (thereby running a concurrent active-controlled trial) or against a placebo (thereby running a concurrent placebo-controlled trial)? It might seem that the former is preferable. Why should we deny to the control group the benefits of the already approved drugs? There are, however, a number of reasons (Appendix 3.4) why placebo-controlled trials are more satisfactory than active-controlled trials. For statistical reasons, trials designed to test the equivalence of the new drug with the older drugs must be larger, and therefore more costly, than trials designed to prove that the new drug works better. Even if equivalence is established in these larger trials, it does not show that the new drug is doing any good. It may be that the equivalence is due to the established drug not doing any good in the trial. This is a particularly troublesome concern when there is a great variability in the effectiveness of the established drug or when the condition often responds spontaneously without the use of any drug. Note, by the way, that these two problems are problems primarily for active-controlled trials designed to test for equivalence; they are not problems for active-controlled trials designed to test whether the new drug is better than the old drug. This type of trial has not, to my mind, received sufficient attention.

The ethical issue in such cases is very clear, although its resolution is often far from clear. From the perspective of getting well-established answers (the perspective of the investigators, of the drug regulatory agencies, and of future patients), the use of placebo-controlled trials may be better. From the perspective of protecting the health of those who will be assigned to the control group (the perspective of the subjects and of their clinicians), the use of active-controlled trials may be better. In cases of testing new drugs for life-threatening conditions that do not resolve spontaneously or in response to placebos (e.g., new antiviral drugs for AIDS patients), the concerns about the control group are far more pressing than the scientific concerns, and we should certainly use an active-controlled trial (e.g., the control group receives AZT). But there are many cases that are far less clear. There are cases in which less is at stake for the patients and the scientific concerns are greater. In such cases, deciding which control group to use can be very difficult ethically. Some of these difficulties can be alleviated if the placebo-controlled trial has a careful plan for monitoring subjects and providing alternative treatment (sometimes called, perhaps too dramatically, rescue medicines) before their condition deteriorates significantly, but this is not always an adequate solution.

Some guidance about these problems can be found both in various official policies and in the statements of professional groups. This is one example of attention being paid to the special ethical issues posed by clinical trials.

The Declaration of Helsinki, which now explicitly accepts that placebo-controlled trials are justified when there are no proven therapies, still asserts that "In any medical study, every patient—including those of a control group, if any—should be assured of the best proven diagnostic and therapeutic method" (Appendix 1.2, Principle II.3). The 1997 proposed Canadian Code[14] asserts that "The use of placebos in clinical trials is ethically unacceptable when clearly effective interventions are available," and that position has been explicitly adopted by the Canadian National Council on Bioethics in Human Research.[15] Similarly, the Australian National Health and Medical Research Council said that "Patients in control groups should receive what is considered to be the best treatment currently available; in some cases this may be simply observation or administration of placebo" (Appendix 4.12, Supplementary Note 3). These statements seem too absolute in their opposition to placebo-control groups when there are effective therapies available, no matter how serious the scientific problems of an active-controlled trial and no matter how modest would be the possible losses to those in the proposed placebo-controlled group.

A quite different approach is found in guidelines issued in 1989 by the United States Food and Drug Administration (Appendix 3.4). These guidelines stress the problems with active-controlled trials designed to establish equivalence, concede that placebo-controlled trials are sometimes ethically unacceptable but seem to confine that concession to cases in which existing treatments are life-prolonging, and urge the use of placebo-controlled trials with mechanisms (such as early rescue and minimization of study duration) designed to limit the losses to those in the placebo-control group. I am not convinced, however, that this approach places sufficient emphasis on the seriousness of the placebo group's losing the benefits of established therapy even when life prolongation is not at stake. No matter what trial design measures are taken to limit the losses to those in the placebo-control group, the remaining losses from not receiving established treatments that effectively limit morbidity and/or discomfort may be too great to allow for the use of a placebo-control group.

A 1996 statement by the American Medical Association (AMA) offers a useful balance between these two more extreme positions.[16] It goes beyond the FDA in discouraging the use of placebo-control groups for trials concerning illnesses that produce severe or painful symptoms when effective treatments are available. At the same time, it is more permissive than the Declaration of Helsinki, the Canadian Code, and the Australian guidelines in allowing such placebo-controlled trials when the standard therapy has a bad profile of side effects. Finally, while recognizing that informed consent does not justify all placebo-controlled trials, it does emphasize the importance of good consent processes.

Where does all of this leave the investigator? Certain conclusions are clear:

1. From a scientific perspective, concurrently controlled trials are better than historically controlled trials.
2. From a scientific perspective, placebo-controlled trials and active-controlled trials designed to test the superiority of a new intervention are superior to active-controlled trials designed to test the equivalence of the new intervention with the treatment received by the control group.
3. In some cases, it is ethical to achieve those scientific benefits by using a placebo-control group and by withholding from the control group an established effective therapy. These include cases in which the established therapy has significant side effects and cases in which the disease process being treated is not that important. It is particularly important to achieve those benefits when the scientific issues about trials to test equivalence are particularly pressing.
4. The more serious the disease process and the less likely that the established therapy will produce bad side effects, the more problematic is a placebo-controlled trial. Investigators should then consider measures (e.g., early rescue, limitation of study duration) that would make the placebo-

controlled trial acceptable or should consider the possibility of an active controlled trial designed to test the superiority of the new intervention.

5. There will be cases in which the only way to adequately protect the subjects is to run a historically controlled trial or an actively controlled trial designed to test equivalence, even if the results of such trials are not as well established as one would like.

There is one additional issue about control groups in a special context that deserves to be mentioned. The special context is clinical trials of inexpensive but promising therapies run in less developed countries when there already exists an expensive but clearly efficacious treatment generally used in more developed countries but not available in the less developed countries because of the cost. May these trials be run as placebo-controlled trials? It could be argued both that the subjects are not being unfairly denied by the trial the expensive therapy, because they would not have received it anyway because of its cost, and that this approach is the scientifically best way of quickly obtaining clear answers to a vital public health question. Or it could be argued that this would be an inappropriate exploitation of these poor subjects. This issue arose in the spring of 1997 when it was revealed that the United States was sponsoring trials in third world countries of inexpensive approaches to minimizing maternal-fetal transmission of HIV, where the control group was receiving a placebo rather than the expensive AZT treatment common in the United States and other developed countries.[17] This question of cross-national research ethics will continue to be debated as long as the disparities in health care expenditures between countries persist.

Issues in Randomization. As indicated above, there are many scientific advantages that result from randomly assigning subjects to the treatment group or the control group. Providing that the patients are informed about the basis of the assignment, and assuming that the trial has an appropriate control group and is taking place under appropriate equipoise, there seems to be nothing wrong ethically with randomization.

Nevertheless, serious ethical issues have arisen in connection with randomization. They grow out of problems with enrollment encountered by a number of major clinical trials, perhaps the most important of which was a trial that began in 1977 to study the comparative efficacy of total versus segmental mastectomy with or without radiation therapy for the management of breast cancer. In the first two years, accrual of subjects to this very important trial was very slow, and this threatened the possibility of the trial being concluded. Clinicians were finding it very difficult to ask their patients to agree to be randomized and patients were balking at the idea of randomization. Various alternatives to the standard type of randomization were adopted in this and a number of other trials, and it is these alternatives that have given rise to the ethical controversies.[18]

Why did these trials encounter these problems with accrual? A number of features could be mentioned. These trials involved very serious medical issues, invasive treatments that were radically and obviously different, and significant differences for the quality of life of the patient/subjects involved from the different treatments. In this setting, clinicians were often reluctant to discuss randomization, with its accompanying admission about uncertainty, and patients were reluctant to be randomized.

Not all such trials have encountered enrollment problems. These features were present in the above-discussed British Neonatal ECMO Trial, and many suggested that it would need to modify the usual consent to randomization process. It did not modify the consent process, encountered only a 10% refusal rate, and was able to enroll the needed number of subjects in a reasonable period of time. The results of that experience may not be fully generalizable, however, because of the unavailability of ECMO in Great Britain outside of the trial and because that trial utilized parental consent rather than subject consent.

In 1979, Zelen suggested for the breast cancer study an alternative approach called prerandomization. On this approach, potential subjects, without being notified, would be randomized to the group receiving the new intervention or to the control group that received the standard therapy. Consent to participate in the trial would not be obtained from those who were assigned to the control group, because they were getting standard therapy. Those in the new intervention group would, however, be asked to consent to receiving that new intervention, but would not necessarily be told about the prerandomization. Objections were raised to this approach, in part because of the nondisclosure of the randomization to the treatment group and in part because those in the control group would never know that they were in the trial. In addition to these ethical problems, prerandomization made it difficult to do follow-up studies involving the control group. Zelen then suggested as an alternative an approach called the double-consent randomized design. On this approach, subjects would first be randomized to one or the other arm, and would be told this, but they would only be asked to consent to receiving the treatment in the arm to which they had been assigned; they were not asked to consent to the randomization. It was thought that not having to consent to being randomized would make a big difference psychologically. This double-consent randomized design was adopted by the breast cancer trial, improved accrual sixfold, and led to the publication of important results that have significantly modified the management of early breast cancer.[19] Although this second methodology avoids the above-mentioned ethical problems, it does raise the ethical concern that enrolling physicians/researchers, approaching potential subjects knowing the arm to which they have been assigned, will (perhaps only subconsciously) bias the presentation of information to favor the arm to which the subject has already been assigned, thereby making the consent less than fully informed. In addition to this ethical concern, there is a scientific concern that this advance knowledge of the assignment might also result in the assignment being not fully randomized.[20]

The fullest discussion I have found in official policies on these issues is in the British Royal College of Physician's report *Research Involving Patients*.[21] While not absolutely opposing either prerandomization or double-consent randomization, the Royal College confines the former to "exceptional circumstances"; it also discourages the latter for both scientific and ethical reasons, while recognizing that it might be "occasionally acceptable" provided that the patient is told of the other option.

Nevertheless, double-consent randomization continues. In 1990, a study of arthroscopic surgery for osteoarthritis of the knee was published.[22] Because of accrual problems, the study switched from classical randomization to double-consent randomization, and accrual increased sixfold. The report concluded that the improvement was primarily due to the increasing comfort of the enrolling physicians. Although all patients were told about the randomization, the study authors conceded that the consent process deemphasized this fact. It is, of course, this deemphasis that is the basis of the ethical concern.

There is much merit in the position of those who oppose these new techniques, both because of scientific concerns about less than real randomization and about follow-up studies and because of ethical concerns about their impact on honesty and upon informed consent. No doubt, double-consent randomization is less objectionable than complete prerandomization, but the objections to it are still weighty. Is there really no alternative to dealing with the accrual problem? I believe that part of dealing with it is correcting a mistaken attitude toward communication about uncertainty. The clinicians who are unwilling to approach their patients to be randomized feel that the discussion of uncertainty undercuts the patient's trust and the patient-physician relationship. But uncertainty is a reality of less-than-perfect medical knowledge and part of the reason why clinical trials are needed. As an alternative to changing the randomization process and the process of obtaining informed consent, physician-researchers and treating physicians in general might want to consider a more open and frank communication with patients/subjects about the reality of medical uncertainty and about the need for clinical trials.

Issues in Blinding. The advantages of blinding in limiting the potential for various biases have been described above. Although not as crucial as randomization, the blinding of subjects and of treating physicians is certainly important. At the same time, blinding gives rise to ethical concerns, both in the design of the trial and in its implementation, concerns that deserve attention.

The first ethical concern is the limits of the burdens to be imposed on the subjects in order to maintain the blind. As noted above, this issue was already raised by Hill's 1948 study of streptomycin, which was not a blinded study because it was felt that it would be unethical to make the subjects in the placebo control group receive regular sham injections for an extensive period of time so as to prevent them and their doctors from knowing that they were not in the treatment group.

The burden of maintaining the blind varies according to the nature of the trial. In placebo-controlled drug trials, the patients in all the arms must take the same number of pills, which must look, feel, and taste the same. This often requires the manufacturers to cooperate in producing placebo pills to match the active drug pills, but the burden on the subjects is not that great. At the other extreme are trials of new surgical techniques against standard medical management. Maintaining a blind in such cases requires performing sham surgery on all the patients in the medical treatment group, exposing them unnecessarily to the risks of anesthesia and of surgery. Such blinded trials have been run in the past. In the late 1950s, Cobb and Dimond[23] conducted studies that demonstrated that a then popular surgery, internal mammary artery ligation for patients with angina, was inefficacious. In these trials, the chests of all the patients were opened, even those who did not undergo the procedure. Such a trial would never be approved today. But the trials of transplantation of fetal tissue for Parkinson's disease, discussed in Chapter Five, were approved even though the placebo group underwent sham surgery (burrhole penetration of the skull only).[24] Was that appropriate? Similar difficulties are raised by nonsurgical trials requiring more difficult shams than merely ingesting dummy pills (e.g., sham injections).

For some, this issue is resolved by the informed consent process. As long as subjects knowingly consent to being randomized into a trial with a sham arm, the research is acceptable. This is a mistake. As pointed out in Chapter Two, obtaining informed consent is only one of the requirements of contemporary research ethics; ensuring that the risk-benefit ratio is favorable and that risks to the subjects are minimized are others, and some trials with a sham arm clearly violate those standards. Unfortunately, little guidance exists on these issues, and the burden falls on investigators and their independent review boards to make a judgment on these difficult design issues.

As noted above, an alternative in cases in which the burdens of blinding are judged to be ethically unacceptable are measures designed to limit the opportunity for biases to make a difference. Among the measures that can be employed are the adoption of end points that are objectively ascertainable and the development of protocols that clearly define the conditions under which concomitant treatments can be provided. Although not perfect, this alternative becomes more attractive as the burdens on the subjects in the control group due to maintaining the blind become greater.

Another ethical issue arises in the course of the trial when a subject experiences a clinical event of concern. The proper treatment may depend upon knowing which arm the subject is in, so some amount of unblinding may be required. Here, the ethical approach is well understood. The research protocol is supposed to contain plans for dealing with such problems as they arise. The plans must ensure that the subject receives appropriate treatment, and should also minimize the unblinding where possible. Where possible, the information can be conveyed to a physician other than the investigators who can then manage the problem as appropriate without the investigator's being unblinded. If the investigator and the subject must be unblinded, the protocol should then specify what will happen once the subject's problems have resolved. Will the subject be continued in the trial? How will data about that subject be analyzed? In short, careful planning can protect the subject while minimizing the damage to the trial.

The Choice of End Points. There are two rather different issues that need to be discussed under this heading. One, the use of surrogate end points, will be very extensively analyzed in Chapter Eight's discussion of ethical issues in drug approval, so I will just introduce it here. The other, the choice of clinical end points, is an issue whose ethical components have not received much attention, and I would like to briefly begin a discussion of it here.

The surrogate end point issue can be summarized as follows: Traditionally, the end points studied in a clinical trial are those clinical events (e.g., mortality, major morbidities) which it is hoped the new intervention will reduce. Such trials can often take a long time, in part because one may be looking at the rate of occurrence of these events at a later time (e.g., trials of new treatment modalities to see whether they increase five-year survival rates in patients with a certain type of cancer) and in part because the difference may only be establishable by looking at a large number of subjects (if, for example, the base rate of occurrence is not that high to begin with). Such a lengthy trial may be troublesome to those paying for it and/or to those potential users of the intervention eager to know the results. Can one identify an alternative end point (the surrogate end point) whose differential occurrence could be established quickly in a smaller number of patients and whose differential occurrence is adequate to justify the claim that there would be a similar difference in the outcome of the clinical events about which you care? This issue, which has both scientific and ethical components, will be addressed more fully in Chapter Eight, because it is now one of the central value questions in designing trials to secure regulatory approval for the use of new drugs.

The other issue relates to the choice of basic clinical end points. Consider, for example, trials of antihypertensive drugs, where the end point usually studied is reduction in blood pressure. It is only recently that trials have paid attention to such quality of life issues as reduction in sexual functioning, and data are now accumulating on the differential influence of equally efficacious antihypertensive medications on quality of life. Surely, in advising patients and in obtaining their informed consent to taking a particular antihypertensive medication, treating clinicians will need to pay attention to the full side effect profile of interventions, particularly their impact on aspects of the patient's quality of life. If this is true, and if the goal of clinical trials is to provide the scientific information needed to guide informed clinical practice, is there not an obligation on the part of those who design clinical trials to ensure that a fuller set of clinical end points are examined? I believe that the answer to this question is yes, and that increasing attention needs to be paid to these questions.

There is, however, a special issue that arises if one accepts this perspective on clinical trials. How shall the quality of life end points be identified? Patients differ considerably about the importance of the different impacts of interventions on their quality of life, and the impacts they judge to be of greatest importance may not be the same as the impacts that researchers and/or clinicians think are the most important. If researchers are to adopt this mandate to incorporate quality of life end points into clinical trials, they need to develop better techniques for involving the population of future possible users of the intervention being tested in the decision as to which end points should be studied.

Independent Monitoring and Stopping of Clinical Trials. In the course of a clinical trial, it may be necessary, as a result of interim data from the trial or data from other trials, to stop the trial either because one treatment has turned out to be unsafe or because the question of the efficacy of the new treatment has been settled. It has now become customary for large clinical trials to be monitored by an independent monitoring board that examines interim data from the trial and data from other trials to decide whether or not the clinical trial should continue. Unlike the investigators or the sponsors, who may face conflicts of interest in making these decisions, the independent monitoring board can approach these difficult questions with greater objectivity. Moreover, there is less risk from unblinding interim results, which may be necessary to make the decision, if the investigators remain blinded, because they are not involved in making this decision.

This common practice is not formally required by the relevant official policies, with the exception of the Australians, who in general require independent monitoring (Appendix 4.12, Supplementary Note 3). The U.S. regulations (Appendix 3.1, section 46.111) merely require, as a condition for IRB approval of a research protocol, that the protocol makes "adequate provision for monitoring the data collected to ensure the safety of the subjects." Nothing is said about who will do the monitoring, about monitoring for sufficient proof of efficacy, and about monitoring the results of other research. However, the 1993 *Institutional Review Board Guidebook* does suggest that IRBs seriously consider requiring both independent review of safety and of sufficient proof of efficacy.[25] The British Royal College of Physicians[26] recommends that arrangements be made from the outset to monitor results and adds that "In the case of some multicentre studies it will be necessary to set up an independent committee to review progress of the trial and to advise termination." Moreover, a 1992 symposium at the NIH makes it clear that having such an independent monitoring committee has become quite common. In the United States, the practice began at the National Heart Institute in the 1960s, and has spread to some of the other institutes (especially those dealing with cancer, AIDS, and ophthalmology). Since 1991, it has become the standard practice for important cancer trials sponsored by the British Medical Research Council and it is being considered for other trials as well. Increasingly, such independent monitoring is being adopted in Canada and in Europe.[27] An interesting set of issues about independence is raised by the use of such boards in industry-sponsored trials of new drugs, which is also an increasing practice. In short, the increasingly common practice to appoint such monitoring boards is an example of the actual conduct of research being more sensitive to an ethical issue than the formal regulations or guidelines.

One issue that such independent boards regularly consider is whether there is sufficient evidence to establish the efficacy of the new intervention being tested to stop the trial. If there is, it would be unethical to deny that intervention to the members of the control group or to patients not in the trial whose treatment will be modified by their physicians when the data is released, and the trial should be stopped to avoid the intervention's being withheld any further. At the same time, it would be unethical for the trial to be stopped prematurely, when the evidence is insufficient, because this might lead to many future patients receiving an unnecessary intervention. This type of decision involves both statistical and ethical considerations.

The statistical considerations reflect the fact that the more often one looks at interim data, the more likely one is to find by chance data of efficacy that reaches a level of significance. Unless one takes this into account, one will draw false conclusions about the efficacy of the intervention being studied. If, for example, one looks at the data five times in the course of a trial, the probability of finding by chance a result that is significant at the .05 level is 14%, and that is too high (it should be 5%). So when a monitoring board reviews interim data for efficacy, it must adopt a strategy that avoids this problem. One standard strategy is to plan a series of interim reviews, and to plan to stop the trial at an interim review only if the data are sufficiently significant. A number of different interim stopping rules have been developed to define what makes the data sufficiently significant.[28] The crucial idea is that the overall level of significance for the trial should remain .05. Although these different rules impose very stringent requirements on the early stopping of trials, they are requirements that can be met. In early 1994, I participated in a monitoring board meeting that recommended stopping a trial (ACTG 076)[29] to see whether the administration of AZT lowered the incidence of the transmission of HIV from pregnant women to their newborn children. There was a 67.5% relative reduction in the risk of transmission in the 364 infants evaluated, and this result was highly significant (p=0.00006).

It might seem that these statistical considerations are all that are relevant. This, however, is a mistake for a number of reasons. First if there are concerns about safety issues or about whether the benefits that have been established endure over longer periods of time, then it may be appropriate to continue the trial to settle those concerns. The latter concern was not relevant in the HIV vertical transmission trial, because a lack of maternal-fetal transmission by birth meant that there would never be any maternal-fetal transmission. The former concern was, however, relevant, but we were reassured by the lack of observed morbidities and (perhaps even more importantly) by the reflection that stopping transmission of a lethal virus would in any case outweigh most morbidities. In any case, the statistical stopping rules did not settle these broader ethical concerns. Second, there may be cases where one is willing to stop the trial on the basis of substantial evidence of efficacy at an interim look even if that evidence is not quite as impressive as is demanded by the interim stopping rules. This is particularly true when the suggested benefit of the new intervention is very important and the risks of its use are minimal and/or when there is other evidence supporting the claim of efficacy. Obviously, great caution must be exercised in such cases so as to avoid the stopping of the trial leading to the use of an intervention that is really not beneficial, but such cases cannot be ruled out. Third, the stopping rules are totally irrelevant to the issue of whether one should stop a trial on the basis of data of efficacy from other trials, on their own or in combination with interim data from the trial being monitored.

If the stopping rules are only part of the answer, what are the full set of guidelines that monitoring boards should adopt when deciding whether or not to stop a trial because efficacy has been established? I would suggest, as a guideline for thought rather than as a strict rule, the following principle: It is permissible to continue a trial, given the evidence now available both from the interim data and from other trials, only if it would have been ethical to commence the trial given that data. In other words, I would suggest that the same criteria of equipoise be employed here as are employed in the question of starting trials.

These criteria are, of course, equally relevant to the other major task of the data monitoring board, monitoring the trial for safety. Here, it is even harder to plan for systematic interim analyses, given that the safety issues that could emerge may have been totally unexpected. For this additional reason as well as the above reasons, it may be hard to specify much more than the use of judgment based on the criteria of equipoise.

One other observation is in place here. If a decision is made to continue the trial even when there are serious reasons for stopping it, it may be appropriate to provide the information about the new data to the subjects and get their consent to continue in the trial. This was done when the AIDS Clinical Trial Group stopped a series of trials of AZT against placebo in asymptomatic HIV-infected patients because of impressive results. For a variety of reasons (including divergences in the patient populations), the monitoring board of a similar trial being run by the VA decided that it was appropriate to continue their trial, but that the subjects should be given the updated information and given the choice to continue in the trial or to receive unblinded treatment. It is of interest that 74% chose to continue in the trial.[30] Obtaining the subjects' reconsent may be a good strategy for resolving an ethical dilemma when it is uncertain whether or not a trial should continue.

Certain conclusions emerge very clearly:

1. The protocol for a clinical trial should contain a plan for monitoring the trial by some independent board, a board that has the authority to recommend when appropriate that the trial be stopped;
2. In monitoring the trial, that board must consider both interim data from the trial and data from other trials;
3. In deciding whether to stop the trial, the board must consider issues of safety and of efficacy;
4. While it can be guided by certain statistical rules, at the end it must make a judgment about the continued existence of sufficient equipoise;
5. An option in cases where there is no clear conclusion is to continue the trial in those subjects who, given the updated information, consent to continue in the trial.

Conclusion

As noted at the beginning of this chapter, clinical trials raise a significant number of ethical issues beyond those raised by human subjects research in general. We have explored those issues in this chapter and have reached a series of conclusions. Both the initiation and continuation of such trials requires an equipoise that is not easy to define, although some guidelines can be provided. The study population needs to be carefully defined so as to avoid inappropriate exclusions of women or members of various groups. Similarly, the end points need to be defined so as to include quality of life end points of importance to future patients. While concurrent placebo-controlled trials are scientifically superior to other trials, there are occasions where one must be content with data from active controlled trials or historically controlled trials; some guidelines for when such trials are more appropriate can be provided. Randomization is ethically unproblematic, and it is best to deal with accrual problems by being honest about the uncertainty that requires a randomized trial. The benefits of blinding are considerable, but they are sometimes outweighed by the necessary burdens or by the need of treating clinicians for information; careful planning can minimize the problems of not maintaining the blinded nature of the study. Finally, the increased use of independent monitoring boards to address these issues in the course of the trial seems justified.

In reaching these conclusions, we have occasionally been able to draw upon official policies. Several provided useful ideas on the placebo control issue, on independent monitoring, and on the ethical character of Zelen's different proposals. But on many of the most important issues (defining the window for running concurrently controlled trials, limiting the burdens imposed to maintain the blind, choosing the right end points, and deciding when to stop a trial), they were silent. This is one of the few examples we have seen of a failure of official policies to even address central issues of research ethics. Why this failure?

As we review the earlier chapters, we can see that official policies for research ethics emerged either in response to well-publicized questionable cases of research or in response to extensively discussed public concerns about the implications of new technologies. Neither of these factors is present for these issues. Moreover, they have quite technical aspects, and it is easy to mistakenly suppose that they need technical resolutions rather than ethically informed policies. I would suggest that these factors explain the failure of the official policies. This is a failure that should be rectified. The independent scholarship done on these issues has certainly not fully resolved them, and it may well be that a lack of official policies and a resulting lack of adequate evaluation has permitted the running of morally questionable trials.

Chapter eight

RESEARCH AND THE DRUG/DEVICE APPROVAL PROCESS

All medical research is designed to answer scientific and clinical questions, but some is also designed to play a role in securing approval from a regulatory agency to produce and sell a drug or a medical device. Research designed to play that role must meet the ethical standards discussed in Chapters One through Six for all animal and human subjects research. If this research involves a clinical trial, it must also meet the ethical standards discussed in Chapter Seven for all clinical trials. The design and conduct of research relating to securing regulatory approval raises, however, a number of additional ethical issues that will be analyzed in this chapter.

In order to understand those issues, it will first be necessary to present an overview of the history and the resulting structure of the various national policies on drug/device regulation and approval. Although there are important differences between them, there are major similarities that will be the center of attention. Emerging out of the overview will be the identification of a fundamental issue about the standards for approval; the rest of the chapter will be devoted to exploring the implications of that issue for other ethical issues about the design and conduct of research related to obtaining regulatory approval.

One preliminary point. There are official policies covering the introduction of new medicines and new devices, but there are no analogous policies governing the introduction of new procedures. As noted in Chapter Seven, this is one of the reasons why fewer clinical trials are run on new procedures. To some degree, this difference is appropriate. Procedures are not manufactured and sold, in the way that drugs and devices are, so their introduction cannot be easily regulated. But to some degree, this difference is problematic. If drug and device regulatory schemes emerged as necessary to protect the public health, are there not equally good public health reasons for a regulatory scheme for new procedures? This is certainly a question deserving further thought.

The History of Official Policies on Drug/Device Regulation and Approval

The history of the United States drug regulatory policies, the policies that have received the most attention (in part because they cover the largest source of new drugs), can be divided into three periods.[1]

The first period extends from 1906 to 1962 and is really the prehistory of the current policies. In 1906, in response to a growing awareness of the fraudulent claims made for various patent medicines, the U.S. Congress passed a law prohibiting the adulteration or mislabeling of drugs. In 1938, in response to the death of more than 100 children from a liquid form of sulfanilamide, the U.S. Congress required that no drug could be sold without the seller submitting a new drug application (an NDA) to the Food and Drug Administration (the FDA) that demonstrated that the drug was safe for its intended use. This requirement gave rise to the need for clinical research to demonstrate safety.

The second period extends from 1962 to the rise of the AIDS crisis in the mid-1980s. It began with new legislation in 1962, passed in response to the thalidomide tragedy, in which children born to mothers who had received thalidomide, a drug that was being tested, developed phocomelia (short stumps rather than proportionately sized arms or legs). The new legislation mandated that the clinical research to demonstrate safety and effectiveness could not commence until the sponsor submitted an investigational new drug (IND) application to the FDA that justified running the trials in question. Moreover, the new legislation required that drugs be shown by the information provided in the NDA to be effective for their intended use, and not merely safe, before they could be sold. This additional requirement gave rise to the need for further clinical research to demonstrate effectiveness.

The third period extends from the mid-1980s to the present. During this period, in response to those suffering from AIDS and other diseases who demanded quicker access to new drugs that might help them, the FDA changed the process for drugs treating serious or life-threatening illnesses in two major ways: (1) The FDA introduced expanded access programs such as the Treatment IND Program (1987)[2] and the Parallel Track Program[3] (1992). In both of these programs, drugs being tested in clinical trials are also made available for use by others ineligible to participate in the trials. The former program, which applies to a wide variety of life-threatening or serious illnesses, requires more preliminary evidence of safety and of effectiveness than does the latter program, which is confined to drugs for treating AIDS patients. In early 1996, these two programs were supplemented by a program[4] that allowed access to cancer-fighting drugs approved in other countries while research is being conducted to justify U.S. approval under regular or accelerated approval programs. (2) The FDA introduced accelerated approval programs (Subpart E and Subpart H Programs). In both of these programs (the first dating from 1988 and the second from 1992), which differ in technical details but which apply to a wide variety of life-threatening or serious illnesses, final approval for general use of the drug is given on the basis of less evidence than is generally required (Appendix 3.5). At the same time, the FDA may require additional postapproval surveillance to protect against errors resulting from the drugs being approved too quickly.

As a result of these changes, there has emerged in the United States a complex set of policies for research designed to secure approval for the sale of a drug. The first step is that the sponsor must submit an IND notice to the FDA before testing in humans can begin. The IND must contain information about the composition of the drug, about preclinical testing (including animal studies) of its safety, about the protocol for the proposed tests (including the provisions for obtaining informed consent), and about the qualifications of the investigators. If the FDA does not object, clinical trials on human subjects can commence. These trials are often divided into three phases. Phase I trials test for toxicities and safe dosage ranges. Phase II trials test for effectiveness in a limited number of patients. Phase III trials test for both safety and effectiveness in a randomized controlled trial involving a much larger number of subjects, using the dosage for which approval will be sought. If the results are satisfactory, the sponsor submits an NDA to the FDA, which must contain information about the results, about the proposed way for producing the drug, and about its proposed labeling. The FDA normally submits the application to an advisory committee, but the final decision belongs to the staff.

The FDA has done a great deal (Appendix 3.4) to articulate the stringent standards on the evidence that the staff should use in making its decisions. The primary evidence must be from randomized controlled clinical trials, involving well-defined inclusion and exclusion criteria and maximal blinding, and analyzed according to strict statistical criteria. It has also made it clear that the evidence must show that there is a proper risk-benefit ratio in the use of the new drug, but it has said less about what is the appropriate ratio. Some of these standards have been relaxed in the expanded access and accelerated approval programs.

As might be suggested by this description, the FDA approval process (from the submission of an IND until final approval) can be a very lengthy process; the changes generated by the AIDS crisis, but applied in other areas as well, were an attempt to shorten that process so that the benefits of new drugs would be available sooner to those who desperately needed them.

The regulation of devices was not seriously undertaken until the mid-1970s. Until then, the FDA had sometimes treated them as drugs. Thus, it ruled that the Copper-7 IUD was a drug because its contraceptive action was a result of the chemical action of the copper filament, and that the manufacturer would have to go through the entire drug approval process before it could be marketed. In 1976, the U.S. Congress introduced a device regulatory policy.[5] This was done in response to problems with the Dalkon Shield contraceptive device, with some pacemakers, and with some intraocular lenses.

Under this new policy, the FDA classifies devices as Class I devices (requiring neither meeting standards nor premarket approval), as Class II devices (requiring meeting certain standards), or as Class III devices (requiring premarket approval). Since 1976, new devices can be introduced if they are classified as being in Class I or Class II, if they are equivalent to a pre-1976 device, or on the basis of a premarket approval application. In fact, most devices have been approved under the first two mechanisms.

In 1992, wrestling with issues raised by silicone breast implants (which were mostly pre-1976 devices), the FDA constituted a committee (the Temple Committee) that recommended that device premarketing approvals should be based on the same standards as drug approvals and that the studies to prove equivalences with pre-1976 devices must show comparability of function and performance and must also be subject to these standards.[6] This suggests that the FDA will increasingly be requiring the same sorts of trials for devices that it requires for drugs.

We turn from this history of the U.S. experience to the experience of other countries, particularly those with large pharmaceutical and device industries, starting with Great Britain. Until 1963, the British had no policies governing the introduction of new drugs. This changed in response to the thalidomide disaster. From 1964 to 1971, the major pharmaceutical companies voluntarily agreed not to test or market new drugs without the prior approval of a Committee on the Safety of Drugs. Since 1971, this voluntary scheme has been replaced by a mandatory scheme.[7]

How does the system work? Physicians or companies can run trials of new drugs by submitting an application (a clinical trial exemption) signed by the physician (or, in the case of companies, by a medical adviser) certifying that he believes that the proposed trial is reasonable. At the end of the trials, applications for approval are submitted to the Medicines Control Agency, whose staff oversees three assessments, pharmaceutical (primarily related to the quality of production), preclinical (primarily related to safety), and clinical (primarily related to efficacy). If these assessments are satisfactory, a license is issued by the Licensing Authority. In contrast to the FDA approach, the British system is far more informal (in not specifying detailed standards for the evidence, relying on the expert assessment), places more emphasis in the initial approval on the demonstration of safety than on the demonstration of efficacy, and relies more upon postapproval monitoring to catch mistakes.

Both the U.S. and the British policies are designed to allow drugs to be sold only after their safety and efficacy have been established. But while the goals are the same, the U.S. policies are often seen as far more demanding. A whole literature, the "drug lag" literature,[8] demonstrated that at least until recently these more demanding standards resulted in drugs becoming available in the United Kingdom and elsewhere before they were available in the United States. There was a great controversy about whether this meant that citizens of the United States were being offered better protection against unsafe or inefficacious drugs or whether this meant that they were being unnecessarily denied for a period of time access to valuable drugs, with the critics insisting that as late as 1991–92, U.S. citizens were suffering from the delay. In 1996, the debate was transformed by FDA[9] data that suggested that there was no longer any difference in approval time between the United States and the United Kingdom and that approval in the United States now often preceded approval in the United Kingdom. This conclusion has been attacked by critics of the FDA.[10] We shall return to all of these issues below.

Great Britain is, of course, part of the European Union, and there are other countries (e.g., Germany) in that community that are very important in pharmaceutical research and development. Moreover, that group of countries is a major market for all new drugs. Consequently, attention needs to be paid to other European policies on securing approval to market new drugs.

Since the mid-1960s, most European countries have required that safety and efficacy be demonstrated before new drugs can be approved for sale. Nevertheless, there have been important differences between the countries. None have the detailed standards of the FDA, preferring to rely, as the United Kingdom does, on the specification that there be an assessment by experts. Some place greater emphasis on assessments within the regulatory agency whereas others place greater emphasis on assessments by outside experts. Some place more emphasis on large-scale controlled clinical trials; others place more emphasis on case series and/or on pharmacological analyses. Some place primary emphasis on the demonstration of safety whereas others insist on more evidence of efficacy as well. All of this means that the studies required for approval in the different countries may differ considerably.

The countries that are part of the European Union are moving toward greater economic integration; there are therefore increasing pressures to produce a standardized European approach, through a combination of having approvals issued by a single community-wide authority and of mandating that all members must recognize the approval given by any single member's regulatory agency.

One final observation. As the pharmaceutical industry increasingly becomes a multinational industry, with multinational companies developing and testing drugs for sale throughout the world, and as the research community increasingly becomes a multinational community with the same standards for scientific validity of evidence, there is increasing pressure for the international harmonization of policies for the approval of new drugs. The International Conference on Harmonization now involves the European Union, Japan, and the United States; we have referred to its 1996 Guidelines for Good Clinical Practice (Appendix 1.5) at many points in earlier chapters. As more harmonized policies are developed, the research community will find it easier to conduct studies that are both scientifically valid and meet the policies of all the regulatory agencies. Given that many studies are run for those regulatory purposes, international harmonization will certainly benefit the research community.

In short, then, clinical research to meet regulatory needs for new drug or device approval usually begins with notification of, or securing approval from, the national regulatory agencies in the countries in which the trials are to be run. These studies may be randomized controlled trials progressing through the traditional three phases, or they may be less formal studies. In any case, they are designed to provide sufficient evidence of safety and (at least to some degree) of efficacy to meet the drug approval policies of the relevant drug regulatory agencies.

Many value questions are raised by such research. One is our fundamental policy issue: What should be the standards required to secure approval of the sale of new drugs and devices? This question will be discussed in the next section. Others relate more directly to the conduct of the studies: Are there special problems with some of the traditional required studies, such as phase I studies? What are the respective responsibilities of those who secure the approval to run the studies (the sponsor) and those who actually run the studies (the investigator) to ensure safety? What subjects should be studied? What end points should be chosen? The remainder of this chapter will deal with these issues, relating them where appropriate to our fundamental issue.

The Fundamental Policy Issue: Setting Standards for Approval

There really are two fundamental questions about standards that any policy must address:

1. How should the goals of effectiveness and safety be balanced in the drug/device approval process?
2. How should the demands of adequate evidence and of speedy approval be balanced in the drug/device approval process?

As these two questions are different even though interrelated, we need to look at each of them separately.

The first question, which we shall refer to as the content question, relates to the content of what must be established before a drug/device is approved for marketing. We want drugs/devices that are effective. We want drugs/devices that are safe. In many cases, however, the more effective drugs/devices carry with them more substantial risks. In deciding whether to approve the drug/device for use for a given indication, these risks must be balanced against the benefits, taking into account the seriousness of the medical problem being treated. The content question asks what is the appropriate balance between risks and benefits, the appropriate risk-benefit ratio, in order for a drug/device to be approved.

The second question, which we shall refer to as the epistemic question, relates to the evidence for that appropriate risk-benefit ratio that must be provided before a drug/device is approved for marketing. We want firm evidence of a favorable ratio before approval so that users are not harmed by a drug/device that turns out with more evidence to be more dangerous than beneficial. We want good drugs/devices to be approved as soon as possible so that we can get the benefits of using them as soon as possible. In many cases, getting sufficiently firm evidence requires waiting for more studies to be conducted, thereby delaying obtaining the benefits. In the extreme case of those with serious life-threatening illnesses, that delay may be fatal. So we must balance the desire for firm evidence with the desire for speedy approval. The epistemic question asks what is the appropriate balance between these two desires in the approval process.

We have discussed above criticisms of the FDA for extensive delays in the approval process in comparison with other countries. It has been claimed that the FDA was insensitive to the need to balance these various goals. A whole literature, the "drug lag" literature, emerged that attempted to quantify both the extent of this problem and the extent of the resulting losses suffered by American patients because of the unavailability of good drugs. Defenders of the FDA insisted, of course, that the other countries were too lax in the balances they drew, and that patients in those countries paid the price of using unsafe drugs approved too quickly. A critical assessment of the claims made by both sides in this often very heated debate lies beyond the scope of this book, but its existence is firm evidence for the importance of our two questions.

One of the results of this controversy has been the emergence in the United States of a whole new set of regulations allowing for accelerated approval, with less evidence, of drugs with serious side effects for use in patients with life-threatening or other serious illnesses, particularly those illnesses that lack alternative treatments (Appendix 3.5). With a greater sensitivity to the trade-off issues as a result of the drug lag discussions and as a result of the strong demands of desperate AIDS patients for quicker access to promising drugs, these new programs also allowed for expanded access during the trials. These new programs, and other procedural changes adopted by the FDA, have led to improvements that have been summarized by the above-discussed controversial claim that the drug lag has disappeared. The emergence of these programs is further evidence for the importance of our two questions.

In the rest of this section, I want to raise a problem about striking the proper balances, a problem that relates our policy issue to difficult philosophical questions about our understanding of the relation between citizens and the social order under which they live.[11]

Perhaps the best way to understand this problem is to consider the following argument illustrated by an example (the use of silicone gel breast implants)[12] that provoked a heated debate.

Developing an answer to the content and to the epistemic questions calls for a balancing of certain goals, and different people will, in light of their different values, balance those goals differently. Consider, for example, the debate about the use of silicone gel breast implants for cosmetic purposes. When questions about safety arose, approval for their use (except for postmastectomy patients) was withdrawn in the United States. What evidence of what degree of safety should be required for reapproval? The level of acceptable risks would obviously be higher for those who wanted access to these implants because they are very concerned with a certain conception of body image than for those who find that conception and the ensuing breast augmentation procedure pointless, if not offensive. The same observation could be made about the degree of evidence required.

Any drug/device regulatory policy will involve some society-wide balancing of these goals, a balancing that will be appropriate in the light of the values of some citizens but inappropriate in the light of the values of others. Any drug/device regulatory policy involves an answer to both the content and the epistemic question, an answer that presupposes a certain balancing of various values. The adoption of any policy means the adoption of a certain balance, one that will be seen as inappropriate by those who have different values that call for a different balancing. If, to return to our example, our policy demands very firm evidence of a very low level of risk before breast implants are reapproved, those who want access to silicone implants will find those standards inappropriate, whereas those who place little value on breast size or shape may find these standards very appropriate.

Any drug regulatory policy will therefore violate the liberal mandate that society not adopt policies that favor the values of some citizens over the values of others. This principle of value neutrality is seen by many as one of the fundamental moral commitments of a modern liberal society. The major exception to that commitment, that we may favor certain values in order to protect nonconsenting third parties from being harmed, is irrelevant here, because the use of drugs/devices such as silicone implants imposes risks of harm on the user, rather than on third parties. So, concludes the argument, there is no way to have a drug/device approval policy in a tolerant liberal society.

These type of reflections have led some commentators to conclude that we should do without drug/device regulatory policies.[13] On their approach, researchers should do research on the safety and efficacy of drugs and should make that information available to clinicians and their patients, who should be free, without any governmental approval, to use whatever drugs/devices they think are appropriate in the light of their values. Although such a conclusion is rejected by most, no clear understanding has emerged about how societal drug/device regulatory policies should deal with the implications of the existence of a diversity of values among those who might use the drug/device in question. Resolving this question, and tracing the implications of the resolution for the type of research that should be done before approval, remains a fundamental policy issue for those who want ethically sensitive regulatory policies.

Four Issues about the Conduct of Research

The Conduct of Phase I Trials. Traditionally, the first step in the clinical testing of new drugs is the conducting of phase I trials. These trials may be conducted in healthy volunteers or they may be conducted in patients with the disease that the drug may eventually be used to treat. In the latter case, these trials are sometimes called phase I/II trials. The primary goal of a phase I trial, in either case, is to identify the maximum tolerated dose of a new drug. The traditional approach is to administer the drug at a very low dose to an initial cohort of subjects and then to give ever-increasing doses to later subjects. Eventually, a dose is reached at which the level of toxicities is sufficiently severe so that it is treated as the maximum tolerated dose. The previous dose level becomes the recommended dose, which is tested for efficacy in a subsequent phase II trial. Given both the goal and the design of such trials, it is not surprising that the therapeutic response rate in phase I trials involving patients is very low.

A recent report[14] from the M. D. Anderson Hospital, one of the country's leading oncology centers, gives a good picture both of how these trials are run and about their results. The report surveyed all 23 published phase I trials conducted at that institution in the period 1991–93. For the trials of drugs not previously tested in humans, a median of ten dose levels were required before the maximum tolerated dose was reached, and the median resulting recommended dose was 40 times the initial dose given. For the trials of drugs or biologic agents previously tested in humans, a median of five to six dose levels was required, and the median resulting recommended dose was less than three times the initial dose given, except for the trials of some of the biologic agents. Of the 610 patients enrolled, 19% got more than 110% of the recommended dose; at the other extreme, 29% got less than 70% of the recommended dose. There was some response in 19 patients (3%), with 4 being complete responses and 15 being only partial responses. This is at the lower end of what is usually reported. In reviews of both adult and pediatric phase I oncology trials from the early 1990s, the response rate was 4% to 6%, with more than half coming only at the end of the phase I trials, where the doses are higher.[15]

Three related ethical issues have been raised. The first has to do with informed consent for phase I trials. Are the patients/subjects adequately informed about the realities of these trials? Even if they are, do they agree based on an under-standing of the information, or is their agreement based on a failure of under-standing, perhaps related to their vulnerability, that undercuts the validity of the consent? The second has to do with the risk/benefit ratio for these trials. Given the substantial toxicities experienced by the subjects, especially those that are close to the end of the trial, and given the low response rate, even near the end of the trial, is there an acceptable risk/benefit ratio? Or is that ratio unacceptable and reflective of the exploitation of these vulnerable subjects? The third has to do with the legitimacy of phase I trials in the pediatric population. As discussed in Chapter Six, there are special protections governing pediatric research both in terms of consent of the parents/assent of the children and in terms of limi-tations on risks undergone, especially for nontherapeutic research. Do these spe-cial protections pose special problems for pediatric phase I trials? Let us turn then to an examination of each of these issues.

Two recent studies support the concerns about the informed consent process. One studied 30 patients/subjects in phase I trials to see why they participated.[16] The predominant reasons were the possibility of benefit (100%), lack of a better option (89%), and trust in the oncologist (70%). Only 33% talked about helping future patients, the benefit that is most likely to occur. It is certainly possible to interpret these data as at least suggesting that these desperate and therefore vulnerable subjects were exploited by the oncologists they trusted to participate in a trial in the hopes of securing a benefit that they were very unlikely to attain. This troubling possibility is not the only interpretation of the data; an alternative interpretation is that the patients/subjects clearly understood the situation and knowingly and freely chose to participate with the hope that they might be one of the lucky few who responded. The troubling interpretation is, however, sup-ported by the facts that only one third clearly understood the purpose of phase I trials and that only 30% acknowledged that the no-treatment-except-for-palliation option had been discussed as an alternative to participation in the phase I trial (although it was mentioned in the consent forms they signed). A 1996 U.S. report from the Advisory Committee on Human Radiation Experi-ments also highlighted these issues. As part of its work, it conducted a Research Proposal Review Project and concluded on the basis of it that[17]:

> . . . we reviewed consent forms that appeared to overpromise what research could likely offer the ill patient and underplay the effect of the research on the patient's

quality of life . . . Not surprisingly, this problem was the most acute in the RPRP among phase I trials that, while not being non-therapeutic in the strict sense, appeared to offer only a remote possibility of benefit to the patient-subject . . . desperate hopes are easily manipulated.

These concerns about informed consent are obviously very serious. But they may be manageable if we can find better consent processes for phase I trials. Among the suggestions that can be offered,[18] even without the modifications in the trial designs we will be discussing below, are the following:

1. Patients need to be told very explicitly that the likelihood of any response is very low and that the few responses are not particularly significant.
2. Patients need to be told very explicitly that the purpose of the trial is to learn about toxicities so that better trials can be run for future patients that might help them.
3. Patients need to be told very explicitly that the trial is designed to keep on escalating the doses until significant toxicities are reached so that they are at risk of suffering those toxicities.
4. Patients need to be explicitly told which cohort they are in and what is the significance of that fact both for the slim likelihood of benefit and the much larger risk of suffering toxicities.
5. Patients need to be told very clearly about good palliative care as a legitimate alternative.
6. Finally, patients need to be encouraged to think about the relative importance to them at this point near the end of their life of altruistic motives, even if that is not their major reason for enrolling.

If all of this information could be conveyed so that it was understood, then the ethical concerns about informed consent would be alleviated. It remains to be seen what would be the enrollment rate in phase I trials for which such consent was obtained.

I turn to the more difficult issues about the acceptability of the risk-benefit ratio. As pointed out in Chapter Two, even if subjects consent to participation in a research protocol, that protocol is illegitimate and against all the international standards for research ethics if the risk-benefit ratio is sufficiently unfavorable. Even when informed consent is necessary for legitimate research, it is not sufficient. Are the risk-benefit ratios in phase I trials acceptable?

The traditional design of phase I trials is quite conservative, emphasizing the protection of the research subjects from excessive toxicities. For example, the starting dose is chosen, based on animal toxicology data, to be at a level considered to be minimally toxic. As a result of that policy and similarly conservative policies governing the escalation of dosages, many subjects receive dosages that are way below the dosage ultimately recommended for study in the succeeding phase II trial. Although these dosages are safer, they are also more likely to be nontherapeutic. On this traditional approach, an acceptable risk-benefit ratio is achieved for many subjects by protecting them from toxicities, but at the cost of lowering an already low likelihood of receiving a therapeutic benefit. Given what we know about why these subjects are enrolling in the phase I trial, is that way of obtaining a favorable risk-benefit ratio appropriate? Is this approach downplaying the desired access to dosages that are more likely to be therapeutic?

Several alternative approaches to the design of phase I trials have recently been advocated. Of particular interest is the continual reassessment method (CRM).[19] The basic ideas behind that method are to treat the subjects from the very beginning at the dosage anticipated to be recommended for study in the phase II trial and to adjust that anticipation as toxicity data becomes available in the trial. This approach offers the hope of more responses, but at the price of more experienced toxicities. The resulting risk-benefit ratio is acceptable, if it is acceptable, because of the greater chance of benefit, the very chance that motivates enrollment. Access to potential benefit is emphasized more than protection from toxicities.

A recent simulation study[20] has shed much light on these issues, but it has also raised another issue. The goal of running a phase I trial is to produce the data necessary to choose a dosage to be studied for efficacy in later phase II and phase III trials. From the perspective of access for many more subjects to promising therapies, it is important to complete the phase I trial as quickly as possible. The simulations show, however, that the CRM design increases the number of cohorts studied, thereby lengthening the time required to complete the phase I trial. This relates to the fact that the dosage is modified as the data comes in for each subject, making each subject a separate cohort from which one needs data before changing the dosage for the next subject/cohort. An obvious suggestion would be to modify the design so that more than one subject was in each cohort, but that would result in more subjects being exposed to higher chances of toxicities. So there is a real design problem here, one with significant ethical components.

There is obviously a balancing to be done here. We want to protect these vulnerable subjects from excessive toxicities. At the same time, we want to give them a better chance of access to dosages that are more likely to be effective. We also want to complete the phase I trial as soon as possible so that trials of efficacy can begin. All of these values are involved in our fundamental policy issue. How to best balance these three goals in a proper trial design is unclear. However, given what motivates these subjects to enroll, it seems best to get a more favorable risk-benefit ratio in phase I trials by increasing the likelihood of their obtaining a benefit through use of some version of the CRM.

Our two concerns about informed consent and about appropriate risk-benefit ratios have additional implications when considering the ethics of phase I trials involving pediatric patients. In order to understand why, it is necessary to remember two special ethical requirements, discussed in Chapter Six, that are universally imposed upon pediatric research. The first is that the assent of the pediatric subject, as well as the consent of the subject's parents, must be obtained if the subject is old enough. The second is that the risks must be particularly minimal, or the risk-benefit ratio particularly favorable, when research is conducted on pediatric subjects.

For many, the hardest problem in meeting the requirement of obtaining the informed assent of the pediatric subject in a phase I trial will be the presupposed honesty about the subject's prognosis. I have elsewhere discussed the merits of being honest about this point.[21] For me, the harder problem is how to convey the requisite information, listed above as points (1) through (6), to older pediatric subjects in an age-appropriate fashion. Given that it is not easy to convey this information to the parents, conveying it to the subjects will be a special challenge.

There is one additional point to be noted about pediatric assent to phase I trials. The U.S. regulations (Appendix 3.1, section 46.408) allow that the requirement of assent can be waived by the IRB when "the intervention or procedure involved in the research holds out a prospect of direct benefit . . ." This clause has often been invoked to allow pediatric subjects/patients with cancer to be enrolled with parental consent in research trials against the wishes of the subjects. Its use is very problematic in phase I trials when the prospect of direct benefit is so modest. Actual assent will have to be obtained.

This last point leads us directly to the question of risks and benefits in phase I pediatric trials. The regulations discussed in Chapter Six differentiate two types of research, therapeutic research (research that offers direct benefit to the individual subjects) and nontherapeutic research (research that only yields general knowledge about the subject's disease). The former is allowed when the risks are justified by the benefits *to the subjects* and the risk-benefit ratio is as favorable as that of any alternative; the latter is allowed in the United States (Appendix 3.1, section 46.406) when the risks are only "a minor increase over minimal risk" and elsewhere (Appendix 2.3, Article 17.2; Appendix 4.2, Section 6.3.2; and Appendix 4.8, Article 209-6) when they only constitute a minimal risk. Will phase I trials be able to meet these standards?

This problem is illustrated by a major controversy in research ethics that developed in New Zealand in the spring of 1996.[22] A researcher at the Auckland School of Medicine enrolled two children with Canavan's disease in a phase I trial of gene therapy. He had the approval of the local research ethics committee, obtained after submitting primate data, but not of a national advisory committee created by the New Zealand Health Research Council. Critics claimed, appealing to the international standards for pediatric research, that such risky protocols should not be approved in cases of what seems to be phase I nontherapeutic research. Even if that claim is correct, they need to explain what research on treating such terrible diseases should take place between animal research and clearly therapeutic research on children. Answering that question is the crucial issue surrounding phase I clinical trials in the pediatric population.

The threshold question is, of course, whether phase I trials should be classified as therapeutic or nontherapeutic research. To my mind, as traditionally designed, they must be treated as nontherapeutic research. It is not just that the response rate is so low and that the clinical significance of the few responses is so modest. The crucial point is that the traditional design makes no attempt to maximize the possibility of therapeutic response. This design, even more than the results, is clear testimony that what is being conducted is nontherapeutic research, with any therapeutic benefits being welcome side effects. As nontherapeutic research, many traditionally designed phase I trials cannot meet the requirements for pediatric research. They involve a significant risk of serious toxicities, and this is more than a minimal risk or even more than a minor increase over a minimal risk. The situation is quite different when using new designs such as the continual reassessment method. Then, the chance of a therapeutic response is presumably greater. More crucially, the design attempts to maximize that possibility. With such a design, it is possible to argue that the research is therapeutic research justified by the potential benefits to the pediatric patient/subject. So we have in the pediatric population, even more than in the adult population, reason to seek alternatives to the traditional design of phase I trials.

Not all commentators would agree with this analysis of traditionally designed phase I trials. Ackerman, for one, has argued that they should be treated as therapeutic research.[23] He points out that therapeutic benefits are not excluded and, even if modest, may only be available in such trials. Moreover, there may be other side benefits of participation including reduction of symptoms, enhanced attention in the hospital, and maintenance of hope. I am unpersuaded. Mere possibility of benefits do not count as much as the actualities of minimal benefits and of designs not structured to maximize benefits. Moreover, some of his benefits may be spurious; it is arguable, for example, that his "maintenance of hope" is actually a harmful avoidance of helping the child deal with his or her impending demise.[24]

In conclusion, we need to redesign phase I trials so as to better balance protecting subjects with assuring access to promising therapies, both for those in the phase I trials and for those who will be enrolled in the succeeding phase II and phase III trials. How to better balance these values in general is our fundamental policy issue, but in the case of phase I trials, we should be guided by the motives of the subjects. Newly proposed designs may be more successful in achieving this needed balance. Developing better versions of these designs, and shaping an informed consent process that conveys what is involved in phase I trials with these new designs, is a major challenge for research ethics.

Monitoring for Safety. Clinical trials of new drugs/devices being tested for approval purposes always have the potential for unexpected adverse events, and the informed consent forms must always mention that possibility. Moreover, provisions must be made for notifying subjects when such unexpected adverse events emerge so that they have the opportunity to decide whether or not to continue in the trial. But in addition to these consent issues, what can be done to minimize the risk? What is the responsibility of the investigator who conducts the trial, of the sponsor who has secured the permission to run the trial and is funding it, and of the national regulatory agency?

An incident in 1993 heightened awareness of the importance of this issue. A study was being conducted of the use of fialuridine (FIAU) in patients with chronic hepatitis B virus infection. It resulted in five deaths before the problem was identified and the study stopped. Some (the FDA)[25] concluded that the investigators had failed to recognize and properly analyze the problem; others[26] concluded that the result, although unfortunate, was due to a previously unrecognized late drug toxicity that was hard to identify and that the investigators had not failed in their responsibility to monitor for problems.

In 1992–93, the World Health Organization,[27] building on many earlier national policies, developed a set of guidelines on good clinical practice for trials on pharmaceutical products. These guidelines make a number of major points about this issue:

1. The original research protocol must contain a plan for handling adverse events. This plan must cover both the management of patients experiencing unacceptable toxicities (e.g., dosage reduction or withdrawal of therapy) and the investigation of those episodes.
2. The investigator should report the episode and the results of the investigation to the sponsor, and that sponsor, following the relevant national regulations, should report serious episodes to the national regulatory agency.
3. Independent monitoring committees can make an important contribution to this process.

These general guidelines seem perfectly appropriate as far as they go, but the FIAU controversy raises the question of whether further guidance is needed on the design of such safety monitoring in clinical trials if investigators, sponsors, and agencies are to fulfill their ethical responsibilities to research subjects.

One approach is found in regulations proposed by the FDA[28] in late 1994 in response to the FIAU episode. The most important components relate to better planning for safety monitoring. The most crucial points are the following:

1. The protocol should spell out exactly what events should be treated by the investigator as adverse events to be reported to the sponsor. These would normally include any deaths, any life-threatening or serious (e.g., resulting in serious incapacity or hospitalization) events, and any laboratory values that exceed specified limits or are markedly abnormal. Most crucially, these events must be reported even if they might be attributable to the patient's underlying disease or to medications that the patient is taking concomitantly.
2. To help the sponsor differentiate between toxicities due to the drug being tested and those due to other causes, the sponsor should consider use of a formal control group (placebo, active, or historical) even in safety studies and/or should estimate in advance the adverse event rate due to the underlying disease or to concomitant medications and presume that excess events are due to the drug being tested.
3. The sponsor must provide more immediate and more regularly scheduled reports to the FDA in response to these adverse events.

Much of the research community[29] has been very critical of these proposed regulations, seeing them as an overreaction to the FIAU episode. They see these proposals as adding to the burden on investigators without improving subject safety. They feel that at most there should be a careful review of monitoring plans to see whether or not they are appropriate in the light of expected toxicities. The validity of this reaction remains an important open question in research ethics.

It is important to note that none of this material specifies the criteria for stopping new drug/device trials in the light of these reports of adverse events. Even if more serious adverse events are better analyzed and reported sooner, the preliminary data on efficacy may make it advisable to continue to run the trial as the resulting risk-benefit ratio may still be favorable. This point has been missed by many of the critics of the FDA's proposed regulations, who believe that more reporting of adverse events would necessarily lead to inappropriate early stoppings of clinical trials. It is not surprising that the safety-based stopping criteria are not specified. Until our fundamental policy issue about standards is resolved, including the content question about trade-offs between safety and effectiveness, we will have no basis for developing clear criteria for stopping clinical trials because of safety concerns. This is a good example of how issues about the conduct of research cannot be resolved without a resolution of our fundamental policy issue about the standards for drug/device approval.

Choosing Research Subjects. It is often the case that a new drug or device is studied in one patient population, approved for use in that population, and then used by physicians in other patient populations without its use being adequately tested in those other populations. National policies usually give clinicians that freedom, although physicians do face malpractice risks if they exercise it.

This pattern raises a serious problem for children, the elderly, women, and members of minority groups. The concern is that they are not included in the research leading up to approval and that they therefore undergo greater risks when using new drugs/devices that have not been tested for them. We will now consider this issue in connection with children and with the elderly. In Chapter Nine, we will return to this issue as it applies to women and members of various minority groups.

We begin with the case of children. Since 1979, the Food and Drug Administration in the United States has required that approval of drugs for the pediatric population be based on adequate studies in the pediatric population. A 1990 survey by the American Academy of Pediatrics revealed that 80% of the new molecular entities approved by the FDA between 1984 and 1989 were not approved for pediatric use, not because they were necessarily inappropriate for that use but because there were no studies that established appropriateness. A more recent study reveals that the situation in the United States did not improve markedly in the period 1990–95.[30] In large measure this is due to the common standard that trials of new drugs or devices should first be conducted in adults. The major exception is when the disease in question is peculiar to pediatric patients. This standard gives rise to two problems: (1) once a drug or device is approved for the adult population and can then be used by pediatricians if they wish to do so, there is often insufficient economic motivation for the sponsor to run the additional trials in the pediatric population; (2) because these trials would have to be adequately controlled (often, placebo-controlled), clinicians may be unwilling to have their patients randomized to not receiving a treatment that has worked well in the adult population, so accruing subjects to such trials may be difficult.

All of this means that pediatricians must make clinical decisions without appropriate guidance from research, often imposing unnecessary risks on pediatric patients. Children are in this way therapeutic orphans. This is clearly unacceptable. Two approaches to solving this problem have been suggested. The first, the extrapolation approach, involves developing new standards for approving pediatric use on the basis of data from studies in adults. The second, the starting with children approach, involves a shift of attitudes on the ethics of pediatric research. Let us examine both of these approaches.

In late 1994, the FDA adopted the extrapolation approach to approving drugs for pediatric use.[31] According to its new rule, drugs could be approved for such use based upon studies showing an appropriate risk-benefit ratio in the adult population providing that (1) there is evidence that the course of the disease and the effects of the drug, both positive and negative, are the same in the pediatric and the adult populations so that one can reasonably extrapolate from one population to the other and (2) the sponsor provides at least dose-finding and pharmokinetic data about the drug in the pediatric population so that one can determine appropriate dosages.

If one thinks about this proposal from the perspective of the value trade-off raised by our epistemic question, this proposal has some plausibility. Although the level of evidence of an appropriate risk-benefit ratio for children would be higher if it were based on trials in that population, one might have to wait a long time for those trials to be run, and that cost might be too great. It seems a better trade-off to accept the more readily available data from the adult trials providing that conditions (1) and (2) are satisfied. The implication for research, of course, is that studies to help the sponsor satisfy conditions (1) and (2) would need to be conducted.

Although this extrapolation approach seems plausible, some caution about it is also in place. In 1993, the Canadian National Council on Bioethics in Human Research,[32] in a report on research involving children, documented some of the dangers of this extrapolation approach. A typical example was the early use of chloramphenicol for neonatal sepsis at a dosage extrapolated from older children and adults that turned out to be too high (producing cardiovascular collapse) because the system responsible for detoxification is less active in the immediate neonatal period. The requirement to provide dose-finding and pharmacokinetic data is meant, of course, to alleviate such concerns, but we must understand that adopting the extrapolation approach means taking greater risks to get quicker benefits. Whether these concerns are sufficient to rule out the extrapolation approach depends upon what trade-offs we make as a society. The existence of these trade-offs and the need to choose standards for approval in light of them is, of course, the whole point raised by our fundamental policy issue. Until that policy question is resolved, it is hard to come to a definitive conclusion about the FDA extrapolation policy. But there is an alternative that is surely worth considering.

The alternative to the extrapolation approach, the starting with children approach, avoids these problems by calling for a rethinking of the attitudes toward pediatric research. We noted at the end of the section on pediatric research in Chapter Six that at least some of the failure to do research in pediatric subjects was due to an excessive desire to protect such subjects from the risks of research and that children may be paying a high price for being overprotected. The starting with children approach says that the time has come to rethink this classical protectionist view and to include children as well as adults in initial trials designed to obtain approval.

There is evidence of a shifting attitude toward the starting-with-children approach to this issue. The 1993 CIOMS guidelines[33] assert that "The participation of children is indispensable for research into diseases of childhood [the old exception to adult priority] and conditions to which children are particularly susceptible [the broadening clause]." It is very important that this second class of diseases is included in these CIOMS guidelines because the failure to do research on children with these diseases is a central component of the problem we have been discussing. Similarly, the 1997 proposed Canadian Code says[34] that "Children should not be excluded from participating in research which is potentially directly beneficial to them as individual participants and, with appropriate safeguards, indirectly beneficial to them as a group." The FDA has implemented a pediatric studies page in NDAs and a committee has been formed to facilitate pediatric testing in the approval process. This led, in the summer of 1997, to proposed regulation which would lead the FDA closer to a starting-with-children approach.[35] Finally, legislation was introduced in the United States in 1997[36] that would extend the period of patent protection for those drugs tested in children before they were introduced into the market.

It may be that an even stronger starting-with-children stance would be appropriate, so that it be mandated that children as well as adults should be included in trials of new drugs and devices, as long as the disease process to be treated is one that is found in a substantial number of children, even if children are not particularly susceptible. As noted in Chapter Six, the NIH is moving in that direction. This would involve a different answer to our policy issue about standards, one that involves refusing to accept a lesser degree of evidence of an appropriate risk-benefit ratio for pediatric use and one that involves insisting on the appropriate involvement of children in the crucial clinical trials.

Support for this approach can be obtained by contrasting these developments in connection with the pediatric population with analogous developments in connection with the geriatric population. There had been similar concerns that elderly subjects were excluded from research. In response to those concerns, the starting-with-the-elderly approach has clearly won out over any extrapolation approach. In 1989, the FDA issued guidelines[37] that indicated that sponsors should determine whether a drug being studied for approval is likely to be used by the elderly. If it is, older patients should be included in the clinical trials, and data about them should be used to determine if there are any large age-related differences. These guidelines also talk about the need for appropriate pharmacokinetic, pharmacodynamic, and drug-drug interaction studies. An expanded version of these guidelines was adopted in 1993 as part of the International Harmonization effort.[38] This expanded version applies both to diseases of the elderly (e.g., Alzheimer's) and to diseases had by many elderly people (e.g., hypertension). It emphasizes the importance of including the very old (>75). It calls for including enough older subjects (usually, a minimum of 100) in the regular phase III trials to detect clinically significant differences.

It is to some degree understandable that the elderly be treated differently than children. The elderly subjects in question can in most cases be cognitively intact. They require no special protection and there is no need for concerns about the consent of surrogates and about special limits on the risks to be imposed. Nevertheless, these guidelines could appropriately be used as a model for research on children. It could be mandated that they be included in phase III trials of drugs that are likely to be used in the pediatric population in sufficient numbers to detect clinically significant differences. Their inclusion in these clinical trials would be therapeutic research, so it would not raise the issues about inappropriate risks we discussed above in connection with phase I trials. With appropriate parental consent and pediatric assent, their inclusion would pose no ethical concerns. I would conclude, therefore, that the problem of pediatric underinclusion should be solved not by adopting the different trade-off on the epistemic question involved in the extrapolation approach but by insisting that pediatric subjects be included in appropriate phase III trials.

Choosing End Points. The benefit of using a drug/device consists of its use producing favorable clinically relevant end points. It would seem, then, that clinical trials designed to establish the risk-benefit ratio for use in approval decisions should focus on those end points. In recent years, however, there has been considerable discussion of the use of surrogate end points to assess benefits, primarily from the use of drugs. In this final section, we will analyze the reasons for the emergence of this trend and assess the validity of this trend, relating it to our epistemic question.

What is a surrogate end point? It is some end point whose occurrence is closely enough correlated with the clinically relevant end point in which we are interested so that we can use the occurrence of the surrogate end point to study the benefits of the use of a drug. Some have insisted that the surrogate end point must fully capture the effect of the treatment on the clinically relevant end point, but this seems too strict. A weaker correlation would be sufficient, but how much weaker is part of the controversy over the use of surrogate end points.

Why use surrogate end points rather than the clinically relevant end point in which we are interested? Two reasons are often given: (1) the clinically relevant end point in which we are interested occurs much further in the future than the surrogate end point, so that using the surrogate end point enables us to answer the question of benefit more quickly; (2) the potential benefit of the use of the drug is an increase over the baseline of the occurrence of the clinically relevant end point. However, the baseline rate may already be very high, so that establishing a significant increase over the baseline would require a very large number of subjects. Establishing an improvement in the surrogate end point might require far fewer subjects.

It is useful to have an example of each of these reasons. Clinical trials of

AIDS drugs provide us with an example of the former. The benefits of various antiviral drugs have been assessed on the basis of improvements in the CD4 lymphocyte count (the surrogate end point), without waiting for evidence of delay of disease progression or of longer survival (the clinically relevant end points), because those end points come later, and we could establish the benefit using the surrogate end point much sooner. Of course, doing so requires assuming that improvements in CD4 lymphocyte counts are sufficiently predictive of improvements in the clinically relevant end points. Clinical trials of thrombolytic agents designed to increase survival rates after myocardial infarctions provide us with an example of the latter. The baseline survival rate of such patients is already quite high, so we would need to run trials involving a very large number of subjects (tens of thousands) to demonstrate significant improvements. It might be possible to show a significant improvement in the rate of early clot lysis (the surrogate end point) in a much smaller number of patients, and use that improvement as a surrogate end point to establish an improvement in survival rate (the clinically relevant end point). Of course, doing so requires assuming that improvements in the rate of early clot lysis are sufficiently predictive of improvements in survival.

Both of these examples are also illustrative of the controversies about the use of surrogate end points. To illustrate, we turn to an examination of the controversies surrounding CONCORDE and TIMI.

CONCORDE was a study of immediate-versus-deferred use of zidovudine in symptom-free HIV-positive individuals with CD4 counts ranging from 200 to greater than 500.[39] There was both an immediate and a long-term improvement in CD4 counts in the group treated immediately. There were, however, no significant differences in either three-year survival or three-year disease progression rates. There was, however, a significant difference in the one-year disease progression rate, primarily due to the fact that those who started zidovudine earlier had a lesser one year progression to ARC rate. Those who are concerned about the use of surrogate end points emphasize the failure of improved CD4 counts to correlate with improved three-year survival or disease progression rates. Those who advocate the use of surrogate end points emphasize that the improved CD4 counts were correlated with an improvement in one-year disease-free rates. This debate has been transformed by the emergence of decreased viral loads as an alternative surrogate end point for such trials.

TIMI was a trial comparing two thrombolytic agents, streptokinase and tissue plasminogen activator. It was stopped after an interim analysis showed a higher early clot lysis rate for tissue plasminogen activator. Nevertheless, an FDA advisory panel recommended immediate approval for streptokinase (because there was evidence from the GISSI trial that it improved survival over the use of a placebo) but urged delay in the approval of tissue plasminogen activator, despite the fact that use of the surrogate end point suggested that it was a better drug.

Eventually, both were approved. Since then, two very large major trials (GISSI 2 and ISIS 3) failed to show any difference in survival rates after the use of the two drugs, while one very large trial (GUSTO) did, but only with the immediate use of heparin to keep the arteries open. Those concerned about the use of surrogate end points emphasize the failure of the clot lysis benefit to translate into a survival benefit in two of the major trials.[40] Those who support the use of surrogate end points emphasize the survival benefit in GUSTO when measures are taken to preserve the benefits from the improved rate of early clot lysis.

The Accelerated Approval Program adopted by the FDA (Appendix 3.5) clearly represents a decision to emphasize surrogate end points as the basis for the approval of desperately needed drugs. Those who have criticized this approach have argued from many examples that there are real risks in extrapolating from improvements in surrogate end points to improvements in clinically relevant endpoints.[41]

I think that this type of debate illustrates two crucial points: Waiting for clinically relevant end point results certainly provides more secure evidence than relying upon results involving surrogate end points. Less secure evidence from studies using surrogate end points may mean having to rethink issues when more evidence comes in from studies using the clinically relevant end points. But waiting for those results may also mean delay in attaining the benefits of earlier approval. There are real trade-offs to be made here, and both sides are wrong when they focus on the gains of their approach while disregarding the costs. Our problem about different standards being appropriate for different individuals with different values reemerges with increased force as we reflect on these cases. Different clinicians and the patients they advise may be willing to put different degrees of reliance on the evidence to be obtained from studies involving surrogate end points. Is there a socially correct approach to be mandated in the policies of a national drug regulatory agency, as has been presupposed by both sides in the debate about surrogate end points, or must we find better social policies for respecting these differences in values?

Conclusion

In this chapter, we have identified a fundamental policy issue about the standards for the approval of drugs/devices. We have also identified and analyzed four major ethical issues that arise in the design and conduct of clinical trials leading to meeting these standards for regulatory approval: using phase I trials, monitoring trials for unexpected safety issues, enrolling children and the elderly in such trials, and using surrogate end points. Some of these issues (e.g., the monitoring issue and the enrollment issue) have been discussed in at least some official policies, whereas others (most notably the phase I issues) have received very little attention. Moreover, there is far from a consensus in official policies on those issues that have been discussed more extensively.

These results are very much like what we saw in Chapter Seven. The explanations we invoked there, about the lack of attention in official policies being due to a lack of widely discussed questionable cases and/or a lack of widely discussed public concerns about newly emerging technologies, are probably relevant here. But there is an additional point that must be noted here. Most of these ethical issues are intimately related to our fundamental policy issue, and we have seen that there are reasons for being concerned about how that policy issue can be resolved given that the members of our society have such different values. It may be that the development of justified official policies on some of our issues will be severely hampered by the difficulty in resolving the fundamental policy issue.

Chapter nine

RESEARCH INVOLVING WOMEN
AND MEMBERS OF MINORITY GROUPS

In earlier chapters, we encountered a number of problems relating to the involvement of women in clinical research, but left them for later discussion. In discussing research on fetuses in utero in Chapter Five, we analyzed the ethical issues posed by research protocols involving pregnant women devoted to studying issues of fetal health. This left for later discussion the ethical issues posed by research protocols involving pregnant women devoted to studying their health issues. In Chapters Six and Seven, we identified as a crucial issue of justice in research the appropriate inclusion of various groups in clinical research so that they may share in the benefits as well as the burdens of research. That led us in Chapter Six to an extensive discussion of the need to include children and the mentally infirm in clinical research; left out were the ethical issues posed by the need to include women, whether they are or are not of childbearing potential, in clinical research. Finally, in our discussion in Chapter Eight of the ethical issues related to choosing research subjects in trials designed to secure regulatory approval for the use of new drugs/devices, we identified and evaluated from an ethical perspective two approaches to the inclusion of pediatric and geriatric subjects, the extrapolation approach and the starting with pediatric and geriatric subjects approach. We left for later discussion the ethical evaluation of the analogous approaches as they apply to women.

The main focus of this chapter will be on completing those earlier discussions with the needed analysis of the ethical issues related to the inclusion of women in research. We will pay special attention to the clinical trials run to secure regulatory approval of new drugs/devices. We will also examine special ethical issues raised by the inclusion of women of childbearing potential and pregnant women in clinical research.

The first of these ethical issues, related to inclusion in clinical research, has also arisen in connection with members of various minority groups. It deserves more attention than it has received, and the last section of this chapter will be devoted to it.

Our primary focus in this chapter will be on the developments in official policies in the United States, where these issues have been extensively discussed in recent years. However, we will not neglect the official policies of other countries.

The Inclusion of Women in Clinical Research

Two concerns about the inclusion of women in clinical research have been identified. One of these concerns grows out of the underrepresentation of women in clinical trials, either because they are excluded directly or indirectly by the inclusion and exclusion criteria or because the mechanisms for enrolling patients fail to enroll them. The other grows out of the insufficient attention paid to special health issues faced by women. We will examine each of these concerns and the response to them separately.

Considerable attention has been devoted in recent years to quantifying the extent of gender underrepresentation in clinical trials. Perhaps the best-documented area of concern is the failure to include women in cardiovascular trials, including some of the most important cardiovascular disease prevention trials such as MRFIT and the Physician's Health Study. Concern has also been expressed about the documented underinclusion of HIV positive women in the early trials run by the ACTG (AIDS Clinical Trials Group).[1]

These concerns resulted in the early 1990s in a variety of legislative and regulatory policies in the United States relating to clinical research. These include the 1993 NIH Reauthorization Act (Appendix 3.11, section 131) and its implementing regulations in 1994[2] and 1993 FDA guidelines related to drug approval (Appendix 3.6).

The 1993 NIH Reauthorization Act included as a general requirement on NIH-funded research that women be included as subjects in research unless such inclusion is inappropriate with respect to the health of the subjects or the purpose of the research or unless there is substantial evidence demonstrating no relevant gender differences. A remarkable provision in a time of strict budgets is that cost is not relevant in determining whether inclusion is appropriate. The Reauthorization Act also contained a design requirement that when women are included as subjects, the study design must provide for a valid analysis of differential impact of the intervention on women.

Data released by the NIH in early 1997 suggest that the inclusion requirement has produced considerable progress, even if there is more that can be done.[3] By the end of 1994, 57% of the subjects enrolled in phase III extramural trials funded by the NIH were women. Fifty-two percent of the subjects enrolled in all NIH-funded extramural research were women.

The design requirement has been more problematic. Its implementation in a given trial requires that the trial be significantly larger so that it has adequate power to test for these subgroup differences. For example, if one suspects that an intervention that produces a 25% reduction in the hazard of a disease among men will be beneficial in only half as many women, one needs to increase the size of the trial 16-fold to have adequate power to test for that difference. This greatly increases both the difficulty and cost of running such a trial. The NIH regulations,[4] attempting to ameliorate this difficulty, require the full power to test for differences only when there is pretrial evidence strongly indicating the existence of significant differences. When there is no such evidence, the trial must provide for a subgroup analysis but need not be designed to have high power to detect those differences if they exist. This compromise seems reasonable, although it certainly weakens the effect of the design requirement. It may need to be supplemented by the adoption of the suggestions of the Institute of Medicine Science Policy Board[5] that clinical trials without adequate power for full subgroup analyses be supplemented by epidemiological studies, postmarketing studies, outcomes research, meta-analyses, and pharmacokinetic/pharmacodynamic studies to identify differential impact on women. In short, the impact of the design requirement will depend on how the NIH regulations are implemented and upon whether these supplementary studies are conducted.

These policies described until now apply only to NIH-funded research. Much clinical research is, however, funded by private companies. This is particularly true of research designed to secure regulatory approval for the sale of new drugs/devices. In order to influence the conduct of this research, the NIH policies had to be supplemented by FDA policies. The FDA's response to these issues was to reject the extrapolation approach in favor of a testing women first approach, in order to ensure that data on women are included as part of the data required to secure approval for a new drug.

In 1988, the FDA issued new general guidelines governing the clinical and statistical sections of new drug applications.[6] These guidelines called for including in studies the full range of those who would use the drug were it approved and for analyzing variations in responses to the drug among different genders, races, and age groups. There is some controversy about the effectiveness of these 1988 guidelines. A 1992 Government Accounting Office (GAO) report claimed a continued underrepresentation of women, especially in trials of cardiovascular drugs, and a continued failure by sponsors to analyze the data for gender differences. In response, the FDA noted that most of the data analyzed by the GAO came from the pre-1988 period and that the cardiovascular drugs were being tested in a younger population in which cardiovascular disease is primarily a disease of men.[7]

Nevertheless, the FDA issued in 1993 clarifying guidelines on gender differences in the clinical evaluation of drugs for approval (Appendix 3.6). These guidelines require

1. The inclusion of both genders in the trials supporting approval. The requirements are that the subjects in the trial should "reflect the population that will receive the drug when it is marketed" and that there should be adequate numbers of both genders included to allow "detection of clinically significant gender-related differences in drug response."
2. Analyses by gender. Analyses of gender differences, both for safety and effectiveness, should be submitted in the integrated analysis of data from the trials. If there are significant enough differences, additional studies might be required before or after approval.
3. Pharmacokinetic differences. These should be studied in pilot studies before the definitive trials are conducted to determine appropriate dosages for the different genders in the definitive studies.

We noted above that there were two concerns related to women in clinical research. Until now, we have discussed the issue of the inclusion of women in general research. But there is also the issue of the adequacy of research on women's health problems. We turn to a consideration of official developments on that issue.

An important policy decision by the NIH was to ensure that health issues of special concern to women would be adequately studied. An Office of Women's Health Research was created at the NIH to lead the effort on promoting such research. This effort has produced encouraging results, although there is more to be done. In 1994, for example, the NIH funded 514 phase III trials; of the 106 that did not involve both men and women, 92 involved women only and were devoted to studying their health needs.[8] Perhaps the most prominent example of progress in promoting such research is the Women's Health Initiative,[9] which began in 1991. It is a 15-year, $628 million study of osteoporosis, cancer, and cardiovascular disease in postmenopausal women. It involves clinical trials of estrogen replacement therapy, of dietary modification, and of calcium/vitamin D supplements. It also involves a 100,000-woman longitudinal study relating health outcomes to various health-related behaviors. To ensure that minority issues are studied as well, a target of 20% minority women was set, and a number of clinical centers were targeted to recruit minority women.

In short, concern about equity in the distribution of the benefits and burdens of research led the United States in the early 1990s to develop major official initiatives to involve many more women as research subjects and to address more directly their health concerns. Similar developments occurred elsewhere, but to a much lesser degree.

The most important of these developments seems to be the policy, announced in the 1997 proposed Canadian Code, that women cannot be routinely excluded.[10] In addition, an emphasis is placed on the inclusion of women who are economically disadvantaged or who belong to minority groups. This inclusion policy is not, however, supplemented by a design policy. However, it is an advance over what has happened in most countries. It is unclear whether these other countries have simply not yet explicitly addressed this newly emerging aspect of the issue of gender justice or whether their silence relates to concerns about the impact of such policies on fetal well-being. In order to understand this second possibility, we turn to the next of our issues.

Women of Childbearing Potential and Pregnant Women as Research Subjects

Although there is room to disagree about the details of the developments discussed in the last section, their basic ethical appropriateness is clear. Justice in the distribution of the benefits as well as the burdens of research requires that women be included as subjects in clinical research and that their health needs be studied more intensively. Naturally, their inclusion must be based on meeting all the usual requirements on research involving human subjects discussed in Chapter Two. But these developments have been complicated by an additional issue, and resolving it is much more complicated. This issue is the appropriateness of including women of childbearing potential and pregnant women in clinical trials in the light of the risks that such inclusion might pose to fetuses.

We begin our examination of this complicating issue by looking at the developments in the U.S. regulations. The FDA, in guidelines published in 1977, had excluded women of childbearing potential (as interpreted, this meant nearly all premenopausal women) from participating in phase I and phase II trials and from participating in phase III trials unless animal teratogenicity studies had been completed.[11] As these animal studies were not required and were often not run, this meant that most premenopausal women were excluded from most clinical trials. The main exception to this policy was for lifesaving or life-prolonging treatments. This policy, together with the fear of sponsors of liability for fetal injury, seems to have significantly contributed to the underinclusion of women in clinical trials.

The implementation of the above-discussed new policies of inclusion required therefore a reexamination of the FDA guidelines on this topic. In 1993, the FDA reversed its earlier guidelines. On its new approach (Appendix 3.6, section G), women of childbearing potential may be included in all stages of clinical trials. A new set of requirements on protocols offer an alternative approach to protecting against fetal harm: protocols should provide for pregnancy tests prior to enrolling women in the trial and for the use of reliable contraceptive methods during the trial; informed consent documents must discuss all available information about fetal toxicities and the importance of taking precautions against pregnancy while in the trial; reproductive toxicity studies should be concluded before the large-scale exposure of women occurs in phase III studies.

It is clear that the main focus of these modifications is on protecting against fetal risk by not including pregnant women in the clinical trials. Women of childbearing potential are to be tested before being enrolled in the trial to ensure that they are not pregnant, they are to be informed about the importance of taking precautions against pregnancy while they are in the trial, and they should be taking adequate contraceptive measures while in the trial.

An excellent example of this approach is provided by ACTG 251, a phase II/III trial of thalidomide for severe mouth ulcers (oral aphthous ulcers) in HIV-infected women.[12] Thalidomide is of course known for producing devastating results when used during pregnancy. As noted in Chapter Eight, it was these results of the use of thalidomide by pregnant women in the early 1960s that resulted in the strengthening of the drug regulatory mechanisms throughout the world. After considerable controversy, it was nevertheless decided to include women of childbearing potential in ACTG 251, after their being informed of the risks to the fetus if they became pregnant, being subject to pregnancy testing every two weeks (because the main risks posed by thalidomide are in the period of 21–35 days after conception), and agreeing either to be abstinent or to use effective contraceptive techniques.

On this approach, less stringent requirements for testing for pregnancy and for use of contraceptives would be appropriate, if the risks to fetuses were known to be less serious. On this approach, this judgment of the balancing of risks and requirements must be made by the researchers (who should not conduct the research unless they are comfortable with the balance), by the IRB or the Research Ethics Commitee/Research Ethics Board (REC/REB) (which should not approve the research unless it is comfortable with the balance), and by the women in question (who should not participate in the research unless they are comfortable with the balance).

There will clearly be cases in which this approach is inadequate, because of the need to include pregnant women in the clinical trial or to not exclude them if they become pregnant. This need may arise in some cases because the trial is studying the implications of the use during pregnancy of a drug needed for concomitant medical problems. Thus, one of my colleagues at Baylor was, after much opposition, able to run a trial to see if nimodipine improved the treatment of pregnancy-related seizures.[13] In other cases, this need may arise because inclusion in the trial may be the best way of getting access to the most promising new drugs. This is regularly the case in the trial of new drugs for controlling HIV.

The traditional U.S. regulations for involving pregnant women in clinical research were the HHS regulations of 1981. Their implications for research devoted to studying issues of fetal health were discussed in Chapter Five. Here, we are concerned with their implications for research devoted to studying issues of maternal health.

The relevant HHS regulation asserts that:

> No pregnant woman may be involved as a subject in an activity covered by this subpart unless: (1) The purpose of the activity is to meet the health needs of the mother and the fetus will be placed at risk only to the minimum extent necessary to meet such needs, or (2) the risk to the fetus is minimal (Appendix 3.1, section 46.207).

In addition, there is a requirement of the consent of the father of the fetus. This latter requirement has already been criticized as nonrespective of the mother's decisional rights in Chapter Five, and it should be dropped. I want to focus on the basic standard.

The first part of this standard is really quite permissive. When the research is therapeutic research (the purpose being to "meet the health needs of the mother"), there is no requirement that maternal and fetal interests be balanced. The only requirement is that the fetus not be placed at more risk than is necessary to meet the maternal health need. As it is hard to see why unnecessary risks should be imposed upon the fetus, this standard is certainly as permissive as possible. The requirement that the risk to the fetus be minimal, which is a more demanding requirement, is only imposed for nontherapeutic research. It seems to be too demanding. In a country whose regulations allow, as noted in Chapter Six, for nontherapeutic research on children as long as the risks are only a minimal increase over minimal risk, it is hard to see why the same permissiveness should not be allowed for fetal research.

Many have been quite critical of this 1981 HHS standard, insisting that it is responsible for much of the unwillingness to include pregnant women in research.[14] I agree that the paternal consent requirement should be dropped and that nontherapeutic research should be allowed in a few more cases. But the basic standard for therapeutic research involving pregnant women is as permissive as it can be, unless one claims that fetal interests should not be considered at all. I suspect that many who have criticized the 1981 regulations have misunderstood them, and have thought that they require that the risks to the fetus be minimal even if the research involving the pregnant woman is therapeutic research.[15]

With this misunderstanding corrected, I think that we can say the following by way of summation about the U.S. official policy in 1997 on the inclusion of women of childbearing potential and of pregnant women in clinical research: women of childbearing potential can be included in clinical research so long as they are not pregnant, are taking adequate contraceptive measures, and have been informed about any potential risks to them and/or to the fetus if they become pregnant. The burdens of meeting these requirements should be proportional to the seriousness of the risks. Alternatively, such women can be included if they are pregnant, and can remain in the study if they become pregnant, if the research is therapeutic research related to their health needs and the fetus is not placed at more risk than needed to meet the maternal health need.

What other official policies exist? Most of the others are far less detailed on these issues. The CIOMS guidelines (Appendix 1.8, Guideline 11) and the Council of Europe directive (Appendix 2.2, Principle 6) allow needed therapeutic research on pregnant women and nursing women, without discussing the issue of risk minimization and without addressing the issue of women of childbearing potential. CIOMS seem to prohibit any nontherapeutic research unless the risks are minimal; the Council of Europe seems to be more permissive.

The 1997 proposed Canadian Code does offer a more substantial discussion, and the policies it adopts seem to differ in important ways from the U.S. policies. While it shares with the U.S. policies the intention of promoting the inclusion of women of childbearing potential and pregnant women in clinical research, its standards for the permissibility of that inclusion seem to differ.

In connection with research involving pregnant women, the 1997 proposed code calls for a balancing of fetal and maternal interests.[16] Therapeutic research is clearly permissible when the potential therapeutic benefits for the woman are substantial and the risks to the fetus are minimal. The harder case, of course, is when both the potential benefits and the risks are substantial. Such research, it is said, ''can sometimes be justified.'' All of this may be somewhat more restrictive than the HHS policy, which involves no balancing and merely requires that unnecessary fetal risks be avoided.

In connection with research involving women of childbearing potential, the earlier version of the proposed Canadian code emphasized the woman's informed consent rather than the negative pregnancy tests and the contraception that are required in addition by the FDA. The latter requirement was specifically rejected on the grounds that ''contraception is a morally sensitive issue.'' There was also the observation that requiring hormonal contraception can sometimes— because of drug interactions—invalidate the scientific validity of the research.[17]

In short, there may be real differences between the two most developed policies. The Canadian policy seems to be somewhat more protective of fetal interests in maternally oriented therapeutic research and was, in its earlier version, much more cognizant of the sensitivity of the contraception issue. The former difference is particularly important as it may foreshadow the emergence of a major international difference.

We saw in Chapter Five, in our discussion of research involving preimplantation zygotes, that the development of official policies becomes very complicated when the issue of the moral status of fetuses becomes relevant. That seems to be happening here. Both policies recognize that fetal interests need to be protected. But how do they compare to maternal interests? The Canadian policy seems to ascribe more significance to the moral status of fetuses and to their interests than does the U.S. policy. As other countries address this issue more carefully, varying views about that question of moral status are likely to lead to even sharper divergences in official policies.

This complicating issue obviously cannot be disregarded. It must not be forgotten, however, that the different ways of resolving it are all compatible with policies that are much more inclusive than previous policies on the inclusion of women, even if of childbearing potential or pregnant, in clinical research.

The Inclusion of Minorities in Clinical Research

The issue of the inclusion of minorities in clinical research has in recent years attracted considerable attention, similar to the attention devoted to the inclusion of women in clinical research. Some of these minorities (in the United States, Canada, Australia, and New Zealand) are members of native populations whereas others (particularly in the United States) are members of nonnative racial or ethnic groups (e.g., blacks and Hispanics in the United States). There are important similarities and differences between these two issues, however, and it is helpful to begin by noting them.

The most important of the similarities is that the basic problem in both cases is one of justice. Just as in the case of women, underinclusion of minorities in clinical research means that they may be denied their fair share of the benefits from clinical research. Health issues of particular relevance to them may not be addressed. The data obtained from clinical trials in which they are not included cannot necessarily be extrapolated to them. Finally, they may be denied access to the most promising interventions, which may be available only in clinical trials.

There are, however, important differences between these issues. The most obvious difference is that policies to more adequately include minorities in clinical research do not have to struggle with fetus-related issues. This, of course, makes correcting the problem of minority underinclusion easier. There are also subtler differences, and they unfortunately make it harder to correct that problem. The first is an issue of mistrust. As a legacy of unfavorable encounters with the health care system in general, and with health care research in particular, members of minority groups are often reluctant to participate in clinical research. For example, researchers in the United States attempting to enroll black subjects in clinical research have reported encountering a legacy of suspicion created by the revelations about the Tuskegee syphilis study discussed in Chapter Two. The other is an issue of lack of contact. Members of minority groups, especially those of lower socioeconomic status, often do not get their health care at the major medical centers at which clinical research is usually conducted, so enrolling them and getting them to stay in clinical research over extended periods of time pose special challenges. U.S. researchers at public hospitals and VA hospitals have been more successful in dealing with this second problem, because the patient population at those hospitals includes a large percentage of minorities.

This is not to say that these problems cannot be overcome. A special program created by the NIH, the Community Program for Clinical Research on AIDS (CPCRA), has demonstrated important lessons for dealing with these challenges.[18] The sites for the research are chosen to include sites that provide health care for significant numbers of minorities. Funding is included for community outreach workers, health educators, social workers, and other professionals needed to adequately inform, enroll, and retain the needed minority subjects. Their work is based on culturally sensitive education about the research that explicitly attempts to overcome the trust issue. Funding is also provided for such services as child care and transportation needed to facilitate participation by minority members of lower socioeconomic status. The success of such programs is evidence that this approach works.

At the level of official policy, the U.S. response to the minority inclusion issue has many parallels to the official response to the inclusion of women issue. An Office of Research on Minority Health has been created at the NIH to encourage research on health issues of special relevance to minorities, although no research project on minority health comparable to the massive Women's Health Initiative has been funded. Still, it should be remembered that that initiative did provide for the significant involvement of minority women. The 1993 NIH Reauthorization Act (Appendix 3.11, section 131) required that minorities be included in NIH-funded research and that the research be designed to investigate differences in minority responses to the interventions being studied. The FDA's 1988 mandate required including in the trials leading to approval members of minority groups if they are likely to use the drug when approved and analyzing differences in responses by the members of minority groups.[19] All of these changes in policies have produced important results, even if more progress could be made. In extramural trials funded by the NIH in 1994, at least 23% of the subjects were black and at least 13% were members of other minority groups.[20]

The other major treatment of these issues is in the 1997 proposed Canadian

Code, which develops these themes very well.[21] It emphasizes the need for inclusion of minorities (especially from disadvantaged social, ethnic, racial, and disabled groups), both to ensure justice in receiving the direct benefits of inclusion and to make sure that the results of the clinical research are applicable to the entire population. It emphasizes, moreover, the importance of culturally sensitive communication to potential research subjects.

There is one other issue raised in the proposed Canadian Code that deserves notice. This has to do with the status of a minority group as a collective. This issue is particularly important in the Canadian context where native tribal collectives are one of the central minority groups. Drawing on ideas developed by CIOMS (Appendix 1.7, sections 5–8), and reflecting the reality that Canadian Native American collectives often have well-defined social structures, common customs, and an acknowledged leadership, the proposed Canadian Code calls for obtaining, in some cases, consent for the research from the leadership of the collective as well as from the individual subjects.[22] The collective is viewed as sometimes having collective interests in the research, over and above the benefits and risks accruing to individuals, so its consent must also be obtained in such cases. The strengths and weaknesses of this approach have already been discussed in Chapter Two.

This concept of the consent of the collective, which has recently emerged in research ethics, is also adopted in the Model Ethical Protocol for Collecting DNA Samples developed by the North American Regional Committee of the Human Genome Diversity Project.[23] The Human Genome Diversity Project is an effort to analyze genetic similarities and differences between communities throughout the world. It is thought that this information will be of importance to historians and anthropologists trying to explain the history of our species as well as to medical scientists trying to explain divergences in the prevalence of diseases in different populations. Naturally, DNA samples will be obtained from many individual members of minority groups, but the interest will be in what this tells us about the genetic makeup of these minority collectives. The Model Ethical Protocol, in accord with the CIOMS Guidelines and the proposed Canadian Code, calls for obtaining consent from the leadership of the collective as well as from the individuals who are sampled.

Conclusion

Official policies have recently been developed primarily in the United States and Canada to ensure that the benefits of participation in research are shared both by women and by members of various minority groups. These policies involve several major components: the inclusion of women and minorities in research, the design of that research to identify crucial subgroup differences, and the presentation of that data to drug/device regulatory agencies when approval is being sought. Both good science and the demands of justice support these policies. Special problems have been identified with the inclusion of women (the problem of including women of childbearing potential and pregnant women) and with the inclusion of minorities (dealing with mistrust and with the lack of prior contact). Policies and/or strategies have been developed for dealing with these issues, but they will certainly need refinement over time.

It is too early to decide whether or not an international consensus will emerge in this area. The issues in question have not yet been sufficiently addressed, for example, by the European countries. Of particular interest will be the policies of countries such as Germany, which have taken strong fetal protection positions on other issues, on the issue of the inclusion of women of childbearing potential and pregnant women in clinical research. We have already noted some subtle but important differences between the Canadian and the U.S. policies on that question.

The emergence of these policies illustrates a new way in which issues of research ethics become of concern to official policy. These new policies result, I believe, neither from a reaction to some problematic cases nor from a professional desire to proactively address issues that are likely to become of public concern. Instead, their emergence is part of a larger social rethinking of issues of gender, race, and ethnicity. Their emergence illustrates the fact that research policy cannot and should not be isolated from broader changing social policies.

Chapter ten

PHILOSOPHICAL REFLECTIONS

In the last nine chapters, we have analyzed a wide variety of official policies from many different sources on a very large number of questions relating to the ethics of research. There can be no doubt that the development of official policies on research ethics has become a major effort throughout the research-intensive regions of the world.

In this concluding discussion, I want to take a broader integrating look at the whole enterprise of developing official policies on research ethics. In the first section, I will discuss the descriptive issues of origins, comprehensiveness, and convergence. In the other two sections, I will fulfill the promise made in the Introduction and return to the question of evaluation, looking both at the methodology employed in developing the official policies and at the content of those policies.

Origins, Comprehensiveness, and Convergence

As we look at the emergence of the many official policies, we see that a number of factors regularly played a role. Official policies on research ethics arose in response to cases of research that generated controversy, in response to public or professional concerns about the research components of dramatic new technologies or about the use of the results of that research, and in response to broader social concerns that had implications for particular types of research. Many examples can be given of each of these patterns, with some examples exemplifying more than one pattern.

There are many examples of controversial cases of research leading to the development of official policies. From the controversies over the work of Magendie, Bernard, and their British followers in the nineteenth century to the controversies over primate research in the 1980s, controversial examples have influenced the development of official policies on the ethics of animal research. The revelations about the Nazi experiments led immediately to the creation of the Nuremberg Code on research on human subjects. Equally importantly, Beecher's article, which gave so many examples of ethically troubling research conducted in nontotalitarian societies, certainly influenced the development of the official policies on the ethics of human subjects research. The revelations about the Tuskegee study and the controversies about unlinked HIV seroprevalence studies have both influenced the development of policies on the ethics of epidemiological research, the controversy about the UCLA schizophrenia study has led in the United States to calls for official policies on the ethics of research involving mentally infirm adult subjects, and the complaints of AIDS activists have led to a refashioning of the official policies about the research results required for the approval of new drugs or devices.

An equally common pattern is the development of official policies in response to public and/or professional concerns resulting from the emergence of research involving dramatic new technologies. The emergence of the ability to produce transgenic animals and of the ability to do xenotransplants are leading to many official policies on new ethical issues about animal research. The ability to transplant fetal neural material and to create zygotes through in vitro fertilization to be used for research purposes led to the official policies on the ethics of fetal research. Genetic engineering and gene therapy are leading to the still emerging official policies on the ethics of genetic research and of the use of information from genetic testing.

Still a third common pattern is the emergence of official policies governing research in response to the recognition that the research in question raises concerns that are part of larger concerns being faced by the society in question. The most obvious example of this is the emergence of the recent U.S. and Canadian policies on the inclusion of women and minorities in research. When their underinclusion was recognized as an injustice similar to many other injustices being confronted by women and minorities in those societies, official policies were developed to deal with this injustice in research. Similarly, the official policies on the ethics of animal research emerged as part of a broader concern about animal rights; the official policies on the ethics of human research, with their emphasis on individual consent, emerged as part of a broader concern about individual rights and about mistrust of authorities; the official policies on the ethics of epidemiological research emerged as part of a broader concern about confidentiality and privacy in a world of accessible, large databases; the official policies on the ethics of reproductive research emerged as part of broader debates about fetal rights and reproductive freedom; and the new policies on accelerated approval of drugs and devices emerged as part of the concern about deregulation of the economy. In all of these cases, the emergence of official policies on research ethics has been part of far broader social movements and not just a regulatory response to controversial cases and new technologies.

When none of these patterns are present, official policies may not emerge even for ethical questions that are very important. We saw this in Chapters Seven and Eight when we looked at the ethical issues surrounding clinical trials and regulatory approval. There are many such issues and they have been extensively analyzed in the scholarly literature. Surprisingly, the official policies do not have much to say about many of these issues. Because of the technical nature of these issues (e.g., the window for running concurrently controlled clinical trials, the proper design of Phase I trials), cases raising these issues have not resulted in the public controversies that often lead to official policies. Moreover, these issues may not be related either to the emergence of new dramatic technologies or to larger social concerns, so the other factors that often lead to official policies are not present. In short, the importance of the ethical issues in question may not be sufficient to prompt the emergence of official policies. Something more, like one of our three patterns, must be present to ensure that their importance is recognized.

We turn from questions of origins to questions of comprehensiveness. Any definitive judgment of the comprehensiveness of these policies requires a careful comparison between the issues raised in the ethics literature and the issues covered by the official policies, to see whether there are important issues raised in the literature that are not covered in the policies. No such comparison has been attempted in this book. Still, in the light of the very extensive range of issues covered, the impression one has is that the official policies are on the whole quite comprehensive. The clinical trials/regulatory approval issues discussed in Chapters Seven and Eight apparently are, for the reasons indicated above, an exception to a general pattern of comprehensiveness. However, even some of those issues (e.g., the choice of control groups) are receiving more attention in the recent policies. This may reflect the capacity of these policies to become more comprehensive over time.

We turn to the question of convergence. As one reviews the various issues we have covered, one sees that there is a remarkable consensus on some issues, an emerging consensus with some uncertainty about applications on other issues, and more substantial disagreements over other issues. Identifying when these different patterns are present may shed some light on the forces leading to convergence, and on the forces hindering such convergence, in official policies.

The general policies on the ethics of research involving human subjects discussed in Chapter Two and the additional policies protecting vulnerable subjects discussed in Chapter Six provide the best examples of a remarkable and stable consensus among official policies. They all agree that such research must be independently reviewed, that consent of competent subjects must usually be obtained, that consent of surrogates and (where possible) assent of the subjects must be obtained when subject consent is not sufficient, that there must be appropriate risk-benefit ratios to justify the research, and that confidentiality must be respected. Even in policies coming from countries such as France and Japan where the paternalistic tradition in medical practice is stronger, these principles are maintained, with at most modest exceptions, in official policies governing research. The major differences among official policies are over the issue of compensation for those injured in research and over the degree of risk to which vulnerable subjects can be exposed in nontherapeutic research. Although these differences and others of an even more modest nature are not unimportant, their existence does not take away from the remarkable consensus on all issues of fundamental policy.

There are other areas in which a consensus exists among the official policies, although it may be more recent and its stability is less certain. Perhaps the most remarkable example is the consensus in the official policies on research using fetal tissue discussed in Chapter Five. Since the 1993 NIH Reauthorization Act, which brought U.S. policies into agreement with policies in other countries, the separation approach, based upon the isolation of the abortion decision from the decision to use the tissue, has emerged as the standard approach in official policies. There are still some disagreements over details (e.g., informing recipients about the source of the tissue), but that does not take away from the achievement of a remarkable official consensus over an issue that had been very contentious.

There are other consensuses that are still emerging and whose full meaning and implications are still being worked out. Epidemiological research provides an excellent example of this. As we saw in Chapter Three, it is now widely, but not uniformly, accepted in official policies that independent review of epidemiology protocols is often necessary, that individual informed consent should be obtained when feasible but that research can proceed without that consent as long as there are adequate protections of confidentiality, and that community consent may be necessary as well but that it cannot replace individual consent. Nevertheless, the continuing official discussions about research on stored tissue samples and about anonymous HIV seroprevalence studies show that there is much work to be done before the meaning and implications of this emerging consensus are fully understood.

I think that a similar pattern emerged in Chapter Four when we reviewed the official policies on genetic research and its use. In the existing and emerging official policies, genetic engineering protocols must provide for appropriate levels of safety, gene therapy protocols must not involve eugenics or germ line modifications, screening programs must be based on voluntarism and must meet stringent additional criteria, individuals must be protected against genetic discrimination, and appropriate intellectual property rights in genetic discoveries must be protected. Still, the continuing debates about whether gene therapy protocols need a special level of review, about the use outside of research protocols of tests for genetic susceptibility for breast cancer and for Alzheimer's disease, and about the extent of discovery required for receiving a patent indicate that elucidating the meaning and implications of these consensus statements will require further work.

There are other areas where there are real disagreements in principle among the official policies so that one cannot talk of a consensus, even one whose meaning and implications remain to be worked out. The two most prominent examples are the official policies on the ethics of animal research discussed in Chapter One and on the ethics of research involving preimplantation zygotes discussed in Chapter Five.

Some official policies on animal research clearly adopt an approach that balances human interests in the results of the research against animal interests in not being harmed by the research, even though these interests are not weighed equally. The most prominent examples of such an approach are the British policy established by the 1986 Act and the Australian policy established by the 1990 *Code of Practice*. Other policies, such as the U.S. Public Health Services policy, avoid such balancing. They give priority to human interests and remain content with limiting animal suffering to the extent compatible with conducting the desired research. More extreme policies in either direction are not incorporated in official policies. But that does not take away from the existence of a fundamental disagreement over basic principles, between the balancing position and the human priority position, in the official policies governing research using animal subjects.

This type of disagreement is even more evident in the case of official policies governing research on preimplantation zygotes. As we saw in Chapter Five, official policies range from the permissive British policy found in the 1990 act that allows for a wide variety of such research and for the creation of zygotes for research purposes to the totally restrictive policy found in the 1990 German Act that bans all such research no matter what the source of the zygotes. The extent of this disagreement is evident both from the reactions in the United States to the report of the NIH Advisory Panel and from the compromises required on this issue so that it would not stop the completion of the European Bioethics Convention.

It might be suggested that an additional example is provided by the official policies on drug/device approval. Even with all of the recent changes in FDA policy described in Chapter Eight, the U.S. policies still seem to demand more by way of formal scientific proof of effectiveness than do the policies in other countries. It might be suggested that this means that the other countries are more willing to let the judgment of effectiveness, as opposed to safety, be made by patients and clinicians. But I have not found this stated in those policies, and the new harmonization efforts may mean that these differences are disappearing. A greater policy convergence is one explanation of the possible disappearance of the drug lag discussed in Chapter Eight. For all of these reasons, I am not sure how to categorize the varying official policies on regulatory approval.

Three general descriptive observations about convergence seem in order. The first is that the greatest disagreement among the policies is found when the issue of the moral status of the subjects is involved. Balancing policies on animal research presuppose that animals deserve more respect than afforded to them by human priority policies. Permissive and restrictive policies on preimplantation zygote research obviously see the moral status of such zygotes differently, even though the permissive policies insist that they respect the human life present in such zygotes. Some social anthropologists have suggested that the greatest differences between the moral codes of different societies relate to who is protected by those codes and the extent to which they are protected.[1] That suggestion is confirmed by our analysis.

The second general observation is that it takes time for the meaning of consensuses to be worked out. It was not until the mid-1990s that there was general recognition that there are cases of legitimate invasion of privacy in unconsented-to epidemiological research. Why then should it be surprising that official policies on stored tissue sample research were still controversial in 1997? Similarly, the official policies on genetic screening programs are a product of the mid-1990s. Why should it be surprising that their implications for those who want still experimental screening tests outside of research protocols are controversial in 1997?

The third general observation is that it is misleading to classify the official policies of different countries on research ethics as generally permissive or generally restrictive. The British policies are among the most restrictive on animal research but among the most permissive on preimplantation zygote research. By contrast, the U.S. policies are far more permissive on animal research but are at least for now far more restrictive on preimplantation zygote research. Canadian policies seem to be somewhat in-between on both issues. German policies are the closest to being consistently restrictive. German legislation is completely restrictive on preimplantation zygote research and seems to have incorporated a restrictive balancing approach to animal research. But German official policy contains less formal regulation of general research on human subjects than the official policies of other countries. We are not dealing, therefore, with national differences that are consistent across issues. Differences between official policies are issue specific.

Evaluation of Methodology

We turn from these descriptive issues to issues of evaluation. In doing our evaluation, we need to distinguish the issue of the theoretical soundness of the official policies from the issue of their practical implications for the conduct of research. As noted several times in the text, we know very little about the impact of these policies on the actual conduct of research—a topic that demands detailed studies, which have not yet been performed. We cannot therefore address that question in this book; we can only look at the issue of theoretical soundness. And as we attempt to evaluate the theoretical soundness of these policies, we need to separate the question of the soundness of the methodology by which they were developed, which will be discussed in this section, from the soundness of their content, which will be discussed in the next section.

One thing that is almost never present in the development of these policies is an attempt to ground them in some fundamental moral theory involving a single basic value such as the utilitarian maximization of general utility or the Kantian treatment of persons as ends. The discussion is always about difficult cases, about the balancing of a variety of moral principles relevant to the cases, and about the policies needed to carry out the appropriate balancing. This avoidance of fundamental theories employing single values has been noted by others in the case of development of the U.S. policies on human subjects research.[2] Our survey shows that this is a much more general pattern.

The clearest example of policies providing explicit moral justification by appealing to a variety of principles occurs in the general policies related to research on human subjects. The 1979 Belmont Report, on which the DHHS regulations were based, identified as the fundamental principles of research on human subjects the principles of respect for persons (respecting autonomy and protecting the nonautonomous), of beneficence, and of justice. These principles are also explicitly invoked in the 1992 CIOMS guidelines and in the proposed Canadian Code. They have led directly to the requirements of informed consent by subjects or their surrogates, of a balancing of risks and benefits, and of ensuring equitable access to the benefits of research. As we saw in Chapter Nine, that last requirement has in turn led in the United States and Canada to a rethinking of the role of women and minorities in clinical research. It may well be that this firm basis in mutually compatible principles has contributed to the remarkably stable consensus noted above among the policies on human subjects research.

The situation is somewhat different in the policies governing animal research. Those policies incorporating a human priority approach are often quite clear on their ethical basis. The Canadian Council on Animal Care policy explicitly endorses the 3R principles (replace, reduce, and refine). The U.S. Public Health Service policy incorporates a set of principles adopted by the Interagency Research Animal Committee that contain the 3Rs, although they are not explicitly referred to by that name. These principles lead to the various requirements imposed by the policies. On the other hand, those policies that contain a balancing component, such as the British and the German policies, have done less to ground themselves in a set of principles justifying the balancing requirements. This is unfortunate. As we noted in Chapter One, the balancing approach seems theoretically superior to the human priority position, but that judgment would be firmer if there was a clearer statement of its principles and of the resulting requirements on research.

There are many additional principles invoked by the policies on genetic research and its uses. Among the principles encountered in the policies analyzed in Chapter Four are principles on the use of gene therapy (no enhancements and no germ line therapy), on screening programs (the principle of voluntarism), and on the use of genetic information (no discrimination based on genetic susceptibility to disease). Some of these principles are clearly related to the general principles on human subjects research; voluntarism is related to the principle of autonomy and nondiscrimination is related to the principle of justice. Others, such as the ban on enhancements and on germ line therapy, are independent deontological constraints.

The principles invoked in the official policies on fetal and reproductive research represent a very special case. The convergent official policies on research involving the use of fetal tissue all incorporate the separation principle. This attempt to totally separate the use of the fetal tissue from the abortion is best seen, as we argued in Chapter Five, as a principle for moral compromise when there is no agreement. In a similar fashion, permissive policies governing preimplantation zygote research attempt to base themselves on principles of moral compromise. The 1993 Canadian report is very articulate about its recommendations being based on principles of moral compromise in pluralistic societies. However, the differences among these permissive policies (e.g., on the creation of zygotes for research purposes) and their repudiation in many cases (e.g., the 1995 Victoria repeal of the earlier permissive law) indicates how difficult it has been to find acceptable principles of compromise upon which to base a permissive policy.

More examples of this explicit grounding of official policies in a variety of principles can be given, but they are not necessary to justify the claim that this is the regular pattern for policy articulation in this area. This conclusion leads us to our first evaluative issue about the methodology of the development of the official policies on research ethics: is the reliance on multiple principles an appropriate way to develop official policies?

There are two ways one can evaluate the methodological avoidance of fundamental theories employing single values. The first evaluation is essentially negative. On this account, moral thought is ultimately incomplete unless it is grounded in such a fundamental single-valued theory. On this account, conflict and/or uncertainty of application is a reflection of this incompleteness. The conflict among some of the official policies we have surveyed (e.g., policies on research on animals or on preimplantation zygotes) reflects this theoretical incompleteness. Similarly, the uncertainties about applications among some of the official policies we have surveyed (e.g., policies on the use of stored tissue samples or on providing genetic screening to those who want to be screened by not yet validated tests) are a further reflection of this theoretical incompleteness. Even when there is a stable consensus among policies with few disagreements about applications, we should have no confidence in the policies because they are not adequately grounded in an appropriate single-valued moral theory.

The other evaluation is far more positive. It sees the avoidance of fundamental theories using single values as a reflection of a basic feature of moral thought. On this account, moral thought is based upon balancing many different values, incorporated in many different and sometimes competing principles. On this account, there is no single value such as the utilitarian maximization of general utility or the Kantian treatment of persons as ends to which all of morality can be reduced. When there is agreement upon the principles and when the implications of the various principles are worked out and reconciled through some balancing process, we can articulate policies that will be, as they should be, officially adopted everywhere. We have seen this in the case of the remarkable convergence in the official policies on human subjects research, on research on vulnerable subjects, and on research using fetal tissue. In other cases, there will be continuing disagreement about the principles or about their applications. This continuing disagreement about principles explains the lack of convergence in the policies on animal research and on preimplantation zygote research and this continuing disagreement about the application of principles explains the lack of convergence on the stored tissue issue. Further reflection may lead to some resolution of conflict. This seems to have happened in many aspects of the policies on epidemiological research (e.g., the increasing acceptance of using data without individual consent as long as confidentiality is protected) and on genetic research (e.g., the increasing acceptance of nondiscrimination in insurance). But this will not always be the case. If further reflection does not lead to resolution, we need to understand this as an acceptable reflection of the realities of moral reasoning rather than as a failure due to insufficient attention to moral theories using single values.

My own view is that the latter evaluation is more accurate. This view is based on an approach to moral reasoning that I have advocated elsewhere, called pluralistic casuistry.[3] It is pluralistic in recognizing as legitimate multiple moral values that are not derivable from some fundamental value and that may not be jointly realizable in particular cases. It is casuistic in deriving those values from reflection on the moral intuitions we have about particular cases. This is not the place to repeat the arguments that I have offered for that approach, but it is necessary for the sake of our discussion to explain some of its features.

It is common to talk of modern societies as pluralistic societies. This is meant to be a sociological description of those societies as containing members with different values growing out of different cultural/religious beliefs. The pluralism of my approach is a very different normative claim. It is the claim that particular value systems are plausible only insofar as they recognize as legitimate a variety of different values that are not derivable from some fundamental value. This stands in contrast to those monistic ethical theories such as utilitarianism and Kantianism that would reduce all of morality to a single value, such as maximization of general utility or respect for persons, from which all other values are derivable. Accepting pluralism means accepting the possibility of legitimate values in conflict with each other in particular cases, without the existence of some fundamental value that serves as the basis for the conflicting values and for the choice between them in the particular case in question. It is this fear of the possibility of conflict without an obvious means of resolution that makes monism seem attractive. Nevertheless, I have argued for pluralism as a more accurate account of the realities of moral reasoning.

Pluralism is a thesis about the content of plausible value systems. Casuistry is a thesis about the ways in which we discover the values to be incorporated into a value system. According to the casuistic approach, we begin our value inquiries with intuitions we have about the rightness or wrongness of actions in particular cases. We then develop generalized principles meant to incorporate these intuitions. This stands in contrast to those more traditional approaches that begin value inquiries by the postulation of some theoretical principles from which conclusions are derived about particular cases. Accepting casuistry means accepting the need to continually modify our principles as we reflect on more cases. It is this fear of the tentativeness of our moral framework that makes the more theory-driven approach seem attractive. I have, nevertheless, argued for casuistry as a more accurate account of the realities of moral reasoning.

This then is the moral framework of pluralistic casuistry. If it is correct, it justifies the avoidance of single-valued moral theories, and the emphasis instead on multiple principles, in the development of the official policies. It also justifies two other methodological features of the development of the official policies: the role of cases in justifying the principles and the resulting policies and the balancing of these principles in formulating the policies.

We have noted in the first section of this chapter the prominent role played by controversial cases in motivating the development of official policies. Magendie's demonstrations taught the value of avoiding unnecessary animal suffering even in the name of science. Beecher's examples taught the need to emphasize informed consent, appropriate risk-benefit ratios, and protecting vulnerable subjects when doing research on humans. Recent cases such as the UCLA schizophrenia study and the Auckland phase I gene therapy trial taught the need to be concerned with relying on the consent of the mentally infirm or the desperate parents of seriously ill children. All this is exactly what we should expect if pluralistic casuistry is correct. Controversial cases teach us what principles are needed. But cases have done more in the development of these official policies. They have also taught us when good principles need to be modified. The trials of thrombolytic agents on stroke patients taught that some research may legitimately proceed without informed consent. Legitimate cases of epidemiological research without consent taught that unconsented-to invasions of privacy can be permissible when the need is sufficient and confidentiality is respected. Finally, new cases are now raising new issues for policy development. The tests for genetic susceptibility to breast cancer and to Alzheimer's disease are raising questions about the right of access to very experimental screening tests, and studies on stored tissue samples are raising questions about the extent to which all options need to be discussed when consent to use tissue is obtained. In all of these ways, cases have driven the development of the official research policies and the principles incorporated in them. This prominent role of cases is a second methodological feature of the development of the official policies that can be justified by an appeal to pluralistic casuistry.

The best way to understand many of the official policies is to see them as attempting to balance a variety of legitimate but conflicting values and principles. Sometimes, the policies explicitly call for this type of balancing. The most obvious examples of this are the British and Australian balancing policies on animal research, which call for balancing the importance of the research to humans with the harms caused to animals. Similarly, the Canadian policy on research on the health needs of pregnant women calls for balancing maternal interests and fetal interests. In other cases, the provisions of the policies rest on an already performed balancing of principles and values. The FDA policy on emergency research is justified as a balancing of the value of the research to the patient, of the problem of the lack of informed consent, of the more general need for the research, and of the impracticality of doing the research if consent is required. The CIOMS policies on cultural sensitivity in obtaining informed consent must be understood as balancing respect for individual autonomy with respect for cultural norms. The Canadian policy on anonymous HIV seroprevalence research is based on a balancing of the need to protect confidentiality, the value of the research, and the right of access to voluntary testing. The various drug/device approval policies discussed in Chapter Eight all involve balancing safety with efficacy and rapid approval with scientific certainty. The controversies about some of these policies also show us that balancing conflicting values is not an easy thing to do when there is no single more fundamental value to which to appeal. Balancing of values and principles is a third fundamental methodological feature of the development of the official policies. It too can be justified by an appeal to pluralistic casuistry.

In short, pluralistic casuistry provides the basis for a positive evaluation of the methodology by which the official policies were developed. It is appropriate that these policies have been driven by reflection on cases, that they incorporate multiple values and principles, and that they involve a balancing of these multiple values and principles. These features are not a reflection of the incompleteness of moral reasoning that is not grounded in a single fundamental moral value but a reflection of the realities of moral reasoning in the light of the truth of pluralistic casuistry.

Evaluation of Content

The adoption of pluralistic casuistry leads, as we have just seen, to a very positive evaluation of the process by which the official policies on research ethics were adopted. It needs to be remembered, however, that the very best process does not guarantee the soundness of the results. We therefore turn in this final section, as promised in the Introduction, to a general evaluation of the content of the official policies on research ethics.

There is, however, a problem with doing that. If we were to adopt as our fundamental moral framework a monistic theory based upon a single general value, such as the utilitarian maximization of general utility or the Kantian treatment of persons as ends, then that single value could serve as the basis for a general evaluation of the content of the policies. Would following the policies lead to a maximization of general utility or to a universal respect of persons as ends? But having adopted pluralistic casuistry as a framework, we have no such single value to serve as the basis for a general evaluation of the policies. We can ask whether a particular policy has taken into account principles incorporating all of the relevant crucial values. We can ask whether these principles have been properly balanced (to reflect our intuitions about a variety of related cases) in particular policies. But these are just the policy-specific questions we have been discussing in the first nine chapters. What room is there then for a general evaluation of the content of the policies? Can it be anything more than a systematic review, supplemented by additional reflections, of what we have already done?

I think that there is something else that can be done. It is to reflect on the significance of the remarkable convergence we have found in the official policies on so many of the topics. Does this convergence provide us with any insights about the moral soundness of the policies?

What do I mean by the moral soundness of a policy? For some, moral objectivists, a policy is morally sound if the moral positions adopted in it are objectively true in some person-independent fashion, if they correspond to some person-independent moral reality. For others, moral subjectivists, something very different is meant. A policy is morally sound if the moral positions adopted in it are intersubjectively acceptable. On this position, moral objectivity is nothing more than moral intersubjectivity. For the moral subjectivists, the convergence among the policies is clearly very relevant to their moral soundness. The greater the policy convergence, the greater the intersubjective acceptability, the greater the moral soundness of the policies. The question I want to ask is asked from the perspective of a moral objectivist: does the convergence among the policies teach us something about their person-independent moral soundness?

To ask this question is to go to the very heart of the great modern debate about skepticism. Since at least the beginning of modern philosophy, one of the most fundamental philosophical questions has been the question of the relation between intersubjective acceptability and person-independent objective truth. Given the ever-present possibility of the divergence between the two, how can we infer the latter from the former? The skeptic says that we cannot and therefore becomes skeptical about what is believed. The subjectivist, desiring to avoid skepticism, eliminates person-independent objectivity and remains content with intersubjective acceptability. The nonskeptical objectivist faces the greatest challenge. In our setting, that challenge just is our question as to whether convergence is a sign of person-independent moral soundness.

This book is obviously not the place to attempt a full treatment of this great debate about skepticism. All that I can do is to present the outline of an approach that I have suggested elsewhere[4] and which I hope to develop on another occasion into a full response to the skeptical challenge. The main claims of this approach are the following:

1. There are very serious analogies between the process by which scientists develop generalizations and scientific theories on the basis of empirical observations and the process by which ethicists develop principles and ethical theories on the basis of moral intuitions.
2. Among the crucial analogies are:
    a. both of these are natural processes;
    b. both of these processes begin with information about particulars, but that information may itself be rejected over time;
    c. the resulting development of generalizations/principles and of theories is a fallible process in that there are no guarantees that person-independent objective truth has been reached at any given time and in that there is always the possibility that it will never be achieved.
3. One of the fundamental commitments that we can choose to make, but whose acceptance or denial cannot be rationally proven to be correct, is that our natural cognitive capacities, while fallible in any given case, are on the whole reliable guides to person-independent objective truth.
4. If we do make that commitment, then substantial intersubjective agreement gives us some reason to believe in the truth of what is agreed upon.

If this approach is adopted, then the remarkable moral convergence we have seen among the policies on research ethics is evidence for their person-independent moral soundness.

Four possible objections to this argument are clearly available. The first challenges this whole line of thought as unsupported. The second challenges its emphasis on convergence in the light of the methodology of pluralistic casuistry. The third challenges the existence of a real convergence. The fourth offers an alternative account of the convergence that strips it of its epistemological significance. Let me elaborate on all four.

When, in the last section, I defended the methodological soundness of the process by which the official policies were adopted, I appealed to pluralistic casuistry. Although that approach to ethics is not defended in this book, it has at least been extensively developed and defended elsewhere. This is not true of the approach to skepticism just outlined. Only the earlier parts—steps (1) and (2)—have been developed and defended elsewhere. The crucial steps—(3) and (4)—are the statement of a future research program rather than the conclusion of an argument developed elsewhere. Some may therefore object to the whole approach just outlined on the grounds that it has not been justified. I hope that many readers will find the basic idea of this approach attractive and will to that extent be willing to consider the convergence among the official policies as the basis for a positive evaluation of their moral soundness. But I recognize that others may not find this basic idea attractive and may therefore be moved by this first objection. I must hope to convince them on another occasion.

The second objection raises the issue of the compatibility of this argument with the methodology of pluralistic casuistry. As noted in the last section, pluralistic casuistry accepts nonconvergence as a reflection of the realities of moral reasoning. How can that be compatible with treating convergence as a sign of moral soundness? This objection is understandable, but it is, I believe, incorrect. Pluralistic casuistry offers us an account of why convergence is so hard to obtain and gives us a basis for accepting nonconvergence when it occurs as an expected reality rather than as a failing. All of this is perfectly compatible with the idea, developed in claims (1) through (4), that convergence, when it does occur, may be a sign of the moral soundness of the content of the convergent policies.It is also perfectly compatible with the claim that nonconvergence, even if accepted as a reality, means that at least some (maybe all) of the nonconvergent policies are not morally sound.

The third objection accepts the basic framework just outlined, but argues that its conclusion, step (4), is inapplicable to this case because the convergence is not reflective of any general acceptance of the policies. The basic idea behind this suggestion is simple: the convergence represents nothing more than an agreement in a few, mostly western, countries by people (scientists and government officials) who get appointed to the committees that draft official policies because they are likely to support certain predetermined directions. It is not surprising, argues this third objection, that the resulting policies are convergent, and their convergence teaches us nothing about the moral soundness of the policies.

I think that this third objection raises important issues, but that it is mistaken about the convergence we have observed. To begin with, we are not dealing here with a mere Eurocentric convergence. The convergent policies are found in truly international documents such as the World Medical Association policies and the CIOMS policies. Second, the policies were usually not developed by the scientific community and its regulatory allies in a closed process. To demonstrate this would require a historical investigation into the development of all of the policies, and such an investigation lies beyond the scope of this book. But let me at least provide one example to illustrate how far the objection is from the truth.

When the great debate began about official policies on the use of previously collected data in epidemiological research, some of those who were involved objected to any unconsented-to invasion of privacy whereas others were satisfied as long as confidentiality was protected. Defendants of both of these positions were part of the process of developing many of the official policies. It was realized over a period of time that the values of protecting privacy and of being able to conduct needed epidemiological research needed to be balanced, and this produced the emerging consensus described in Chapter Three. Debate continues on the details of that consensus. All of this was an open process involving such diverse groups as scientists, public officials, journalists, religious leaders, ethicists, and lawyers, and it took place in many countries, in many international settings, and in many types of forums. The claim that the consensus is an artifact resulting from limiting the participants is hard to imagine for this type of open public debate, which is not atypical.[5]

There is an element of truth in this third objection. It would be a mistake to think that the convergence among the official policies means that everybody agrees with them. But that type of universal agreement is not required for the above argument to go through. It is based on substantial intersubjective agreement, not upon universal agreement. It should probably be understood as claiming that the degree of support offered by convergence for moral soundness is a function of the diversity and extent of support for the convergence. On such an account, the convergent official policies on research ethics would be well supported by that convergence.

The fourth objection accepts the reality of the convergence but offers an alternative account for it. On this account, convergent official policies are useful for researchers and for public officials. Multinational collaborative research projects can be undertaken simply by conforming to the same standards found in the different countries' official policies. This makes convergence useful for researchers. Moreover, in a competitive situation, where research is so important for economic development, one country's researchers are not put at a competitive disadvantage by having to conform to far more stringent standards than the standards imposed on researchers in other countries. This makes convergence among official policies useful for public officials in an internationally interdependent economic environment. The fourth objection claims that it is these types of usefulness, rather than the moral soundness of the content, that lies behind the convergence in the official policies. It additionally claims that the convergence has therefore no epistemological significance.

I want to offer two responses to this fourth objection. To begin with, its alternative account fails to explain the broader acceptance of the convergent policies. Like the third objection, it overemphasizes the role of scientists and public officials, and disregards the role of journalists, religious leaders, ethicists and lawyers. Second, it offers no real account as to why the specific policies were accepted. Its alternative account emphasizes the value of there being some convergent policies but offers no account of why one policy was adopted over another.

Obviously, much more needs to be said in response to each of these objections and in defense of this whole approach. I hope to do so on another occasion. For now, however, I just want to say that convergence in the official policies, when it does occur, offers us some basis for belief in their moral soundness, even if we are moral objectivists.

Conclusion

The official policies on research ethics are a remarkable set of documents. They are on the whole quite comprehensive and they contain a remarkable convergence on many topics. For those of us who believe in pluralistic casuistry, their development is testimony to what can be accomplished by appropriate ethical reflection. Moreover, their convergence offers reason for optimism about their ultimate soundness, even for those of us who are moral objectivists.

Appendix 1
INTERNATIONAL RESEARCH ETHICS POLICIES

Appendix 1.1 The Nuremberg Code (1947)

Permissible Medical Experiments

The great weight of evidence before us is to the effect that certain types of medical experiments on human beings, when kept within reasonably well-defined bounds, conform to the ethics of the medical profession generally. The protagonists of the practice of human experimentation justify their views on the basis that such experiments yield results for the good of society that are unprocurable by other methods or means of study. All agree, however, that certain basic principles must be observed in order to satisfy moral, ethical and legal concepts:

1. The voluntary consent of the human subject is absolutely essential.

This means that the person involved should have legal capacity to give consent; should be so situated as to be able to exercise free power of choice, without the intervention of any element of force, fraud, deceit, duress, over-reaching, or other ulterior form of constraint or coercion; and should have sufficient knowledge and comprehension of the elements of the subject matter involved as to enable him to make an understanding and enlightened decision. This latter element requires that before the acceptance of an affirmative decision by the experimental subject there should be made known to him the nature, duration, and purpose of the experiment; the method and means by which it is to be conducted; all inconveniences and hazards reasonably to be expected; and the effects upon his health or person which may possibly come from his participation in the experiment.

The duty and responsibility for ascertaining the quality of the consent rests upon each individual who initiates, directs or engages in the experiment. It is a personal duty and responsibility which may not be delegated to another with impunity.

2. The experiment should be such as to yield fruitful results for the good of society, unprocurable by other methods or means of study, and not random and unnecessary in nature.

3. The experiment should be so designed and based on the results of animal experimentation and a knowledge of the natural history of the disease or other problem under study that the anticipated results will justify the performance of the experiment.

4. The experiment should be so conducted as to avoid all unnecessary physical and mental suffering and injury.

5. No experiment should be conducted where there is an *a priori* reason to believe that death or disabling injury will occur, except, perhaps, in those experiments where the experimental physicians also serve as subjects.

6. The degree of risk to be taken should never exceed that determined by the humanitarian importance of the problem to be solved by the experiment.

7. Proper preparations should be made and adequate facilities provided to protect the experimental subject against even remote possibilities of injury, disability, or death.

8. The experiment should be conducted only by scientifically qualified persons. The highest degree of skill and care should be required through all stages of the experiment of those who conduct or engage in the experiment.

9. During the course of the experiment the human subject should be at liberty to bring the experiment to an end if he has reached the physical or mental state where continuation of the experiment seems to him to be impossible.

10. During the course of the experiment the scientist in charge must be prepared to terminate the experiment at any stage, if he has probable cause to believe, in the exercise of the good faith, superior skill and careful judgment required of him that a continuation of the experiment is likely to result in injury, disability, or death to the experimental subject. . . .

Appendix 1.2   World Medical Association, Declaration of Helsinki (1964, 1975, 1983, 1989, 1996)

Recommendations guiding physicians in biomedical research involving human subjects

Adopted by the 18th World Medical Assembly, Helsinki, Finland, June 1964 and amended in Tokyo, 1975, in Venice, 1983, in Hong Kong, 1989, and in South Africa, October 1996.

Introduction

It is the mission of the physician to safeguard the health of the people. His or her knowledge and conscience are dedicated to the fulfilment of this mission.

The Declaration of Geneva of the World Medical Association binds the physician with the words, "The health of my patient will be my first consideration", and the International Code of Medical Ethics declares that, "A physician shall act only in the patient's interest when providing medical care which might have the effect of weakening the physical and mental condition of the patient".

The purpose of biomedical research involving human subjects must be to improve diagnostic, therapeutic and prophylactic procedures and the understanding of the aetiology and pathogenesis of disease.

In current medical practice most diagnostic, therapeutic or prophylactic procedures involve hazards. This applies especially to biomedical research.

Medical progress is based on research which ultimately must rest in part on experimentation involving human subjects.

In the field of biomedical research a fundamental distinction must be recognised between medical research in which the aim is essentially diagnostic or therapeutic for a patient, and medical research, the essential object of which is purely scientific and without implying direct diagnostic or therapeutic value to the person subjected to the research.

Special caution must be exercised in the conduct of research which may affect the environment, and the welfare of animals used for research must be respected.

Because it is essential that the results of laboratory experiments be applied to human beings to further scientific knowledge and to help suffering humanity, the World Medical Association has prepared the following recommendations as a guide to every physician in biomedical research involving human subjects. They should be kept under review in the future. It must be stressed that the standards as drafted are only a guide to physicians all over the world. Physicians are not relieved from criminal, civil and ethical responsibilities under the laws of their own countries.

I. Basic principles

1. Biomedical research involving human subjects must conform to generally accepted scientific principles and should be based on adequately performed laboratory and animal experimentation and on a thorough knowledge of the scientific literature.

2. The design and performance of each experimental procedure involving human subjects should be clearly formulated in an experimental protocol which should be transmitted for consideration, comment and guidance to a specially appointed committee independent of the investigator and the sponsor provided that this independent committee is in conformity with the laws and regulations of the country in which the research experiment is performed.

3. Biomedical research involving human subjects should be conducted only by scientifically qualified persons and under the supervision of a clinically competent medical person. The responsibility for the human subject must always rest with a medically qualified person and

never rest on the subject of the research, even though the subject has given his or her consent.

4. Biomedical research involving human subjects cannot legitimately be carried out unless the importance of the objective is in proportion to the inherent risk to the subject.

5. Every biomedical research project involving human subjects should be preceded by careful assessment of predictable risks in comparison with foreseeable benefits to the subject or to others. Concern for the interests of the subject must always prevail over the interests of science and society.

6. The right of the research subject to safeguard his or her integrity must always be respected. Every precaution should be taken to respect the privacy of the subject and to minimise the impact of the study on the subject's physical and mental integrity and on the personality of the subject.

7. Physicians should abstain from engaging in research projects involving human subjects unless they are satisfied that the hazards involved are believed to be predictable. Physicians should cease any investigation if the hazards are found to outweigh the potential benefits.

8. In publication of the results of his or her research, the physician is obliged to preserve the accuracy of the results. Reports of experimentation not in accordance with the principles laid down in this Declaration should not be accepted for publication.

9. In any research on human beings, each potential subject must be adequately informed of the aims, methods, anticipated benefits and potential hazards of the study and the discomfort it may entail. He or she should be informed that he or she is at liberty to abstain from participation in the study and that he or she is free to withdraw his or her consent to participation at any time. The physician should then obtain the subject's freely-given informed consent, preferably in writing.

10. When obtaining informed consent for the research project the physician should be particularly cautious if the subject is in a dependent relationship to him or her or may consent under duress. In that case the informed consent should be obtained by a physician who is not engaged in the investigation and who is completely independent of this official relationship.

11. In the case of legal incompetence, informed consent should be obtained from the legal guardian in accordance with national legislation. Where physical or mental incapacity makes it impossible to obtain informed consent, or when the subject is a minor, permission from the responsible relative replaces that of the subject in accordance with national legislation.

Whenever the minor child is in fact able to give a consent, the minor's consent must be obtained in addition to the consent of the minor's legal guardian.

12. The research protocol should always contain a statement of the ethical considerations involved and should indicate that the principles enunciated in the present Declaration are complied with.

II. Medical research combined with professional care (clinical research)

1. In the treatment of the sick person, the physician must be free to use a new diagnostic and therapeutic measure, if in his or her judgement it offers hope of saving life, re-establishing health or alleviating suffering.

2. The potential benefits, hazards and discomfort of a new method should be weighed against the advantages of the best current diagnostic and therapeutic methods.

3. In any medical study, every patient—including those of a control group, if any—should be assured of the best proven diagnostic and therapeutic method. This does not exclude the use of inert placebo in studies where no proven diagnostic or therapeutic method exists.

4. The refusal of the patient to participate in a study must never interfere with the physician-patient relationship.

5. If the physician considers it essential not to obtain informed consent, the specific reasons for this proposal should be stated in the experimental protocol for transmission to the independent committee.

6. The physician can combine medical research with professional care, the objective being the acquisition of new medical knowledge, only to the extent that medical research is justified by its potential diagnostic or therapeutic value for the patient.

III. Non therapeutic biomedical research involving human subjects (non-clinical biomedical research)

1. In the purely scientific application of medical research carried out on a human being, it is the duty of the physician to remain the protector of the life and health of that person on whom biomedical research is being carried out.
2. The subjects should be volunteers—either healthy persons or patients for whom the experimental design is not related to the patient's illness.
3. The investigator or the investigating team should discontinue the research if in his/her or their judgement it may, if continued, be harmful to the individual.
4. In research on man, the interest of science and society should never take precedence over considerations related to the wellbeing of the subject.

Appendix 1.3   World Medical Association, Statement on Fetal Tissue Transplantation

Adopted by the 41st World Medical Assembly, Hong Kong, September 1989

Preamble

The prospect of therapeutically effective fetal tissue transplants for disorders such as diabetes and Parkinson's disease has raised new questions in the ethical discussion on fetal research. These questions are distinct from those addressed in the 1970s that focused on invasive procedures performed by some researchers on living, viable fetuses. They are also separate from the questions that were raised by the development of new techniques for prenatal diagnosis such as fetoscopy and chorionic villus sampling. Although the use of transplanted tissue from a fetus after spontaneous or induced abortion would appear to be analogous to the use of cadaver tissue and organs, the moral issue for many is the possibility that the decision to have an abortion will become coupled with the decision to donate fetal tissue for the transplantation procedure itself.

The utilization of human fetal tissue for transplantation is, for the most part, based upon a large body of research data derived from experimental animal models. At this time, the number of such transplants performed has been relatively small but the various applications are promising avenues of clinical investigation for certain disorders. The demand for fetal tissue transplantation for neural or pancreatic cell engrafments may be expected to increase if further clinical studies conclusively show that this procedure provides long-term reversal of neural or endocrine deficits.

Prominent among the currently identified ethical concerns is the potential for fetal transplants to influence a woman's decision to have an abortion. These concerns are based, at least in part, on the possibility that some women may wish to become pregnant for the sole purpose of aborting the fetus and either donating the tissue to a relative or selling the tissue for financial gain. Others suggest that a woman who is ambivalent about a decision to have an abortion might be swayed by arguments about the good that could be achieved if she opts to terminate the pregnancy. These concerns demand the prohibition of: (a) the donation of fetal tissue to designated recipients; (b) the sale of such tissue; and (c) the request for consent to use the tissue for transplantation before a final decision regarding abortion has been made.

The abortion process may also be influenced inappropriately by the physician. Consequently, measures must be taken to assure that decisions to donate fetal tissue for transplantation do not affect either the techniques used to induce the abortion or the timing of the procedure itself with respect to the gestational age of the fetus. Also to avoid conflict of interest, physicians and other health care personnel involved in performing abortions should not receive any direct or indirect benefit from the research or transplantation use of tissues derived from the aborted fetus. The retrieval and preservation of usable tissue cannot become the primary focus of abortion. Therefore, members of the transplant team should not influence or participate in the abortion process.

There is a potential commercial gain for those involved in the retrieval, storage, testing, preparation, and delivery of fetal tissues. Providing fetal tissue by nonprofit mechanisms designed to cover costs only would reduce the possibility of direct or indirect influence on a woman to acquire her consent for donation of the aborted fetal remains.

Recommendations

The World Medical Association affirms that the use of fetal tissue for transplantation purposes is still in an experimental stage and should only be ethically permissible when:

(1) The World Medical Association Declaration of Helsinki and the Declaration on Human Organ Transplantation are followed, as they pertain to the donor and the recipient of the fetal tissue transplant.

(2) Fetal tissue is provided in a manner consistent with the World Medical Association Statement on Live Organ Trade and that such tissue not be provided in exchange for financial remuneration above that which is necessary to cover reasonable expenses.

(3) The recipient of the tissue is not designated by the donor.

(4) A final decision regarding abortion is made before initiating discussion of the transplantation use of fetal tissue. Absolute independence is established and guaranteed between the medical team performing the abortion and the team using the fetus for therapeutic purposes.

(5) Decision concerning the timing of the abortion is based on the state of health of the mother, and of the fetus. Decisions regarding the technique used to induce abortion, as well as the timing of the abortion in relation to the gestational age of the fetus, are based on concern for the safety of the pregnant woman.

(6) Health care personnel involved in the termination of a particular pregnancy do not participate in or receive any benefit from the transplantation of tissue from the abortus of the same pregnancy.

(7) Informed consent on behalf of both the donor and the recipient is obtained in accordance with applicable law.

Appendix 1.4   World Medical Association, Declaration on The Human Genome Project

Adopted by the 44th World Medical Assembly Marbella, Spain, September 1992

Preamble

The Human Genome Project is based on the assumption that the information contained in the gene will enable us to diagnose a large number of genetic diseases in utero or even before that; it will enable us to make decisions before procreation.

The key to the understanding of genetic diseases is in the identification and characterization of the genes after mutation. Henceforth, one can state that the understanding of all the human biology is enclosed in the identification of 50,000 to 100,000 genes in the human body's chromosomes.

The Human Genome Project can enable us to identify and characterize the genes involved in the main genetic diseases; later on, it would be possible to identify and characterize the genes involved in diseases with a genetic component together with other factors such as Diabetis, Schizophrenia and Alzheimer. In these diseases the gene creates a predisposition to the disease rather than being the cause itself. These diseases cause severe social problems and if it is possible to diagnose the predisposition before the appearance of the disease, it might be possible to prevent it by changes in life-style, by diet modification and periodic check-ups.

In the second half of the 20th century a conceptional revolution has occurred when one started thinking of diseases in terms of biochemistry. A new revolution is happening now which locates in the gene the instructions for all the biochemical processes in the body's cells.

Policy Problems

There are many important ethical reasons to get the genetic information as quickly as possible so that we may better understand many diseases. However, this information may be frustrating unless we develop at the same time therapeutic means and unless we will inform the public of the various genetic options so that the individual may select the best ones.

Another question is whether the invested efforts are justified compared with other ways to reach those objectives with lesser cost. Should the project aspire to a comprehensive inventory or is it preferable to start step by step with less pretentiousness, and progress modularly?

Funding the Project

The Human Genome Project is considered a formidable project, similar to the space program, therefore one may claim that there is no proportion between the investment and its return. The estimated cost of the project is $3 billion during 15 years, i.e. $200 million a year. This cost may not seem extraordinary when we know that the Cystic Fibrosis Foundation, in the USA, only, has spent $120 million in the last four years, for this disease alone. Thus, the financial scarecrow should not prevent the development of the project.

Another disturbing factor stems from the interdiction—in some countries—to allocate funds for clinical research in human embryos. After having spent money on mapping the genes there could be no money allocated for clinical research based on the outcomes.

Conflict between the Protection of Privacy and the Need for Scientific Collaboration

The mapping of the human genes has to be anonymous, but the information acquired will apply to every human being regardless of individual differences, colour or race. The information should be general property and should not be used for business aims. Therefore no patents should be given for the human genome or parts of it.

Genetic Discrimination in Private Insurance and Employment

There is a conflict between the increasing potential of new technologies to reveal genetic heterogeneity and the criterion for private insurance and employment. It may desirable, regarding genetic factors, to adopt the same tacit consensus which prohibits the use of race discrimination in employment or insurance.

Genetic mapping may become a source of stigmatization and social discrimination, and the "risky population" may turn into a "defective population".

The Danger of Eugenics and the Use of Genes for Non-Medical Aims

Eugenics is based on the assumption that the genes have a decisive importance, and the way to change their distribution in the population is to change reproductive behavior. According to this concept the general good justifies the limitations on the individual's liberty. The power of information raises concern about how it will be used. There is still fear of government eugenics programs for "the improvement of the race", and the use of medical technology not for medical purposes.

Recommendations

The ethical issues raised by the Human Genome Project are not linked with the technology itself but with its proper use. Due to the power of this new tool, its ethical, legal and social issues should be examined whilst the program is still at its start.

Some of the opposition stems from the fear that the researcher may tend "to play God" or to interfere with the laws of nature. If we free ourselves from an uncompromising opposition to the Human Genome Project, we can assess the ethical outcomes with the same parameters that guide us whenever we examine a new diagnostic or therapeutic method. The main criteria remain the evaluation of risk versus advantage, the respect of a person as a human being and the respect of autonomy and privacy.

There is a need to state general ethical and legal guidelines to prevent discrimination and the genetic stigma of the population at risk.

The basic guidelines are:

— The genetic service should be easily accessible to everyone in order to prevent its exploitation by only those who have resources which will increase social inequality.

— There is a need for international information and transfer of technology and knowledge between all countries.

— One should respect the will of persons screened and their right to decide about their participation and about the use of the information obtained.

— Full information should be given to the patient or his legal agent. Medical secrecy should be kept and information should not be passed on to a third party without consent. Even if family members of the patient may be at risk, medical secrecy has to be kept unless there is a serious harm and this harm could be avoided by disclosing the information; the confidentiality can be breached only as a last resort when all trials to convince the patient to pass on the information by himself, have failed; even in this case, the relevant genetic information only should be disclosed.

— The disclosure of information to a third party or the accessibility to personal genetic data should be allowed only with the patient's informed consent.

Appendix 1.5   Internation Conference on Harmonization of Technical Requirements for Registration of Pharmaceuticals for Human Use, Guidelines for Good Clinical Practice (1996)

2. The Principles of ICH GCP

2.1 Clinical trials should be conducted in accordance with the ethical principles that have their origin in the Declaration of Helsinki, and that are consistent with GCP and the applicable regulatory requirement(s).

2.2 Before a trial is initiated, foreseeable risks and inconveniences should be weighed against the anticipated benefit for the individual trial subject and society. A trial should be initiated and continued only if the anticipated benefits justify the risks.

2.3 The rights, safety, and well-being of the trial subjects are the most important considerations and should prevail over interests of science and society.

2.4 The available nonclinical and clinical information on an investigational product should be adequate to support the proposed clinical trial.

2.5 Clinical trials should be scientifically sound, and described in a clear, detailed protocol.

2.6 A trial should be conducted in compliance with the protocol that has received prior institutional review board (IRB)/independent ethics committee (IEC) approval/favourable opinion.

2.7 The medical care given to, and medical decisions made on behalf of, subjects should always be the responsibility of a qualified physician or, when appropriate, of a qualified dentist.

2.8 Each individual involved in conducting a trial should be qualified by education, training, and experience to perform his or her respective task(s).

2.9 Freely given informed consent should be obtained from every subject prior to clinical trial participation.

2.10 All clinical trial information should be recorded, handled, and stored in a way that allows its accurate reporting, interpretation and verification.

2.11 The confidentiality of records that could identify subjects should be protected, respecting the privacy and confidentiality rules in accordance with the applicable regulatory requirement(s).

2.12 Investigational products should be manufactured, handled, and stored in accordance with applicable good manufacturing practice (GMP). They should be used in accordance with the approved protocol.

2.13 Systems with procedures that assure the quality of every aspect of the trial should be implemented.

3. Institutional Review Board/Independent Ethics Committee (IRB/IEC)

3.1 Responsibilities

3.1.1 An IRB/IEC should safeguard the rights, safety, and well-being of all trial subjects. Special attention should be paid to trials that may include vulnerable subjects.

3.1.2 The IRB/IEC should obtain the following documents:

trial protocol(s)/amendment(s), written informed consent form(s) and consent form updates that the investigator proposes for use in the trial, subject recruitment procedures (e.g. advertisements), written information to be provided to subjects, Investigator's Brochure (IB), available safety information, information about payments and compensation available to subjects, the investigator's current curriculum vitae and/or other documentation evidencing qualifications, and any other documents that the IRB/IEC may need to fulfil its responsibilities.

The IRB/IEC should review a proposed clinical trial within a reasonable time and document its views in writing, clearly identifying the trial, the documents reviewed and the dates for the following:

- approval/favourable opinion;
- modifications required prior to its approval/favourable opinion;
- disapproval/negative opinion; and
- termination/suspension of any prior approval/favourable opinion.

3.1.3 The IRB/IEC should consider the qualifications of the investigator for the proposed trial, as documented by a current curriculum vitae and/or by any other relevant documentation the IRB/IEC requests.

3.1.4 The IRB/IEC should conduct continuing review of each ongoing trial at intervals appropriate to the degree of risk to human subjects, but at least once per year.

3.1.5 The IRB/IEC may request more information than is outlined in paragraph 4.8.10 be given to subjects when, in the judgement of the IRB/IEC, the additional information would add meaningfully to the protection of the rights, safety and/or well-being of the subjects.

3.1.6 When a non-therapeutic trial is to be carried out with the consent of the subject's legally acceptable representative (see 4.8.12, 4.8.14), the IRB/IEC should determine that the proposed protocol and/or other document(s) adequately addresses relevant ethical concerns and meets applicable regulatory requirements for such trials.

3.1.7 Where the protocol indicates that prior consent of the trial subject or the subject's legally acceptable representative is not possible (see 4.8.15), the IRB/IEC should determine that the proposed protocol and/or other document(s) adequately addresses relevant ethical concerns and meets applicable regulatory requirements for such trials (i.e. in emergency situations).

3.1.8 The IRB/IEC should review both the amount and method of payment to subjects to assure that neither presents problems of coercion or undue influence on the trial subjects. Payments to a subject should be prorated and not wholly contingent on completion of the trial by the subject.

3.1.9 The IRB/IEC should ensure that information regarding payment to subjects, including the methods, amounts, and schedule of payment to trial subjects, is set forth in the written informed consent form and any other written information to be provided to subjects. The way payment will be prorated should be specified.

3.2 Composition, Functions and Operations

3.2.1 The IRB/IEC should consist of a reasonable number of members, who collectively have the qualifications and experience to review and evaluate the science, medical aspects, and ethics of the proposed trial. It is recommended that the IRB/IEC should include:

(a) At least five members.
(b) At least one member whose primary area of interest is in a nonscientific area.
(c) At least one member who is independent of the institution/trial site.

Only those IRB/IEC members who are independent of the investigator and the sponsor of the trial should vote/provide opinion on a trial-related matter.

A list of IRB/IEC members and their qualifications should be maintained.

3.2.2 The IRB/IEC should perform its functions according to written operating procedures, should maintain written records of its activities and minutes of its meetings, and should comply with GCP and with the applicable regulatory requirement(s).

3.2.3 An IRB/IEC should make its decisions at announced meetings at which at least a quorum, as stipulated in its written operating procedures, is present.

3.2.4 Only members who participate in the IRB/IEC review and discussion should vote/provide their opinion and/or advise.

3.2.5 The investigator may provide information on any aspect of the trial, but should not participate in the deliberations of the IRB/IEC or in the vote/opinion of the IRB/IEC.

3.2.6 An IRB/IEC may invite nonmembers with expertise in special areas for assistance.

• • •

4.8 Informed Consent of Trial Subjects

4.8.1 In obtaining and documenting informed consent, the investigator should comply with the applicable regulatory requirement(s), and should adhere to GCP and to the ethical principles that have their origin in the Declaration of Helsinki. Prior to the beginning of the trial, the investigator should have the IRB/IEC's written approval/favourable opinion of the written informed consent form and any other written information to be provided to subjects.

4.8.2 The written informed consent form and any other written information to be provided to subjects should be revised whenever important new information becomes available that may be relevant to the subject's consent. Any revised written informed consent form, and written information should receive the IRB/IEC's approval/favourable opinion in advance of use. The subject or the subject's legally acceptable representative should be informed in a timely manner if new information becomes available that may be relevant to the subject's willingness to continue participation in the trial. The communication of this information should be documented.

4.8.3 Neither the investigator, nor the trial staff, should coerce or unduly influence a subject to participate or to continue to participate in a trial.

4.8.4 None of the oral and written information concerning the trial, including the written informed consent form, should contain any language that causes the subject or the subject's legally acceptable representative to waive or to appear to waive any legal rights, or that releases or appears to release the investigator, the institution, the sponsor, or their agents from liability for negligence.

4.8.5 The investigator, or a person designated by the investigator, should fully inform the subject or, if the subject is unable to provide informed consent, the subject's legally acceptable representative, of all pertinent aspects of the trial including the written information given approval/favourable opinion by the IRB/IEC.

4.8.6 The language used in the oral and written information about the trial, including the written informed consent form, should be as non-technical as practical and should be understandable to the subject or the subject's legally acceptable representative and the impartial witness, where applicable.

4.8.7 Before informed consent may be obtained, the investigator, or a person designated by the investigator, should provide the subject or the subject's legally acceptable representative ample time and opportunity to inquire about details of the trial and to decide whether or not to participate in the trial. All questions about the trial should be answered to the satisfaction of the subject or the subject's legally acceptable representative.

4.8.8 Prior to a subject's participation in the trial, the written informed consent form should be signed and personally dated by the subject or by the subject's legally acceptable representative, and by the person who conducted the informed consent discussion.

4.8.9 If a subject is unable to read or if a legally acceptable representative is unable to read, an impartial witness should be present during the entire informed consent discussion. After the written informed consent form and any other written information to be provided to subjects, is read and explained to the subject or the subject's legally acceptable representative, and after the subject or the subject's legally acceptable representative has orally consented to the subject's participation in the trial and, if capable of doing so, has signed and personally dated the informed consent form, the witness should sign and personally date the consent form. By signing the consent form, the witness attests that the information in the consent form and any other written information was accurately explained to, and apparently understood by, the subject or the subject's legally acceptable representative, and that informed consent was freely given by the subject or the subject's legally acceptable representative.

4.8.10 Both the informed consent discussion and the written informed consent form and any other written information to be provided to subjects should include explanations of the following:

 (a) That the trial involves research.

 (b) The purpose of the trial.

 (c) The trial treatment(s) and the probability for random assignment to each treatment.

 (d) The trial procedures to be followed, including all invasive procedures.

 (e) The subject's responsibilities.

 (f) Those aspects of the trial that are experimental.

 (g) The reasonably foreseeable risks or inconveniences to the subject and, when applicable, to an embryo, fetus, or nursing infant.

 (h) The reasonably expected benefits. When there is no intended clinical benefit to the subject, the subject should be made aware of this.

 (i) The alternative procedure(s) or course(s) of treatment that may be available to the subject, and their important potential benefits and risks.

 (j) The compensation and/or treatment available to the subject in the event of trial-related injury.

(k) The anticipated prorated payment, if any, to the subject for participating in the trial.

(l) The anticipated expenses, if any, to the subject for participating in the trial.

(m) That the subject's participation in the trial is voluntary and that the subject may refuse to participate or withdraw from the trial, at any time, without penalty or loss of benefits to which the subject is otherwise entitled.

(n) That the monitor(s), the auditor(s), the IRB/IEC, and the regulatory authority(ies) will be granted direct access to the subject's original medical records for verification of clinical trial procedures and/or data, without violating the confidentiality of the subject, to the extent permitted by the applicable laws and regulations and that, by signing a written informed consent form, the subject or the subject's legally acceptable representative is authorizing such access.

(o) That records identifying the subject will be kept confidential and, to the extent permitted by the applicable laws and/or regulations, will not be made publicly available. If the results of the trial are published, the subject's identity will remain confidential.

(p) That the subject or the subject's legally acceptable representative will be informed in a timely manner if information becomes available that may be relevant to the subject's willingness to continue participation in the trial.

(q) The person(s) to contact for further information regarding the trial and the rights of trial subjects, and whom to contact in the event of trial-related injury.

(r) The foreseeable circumstances and/or reasons under which the subject's participation in the trial may be terminated.

(s) The expected duration of the subject's participation in the trial.

(t) The approximate number of subjects involved in the trial.

4.8.11 Prior to participation in the trial, the subject or the subject's legally acceptable representative should receive a copy of the signed and dated written informed consent form and any other written information provided to the subjects. During a subject's participation in the trial, the subject or the subject's legally acceptable representative should receive a copy of the signed and dated consent form updates and a copy of any amendments to the written information provided to subjects.

4.8.12 When a clinical trial (therapeutic or non-therapeutic) includes subjects who can only be enrolled in the trial with the consent of the subject's legally acceptable representative (e.g., minors, or patients with severe dementia), the subject should be informed about the trial to the extent compatible with the subject's understanding and, if capable, the subject should sign and personally date the written informed consent.

4.8.13 Except as described in 4.8.14, a non-therapeutic trial (i.e. a trial in which there is no anticipated direct clinical benefit to the subject), should be conducted in subjects who personally give consent and who sign and date the written informed consent form.

4.8.14 Non-therapeutic trials may be conducted in subjects with consent of a legally acceptable representative provided the following conditions are fulfilled:

(a) The objectives of the trial can not be met by means of a trial in subjects who can give informed consent personally.

(b) The foreseeable risks to the subjects are low.

(c) The negative impact on the subject's well-being is minimized and low.

(d) The trial is not prohibited by law.

(e) The approval/favourable opinion of the IRB/IEC is expressly sought on the inclusion of such subjects, and the written approval/ favourable opinion covers this aspect.

Such trials, unless an exception is justified, should be conducted in patients having a disease or condition for which the investigational product is intended. Subjects in these trials should be particularly closely monitored and should be withdrawn if they appear to be unduly distressed.

4.8.15 In emergency situations, when prior consent of the subject is not possible, the consent of the subject's legally acceptable representative, if present, should be requested. When prior consent of the subject is not possible, and the subject's legally acceptable representative is not available, enrolment of the subject should require measures described in the protocol and/or elsewhere, with documented approval/favourable opinion by the IRB/IEC, to protect the rights, safety and well-being of the subject and to ensure compliance with applicable regulatory requirements. The subject or the subject's legally acceptable representative should be informed about the trial as soon as possible and consent to continue and other consent as appropriate (see 4.8.10) should be requested.

Appendix 1.6   CIOMS, International Guiding Principles for Biomedical Research Involving Animals (1984)

Council for International Organizations of Medical Sciences

Basic Principles

I. The advancement of biological knowledge and the development of improved means for the protection of the health and wellbeing both of man and of animals require recourse to experimentation on intact live animals of a wide variety of species.

II. Methods such as mathematical models, computer simulation and *in vitro* biological systems should be used wherever appropriate.

III. Animal experiments should be undertaken only after due consideration of their relevance for human or animal health and the advancement of biological knowledge.

IV. The animals selected for an experiment should be of an appropriate species and quality, and the minimum number required, to obtain scientifically valid results.

V. Investigators and other personnel should never fail to treat animals as sentient, and should regard their proper care and use and the avoidance or minimization of discomfort, distress, or pain as ethical imperatives.

VI. Investigators should assume that procedures that would cause pain in human beings cause pain in other vertebrate species although more needs to be known about the perception of pain in animals.

VII. Procedures with animals that may cause more than momentary or minimal pain or distress should be performed with appropriate sedation, analgesia, or anaesthesia in accordance with accepted veterinary practice. Surgical or other painful procedures should not be performed on unanaesthetized animals paralysed by chemical agents.

VIII. Where waivers are required in relation to the provisions of article VII, the decisions should not rest solely with the investigators directly concerned but should be made, with due regard to the provisions of articles IV, V and VI, by a suitably constituted review body. Such waivers should not be made solely for the purposes of teaching or demonstration.

IX. At the end of, or when appropriate during, an experiment, animals that would otherwise suffer severe or chronic pain, distress, discomfort, or disablement that cannot be relieved should be painlessly killed.

X. The best possible living conditions should be maintained for animals kept for biomedical purposes. Normally the care of animals should be under the supervision of veterinarians having experience in laboratory animal science. In any case, veterinary care should be available as required.

XI. It is the responsibility of the director of an institute or department using animals to ensure that investigators and personnel have appropriate qualifications or experience for conducting procedures on animals. Adequate opportunities shall be provided for in-service training, including the proper and humane concern for the animals under their care.

Appendix 1.7   CIOMS, International Guidelines for Ethical Review of Epidemiologial Studies (1991)

Council for International Organizations of Medical Sciences

Ethical Principles Applied to Epidemiology

Informed Consent

Individual consent

1. When individuals are to be subjects of epidemiological studies, their informed consent will usually be sought. For epidemiological studies that use personally identifiable private data, the rules for informed consent vary, as discussed further below. Consent is informed when it is given by a person who understands the purpose and nature of the study, what participation in the study requires the person to do and to risk, and what benefits are intended to result from the study.

2. An investigator who proposes not to seek informed consent has the obligation to explain to an ethical review committee how the study would be ethical in its absence: it may be impractical to locate subjects whose records are to be examined, or the purpose of some studies would be frustrated—for example, prospective subjects on being informed would change the behavior that it is proposed to study, or might feel needlessly anxious about why they were subjects of study. The investigator will provide assurances that strict safeguards will be maintained to protect confidentiality and that the study is aimed at protecting or advancing health. Another justification for not seeking informed consent may be that subjects are made aware through public announcements that it is customary to make personal data available for epidemiological studies.

3. An ethical issue may arise when occupational records, medical records, tissue samples, etc. are used for a purpose for which consent was not given, although the study threatens no harm. Individuals or their public representatives should normally be told that their data might be used in epidemiological studies, and what means of protecting confidentiality are provided. Consent is not required for use of publicly available information, although countries and communities differ with regard to the definition of what information about citizens is regarded as public. However, when such information is to be used, it is understood that investigators will minimize disclosure of personally sensitive information.

4. Some organizations and government agencies employ epidemiologists who may be permitted by legislation or employees' contracts to have access to data without subjects' consent. These epidemiologists must then consider whether it is ethical for them, in a given case, to use this power of access to personal data. Ethically, they may still be expected either to seek the consent of the individuals concerned, or to justify their access without such consent. Access may be ethical on such grounds as minimal risk of harm to individuals, public benefit, and investigators' protection of the confidentiality of the individuals whose data they study.

Community agreement

5. When it is not possible to request informed consent from every individual to be studied, the agreement of a representative of a community or group may be sought, but the representative should be chosen according to the nature, traditions and political philosophy of the community or group. Approval given by a community representative should be consistent with general ethical principles. When investigators work with communities, they will consider communal rights and protection as they would individual rights and protection. For communities in which collective decision-making

is customary, communal leaders can express the collective will. However, the refusal of individuals to participate in a study has to be respected: a leader may express agreement on behalf of a community, but an individual's refusal of personal participation is binding.

6. When people are appointed by agencies outside a group, such as a department of government, to speak for members of the group, investigators and ethical review committees should consider how authentically these people speak for the group, and if necessary seek also the agreement of other representatives. Representatives of a community or group may sometimes be in a position to participate in designing the study and in its ethical assessment.

7. The definition of a community or group for purposes of epidemiological study may be a matter of ethical concern. When members of a community are naturally conscious of its activities as a community and feel common interests with other members, the community exists, irrespective of the study proposal. Investigators will be sensitive to how a community is constituted or defines itself, and will respect the rights of underprivileged groups.

8. For purposes of epidemiological study, investigators may define groups that are composed of statistically, geographically or otherwise associated individuals who do not normally interact socially. When such groups are artificially created for scientific study, group members may not readily be identifiable as leaders or representatives, and individuals may not be expected to risk disadvantage for the benefit of others. Accordingly, it will be more difficult to ensure group representation, and all the more important to obtain subjects' free and informed consent to participate.

Selective disclosure of information

9. In epidemiology, an acceptable study technique involves selective disclosure of information, which seems to conflict with the principle of informed consent. For certain epidemiological studies non-disclosure is permissible, even essential, so as to not influence the spontaneous conduct under investigation, and to avoid obtaining responses that the respondent might give in order to please the questioner. Selective disclosure may be benign and ethically permissible, provided that it does not induce subjects to do what they would not otherwise consent to do. An ethical review committee may permit disclosure of only selected information when this course is justified.

Undue influence

10. Prospective subjects may not feel free to refuse requests from those who have power or influence over them. Therefore the identity of the investigator or other person assigned to invite prospective subjects to participate must be made known to them. Investigators are expected to explain to the ethical review committee how they propose to neutralize such apparent influence. It is ethically questionable whether subjects should be recruited from among groups that are unduly influenced by persons in authority over them or by community leaders, if the study can be done with subjects who are not in this category.

Inducement to participate

11. Individuals or communities should not be pressured to participate in a study. However, it can be hard to draw the line between exerting pressure or offering inappropriate inducements and creating legitimate motivation. The benefits of a study, such as increased or new knowledge, are proper inducements. However, when people or communities lack basic health services or money, the prospect of being rewarded by goods, services or cash payments can induce participation. To determine the ethical propriety of such inducements, they must be assessed in the light of the traditions of the culture.

12. Risks involved in participation should be acceptable to subjects even in the absence of inducement. It is acceptable to repay incurred expenses, such as for travel. Similarly, promises of compensation and care for damage, injury or loss of income should not be considered inducements.

Maximizing Benefit

Communication of study results

13. Part of the benefit that communities, groups and individuals may reasonably expect from participating in studies is that they will be told of findings that pertain to their health. Where findings could be applied in public health measures to improve community health, they should be communicated to the health authorities. In informing individuals of the findings and their pertinence to health, their level of literacy and comprehension must be considered. Research protocols should include provision for communicating such information to communities and individuals.

Research findings and advice to communities should be publicized by whatever suitable means are available. When HIV-prevalence studies are conducted by unlinked anonymous screening, there should be, where feasible, provision for voluntary HIV-antibody testing under conditions of informed consent, with pre-and post-test counselling, and assurance of confidentiality.

Impossibility of communicating study results

14. Subjects of epidemiological studies should be advised that it may not be possible to inform them about findings that pertain to their health, but that they should not take this to mean that they are free of the disease or condition under study. Often it may not be possible to extract from pooled findings information pertaining to individuals and their families, but when findings indicate a need of health care, those concerned should be advised of means of obtaining personal diagnosis and advice.

When epidemiological data are unlinked, a disadvantage to subjects is that individuals at risk cannot be informed of useful findings pertinent to their health. When subjects cannot be advised individually to seek medical attention, the ethical duty to do good can be served by making pertinent health-care advice available to their communities.

Release of study results

15. Investigators may be unable to compel release of data held by governmental or commercial agencies, but as health professionals they have an ethical obligation to advocate the release of information that is in the public interest.

Sponsors of studies may press investigators to present their findings in ways that advance special interests, such as to show that a product or procedure is or is not harmful to health. Sponsors must not present interpretations or inferences, or theories and hypotheses, as if they were proven truths.

Health care for the community under study

16. The undertaking of an epidemiological project in a developing country may create the expectation in the community concerned that it will be provided with health care, at least while the research workers are present. Such an expectation should not be frustrated, and, where people need health care, arrangements should be made to have them treated or they should be referred to a local health service that can provide the needed care.

Training local health personnel

17. While studies are in progress, particularly in developing countries, the opportunity should be taken to train local health workers in skills and techniques that can be used to improve health services. For instance, by training them in the operation of measuring devices and calculating machines, when a study team departs it leaves something of value, such as the ability to monitor disease or mortality rates.

Minimizing Harm

Causing harm and doing wrong

18. Investigators planning studies will recognize the risk of causing harm, in the sense of bringing disadvantage, and of doing wrong, in the sense of transgressing values. Harm may occur, for instance, when scarce health personnel are diverted from their routine duties to serve the needs of a study, or when, unknown to a community, its health-care priorities are changed. It is wrong to regard members of communities as only impersonal material for study, even if they are not harmed.

19. Ethical review must always assess the risk of subjects or groups suffering stigmatization, prejudice, loss of prestige or self-esteem, or economic loss as a result of taking part in a study. Investigators will inform ethical review committees and prospective subjects of perceived risks, and of proposals to prevent or mitigate them. Investigators must be able to demonstrate that the benefits outweigh the risks for both individuals and groups. There should be a thorough analysis to determine who would be at risk and who would benefit from the study. It is unethical to expose persons to avoidable risks disproportionate to the expected benefits, or to permit a known risk to remain if it can be avoided or at least minimized.

20. When a healthy person is a member of a population or sub-group at raised risk and engages in high-risk activities, it is unethical not to propose measures for protecting the population or sub-group.

Preventing harm to groups

21. Epidemiological studies may inadvertently expose groups as well as individuals to harm, such as economic loss, stigmatization, blame, or withdrawal of services. Investigators who find sensitive information that may put a group at risk of adverse criticism or treatment should be discreet in communicating and explaining their findings. When the location or circumstances of a study are important to understanding the results, the investigators will explain by what means they propose to protect the group from harm or disadvantage; such means include provisions for confidentiality and the use of language that does not imply moral criticism of subjects' behavior.

Harmful publicity

22. Conflict may appear between, on the one hand, doing no harm and, on the other, telling the truth and openly disclosing scientific findings. Harm may be mitigated by interpreting data in a way that protects the interests of those at risk, and is at the same time consistent with scientific integrity. Investigators should, where possible, anticipate and avoid misinterpretation that might cause harm.

Respect for social mores

23. Disruption of social mores is usually regarded as harmful. Although cultural values and social mores must be respected, it may be a specific aim of an epidemiological study to stimulate change in certain customs or conventional behavior to lead through change to healthful behavior—for instance, with regard to diet or a hazardous occupation.

24. Although members of communities have a right not to have others impose an uninvited "good" on them, studies expected to result in health benefits are usually considered ethically acceptable and not harmful. Ethical review committees should consider a study's potential for beneficial change. However, investigators should not overstate such benefits, in case a community's agreement to participate is unduly influenced by its expectation of better health services.

Sensitivity to different cultures

25. Epidemiologists often investigate cultural groups other than their own, inside or outside their own countries, and undertake studies initiated from outside the culture, community or country in which the study is to be conducted. Sponsoring and host countries may differ in the ways in which, in their cultures, ethical values are understood and applied—for instance, with regard to autonomy of individuals.

Investigators must respect the ethical standards of their own countries and the cultural expectations of the societies in which epidemiological studies are undertaken, unless this implies a violation of a transcending moral rule. Investigators risk harming their reputation by pursuing work that host countries find acceptable but their own countries consider offensive. Similarly, they may transgress the cultural values of the host countries by uncritically conforming to the expectations of their own.

Confidentiality

26. Research may involve collecting and storing data relating to individuals and groups, and such data, if disclosed to third parties, may cause harm or distress. Consequently, investigators should make arrangements for protecting the confidentiality of such data by, for example, omitting information that might lead to the identification of individual subjects, or limiting access to the data, or by other means. It is customary in epidemiology to aggregate numbers so that individual identities are obscured. Where group confidentiality cannot be maintained or is violated, the investigators should take steps to maintain or restore a group's good name and status. Information obtained about subjects is generally divisible into:

Unlinked information, which cannot be linked, associated or connected with the person to whom it refers; as this person is not known to the investigator, confidentiality is not at stake and the question of consent does not arise.

Linked information, which may be:

— anonymous, when the information cannot be linked to the person to whom it refers except by a code or other means known only to that person, and the investigator cannot know the identity of the person;

— non-nominal, when the information can be linked to the person by a code (not including personal identification) known to the person and the investigator; or

— nominal or nominative, when the information is linked to the person by means of personal identification, usually the name.

Epidemiologists discard personal identifying information when consolidating data for purposes of statistical analysis. Identifiable personal data will not be used when a study can be done without personal identification—for instance, in testing unlinked anonymous blood samples for HIV infection. When personal identifiers remain on records used for a study, investigators should explain to review committees why this is necessary and how confidentiality will be protected. If, with the consent of individual subjects, investigators link different sets of data regarding individuals, they normally preserve confidentiality by aggregating individual data into tables or diagrams. In government service the obligation to protect confidentiality is frequently reinforced by the practice of swearing employees to secrecy.

Conflict of Interest

Identification of conflict of interest

27. It is an ethical rule that investigators should have no undisclosed conflict of interest with their study collaborators, sponsors or subjects. Investigators should disclose to the ethical re-

view committee any potential conflict of interest. Conflict can arise when a commercial or other sponsor may wish to use study results to promote a product or service, or when it may not be politically convenient to disclose findings.

28. Epidemiological studies may be initiated, or financially or otherwise supported, by governmental or other agencies that employ investigators. In the occupational and environmental health fields, several well-defined special-interest groups may be in conflict: shareholders, management, labour, government regulatory agencies, public interest advocacy groups, and others. Epidemiological investigators may be employed by any of these groups. It can be difficult to avoid pressures resulting from such conflict of interest, and consequent distorted interpretations of study findings. Similar conflict may arise in studies of the effects of drugs and in testing medical devices.

29. Investigators and ethical review committees will be sensitive to the risk of conflict, and committees will not normally approve proposals in which conflict of interest is inherent. If, exceptionally, such a proposal is approved, the conflict of interest should be disclosed to prospective subjects and their communities.

30. There may appear to be conflict when subjects do not want to change their behavior and investigators believe that they ought to do so for the sake of their health. However, this may not be a true conflict of interest, as the investigators are motivated by the subjects' health interests.

Scientific Objectivity and Advocacy

31. Honesty and impartiality are essential in designing and conducting studies, and presenting and interpreting findings. Data will not be withheld, misrepresented or manipulated. Investigators may discover health hazards that demand correction, and become advocates of means to protect and restore health. In this event, their advocacy must be seen to rely on objective, scientific data.

Ethical Review Procedures

Requirement of Ethical Review

32. The provisions for ethical review in a society are influenced by economic and political considerations, the organization of health care and research, and the degree of independence of investigators. Whatever the circumstances, there is a responsibility to ensure that the Declaration of Helsinki and the CIOMS International Guidelines for Biomedical Research Involving Human Subjects are taken into account in epidemiological studies.

33. The requirement that proposals for epidemiological studies be submitted to independent ethical review applies irrespective of the source of the proposals—academic, governmental, healthcare, commercial, or other. Sponsors should recognize the necessity of ethical review and facilitate the establishment of ethical review committees. Sponsors and investigators are expected to submit their proposals to ethical review, and this should not be overlooked even when sponsors have legal power to permit investigators access to data. An exception is justified when epidemiologists must investigate outbreaks of acute communicable diseases. Then they must proceed without delay to identify and control health risks. They cannot be expected to await the formal approval of an ethical review committee. Nevertheless, in such circumstances the investigator will, as far as possible, respect the rights of individuals, namely freedom, privacy, and confidentiality.

Ethical Review Committees

34. Ethical review committees may be created under the aegis of national or local health administrations, national medical research councils, or other nationally representative health-

care bodies. The authority of committees operating on a local basis may be confined to one institution or extend to all biomedical studies undertaken in a defined political jurisdiction. However committees are created, and however their jurisdiction is defined, they should establish working rules—regarding, for instance, frequency of meetings, a quorum of members, decision-making procedures, and review of decisions, and they should issue such rules to prospective investigators.

35. In a highly centralized administration, a national review committee may be constituted to review study protocols from both scientific and ethical standpoints. In countries with a decentralized administration, protocols are more effectively and conveniently reviewed at a local or regional level. Local ethical review committees have two responsibilities:

— to verify that all proposed interventions have been assessed for safety by a competent expert body, and

—to ensure that all other ethical issues are satisfactorily resolved.

36. Local review committees act as a panel of investigators' peers, and their composition should be such as can ensure adequate review of the study proposals referred to them. Their membership should include epidemiologists, other health practitioners, and lay persons qualified to represent a range of community, cultural and moral values. Committees should have diverse composition and include representatives of any populations specially targeted for study. The members should change periodically to prevent individuals from becoming unduly influential, and to widen the network involved in ethical review. Independence from the investigators is maintained by precluding any member with a direct interest in a proposal from participating in its assessment.

Ethical Conduct of Members of Review Committees

37. Ethical review committee members must carefully guard against any tendencies to unethical conduct on their own part. In particular, they should protect the confidentiality of review-committee documents and discussions. Also, they should not compel investigators to submit to unnecessary repetition of review.

Representation of the Community

38. The community to be studied should be represented in the ethical review process. This is consistent with respect for the culture, the dignity and self-reliance of the community, and the aim of achieving community members' full understanding of the study. It should not be considered that lack of formal education disqualifies community members from joining in constructive discussion on issues relating to the study and the application of its findings.

Balancing Personal and Social Perspectives

39. In performing reviews, committees will consider both personal and social perspectives. While, at the personal level, it is essential to ensure individual informed and free consent, such consent alone may not be sufficient to render a study ethical if the individual's community finds the study objectionable. Social values may raise broad issues that affect future populations and the physical environment. For example, in proposals for the widespread application of measures to control intermediate hosts of disease organisms, investigators will anticipate the effects of those measures on communities and the environment, and review committees will ensure that there is adequate provision for the investigators to monitor the application of the measures so as to prevent unwanted effects.

Assuring Scientific Soundness

40. The primary functions of ethical review are to protect human subjects against risks of harm or wrong, and to facilitate beneficial studies. Scientific review and ethical review cannot be considered separately: a study that is scientifically unsound is unethical in exposing subjects to risk or inconvenience and achieving no benefit in knowledge. Normally, therefore, ethical review committees consider both scientific and ethical aspects. An ethical review committee may refer technical aspects of scientific review to a scientifically qualified person or committee, but will reach its own decision, based on such qualified advice, on scientific soundness. If a review committee is satisfied that a proposal is scientifically sound, it will then consider whether any risk to the subject is justified by the expected benefit, and whether the proposal is satisfactory with regard to informed consent and other ethical requirements.

Assessment of Safety and Quality

41. All drugs and devices under investigation must meet adequate standards of safety. In this respect, many countries lack resources to undertake independent assessment of technical data. A governmental multidisciplinary committee with authority to co-opt experts is the most suitable body for assessing the safety and quality of medicines, devices and procedures. Such a committee should include clinicians, pharmacologists, statisticians and epidemiologists, among others; for epidemiological studies, epidemiologists occupy a position of obvious significance. Ethical review procedures should provide for consultation with such a committee.

Equity in the Selection of Subjects

42. Epidemiological studies are intended to benefit populations, but individual subjects are expected to accept any risks associated with studies. When research is intended to benefit mostly the better off or healthier members of a population, it is particularly important in selecting subjects to avoid inequity on the basis of age, socioeconomic status, disability or other variables. Potential benefits and harm should be distributed equitably within and among communities that differ on grounds of age, gender, race, or culture, or other variables.

Vulnerable and Dependent Groups

43. Ethical review committees should be particularly vigilant in the case of proposals involving populations primarily of children, pregnant and nursing women, persons with mental illness or handicap, members of communities unfamiliar with medical concepts, and persons with restricted freedom to make truly independent choices, such as prisoners and medical students. Similar vigilance is called for in the case of proposals for invasive research with no direct benefit to its subjects.

•   •   •

Appendix 1.8   CIOMS, International Ethical Guidelines for Biomedical Research Involving Human Subjects (1993)

Council for International Organizations of Medical Sciences 1993

General Ethical Principles

All research involving human subjects should be conducted in accordance with three basic ethical principles, namely respect for persons, beneficence and justice. It is generally agreed that these principles, which in the abstract have equal moral force, guide the conscientious preparation of proposals for scientific studies. In varying circumstances they may be expressed differently and given different moral weight, and their application may lead to different decisions or courses of action. The present guidelines are directed at the application of these principles to research involving human subjects.

Respect for persons incorporates at least two fundamental ethical considerations, namely:

a) respect for autonomy, which requires that those who are capable of deliberation about their personal choices should be treated with respect for their capacity for self-determination; and
b) protection of persons with impaired or diminished autonomy, which requires that those who are dependent or vulnerable be afforded security against harm or abuse.

Beneficence refers to the ethical obligation to maximize benefits and to minimize harms and wrongs. This principle gives rise to norms requiring that the risks of research be reasonable in the light of the expected benefits, that the research design be sound, and that the investigators be competent both to conduct the research and to safeguard the welfare of the research subjects. Beneficence further proscribes the deliberate infliction of harm on persons; this aspect of beneficence is sometimes expressed as a separate principle, nonmaleficence (do no harm).

Justice refers to the ethical obligation to treat each person in accordance with what is morally right and proper, to give each person what is due to him or her. In the ethics of research involving human subjects the principle refers primarily to distributive justice, which requires the equitable distribution of both the burdens and the benefits of participation in research. Differences in distribution of burdens and benefits are justifiable only if they are based on morally relevant distinctions between persons; one such distinction is vulnerability. "Vulnerability" refers to a substantial incapacity to protect one's own interests owing to such impediments as lack of capability to give informed consent, lack of alternative means of obtaining medical care or other expensive necessities, or being a junior or subordinate member of a hierarchical group. Accordingly, special provisions must be made for the protection of the rights and welfare of vulnerable persons.

The Guidelines

Informed Consent of Subjects

Guideline 1: Individual informed consent
For all biomedical research involving human subjects, the investigator must obtain the informed consent of the prospective subject or, in the case of an individual who is not capable of giving informed consent, the proxy consent of a properly authorized representative.

Guideline 2: Essential information for prospective research subjects
Before requesting an individual's consent to participate in research, the investigator must provide the individual with the following information, in language that he or she is capable of understanding:

— that each individual is invited to participate as a subject in research, and the aims and methods of the research;

— the expected duration of the subject's participation;
— the benefits that might reasonably be expected to result to the subject or to others as an outcome of the research;
— any foreseeable risks or discomfort to the subject, associated with participation in the research;
— any alternative procedures or courses of treatment that might be as advantageous to the subject as the procedure or treatment being tested;
— the extent to which confidentiality of records in which the subject is identified will be maintained;
— the extent of the investigator's responsibility, if any, to provide medical services to the subject;
— that therapy will be provided free of charge for specified types of research-related injury;
— whether the subject or the subject's family or dependents will be compensated for disability or death resulting from such injury; and
— that the individual is free to refuse to participate and will be free to withdraw from the research at any time without penalty or loss of benefits to which he or she would otherwise be entitled.

Guideline 3: Obligations of investigators regarding informed consent
The investigator has a duty to:

— communicate to the prospective subject all the information necessary for adequately informed consent;
— give the prospective subject full opportunity and encouragement to ask questions;
— exclude the possibility of unjustified deception, undue influence and intimidation;
— seek consent only after the prospective subject has adequate knowledge of the relevant facts and of the consequences of participation, and has had sufficient opportunity to consider whether to participate;
— as a general rule, obtain from each prospective subject a signed form as evidence of informed consent; and
— renew the informed consent of each subject if there are material changes in the conditions or procedures of the research.

Guideline 4: Inducement to participate
Subjects may be paid for inconvenience and time spent, and should be reimbursed for expenses incurred, in connection with their participation in research; they may also receive free medical services. However, the payments should not be so large or the medical services so extensive as to induce prospective subjects to consent to participate in the research against their better judgment ("undue inducement"). All payments, reimbursements and medical services to be provided to research subjects should be approved by an ethical review committee.

Guideline 5: Research involving children
Before undertaking research involving children, the investigator must ensure that:

— children will not be involved in research that might equally well be carried out with adults;
— the purpose of the research is to obtain knowledge relevant to the health needs of children;
— a parent or legal guardian of each child has given proxy consent;
— the consent of each child has been obtained to the extent of the child's capabilities;
— the child's refusal to participate in research must always be respected unless according to the research protocol the child would receive therapy for which there is no medically-acceptable alternative;
— the risk presented by interventions not intended to benefit the individual child-subject is low and commensurate with the importance of the knowledge to be gained; and

— interventions that are intended to provide therapeutic benefit are likely to be at least as advantageous to the individual child-subject as any available alternative.

Guideline 6: Research involving persons with mental or behavioral disorders

Before undertaking research involving individuals who by reason of mental or behavioural disorders are not capable of giving adequately informed consent, the investigator must ensure that:

— such persons will not be subjects of research that might equally well be carried out on persons in full possession of their mental faculties;
— the purpose of the research is to obtain knowledge relevant to the particular health needs of persons with mental or behavioural disorders;
— the consent of each subject has been obtained to the extent of that subject's capabilities, and a prospective subject's refusal to participate in non-clinical research is always respected;
— in the case of incompetent subjects, informed consent is obtained from the legal guardian or other duly authorized person;
— the degree of risk attached to interventions that are not intended to benefit the individual subject is low and commensurate with the importance of the knowledge to be gained; and
— interventions that are intended to provide therapeutic benefit are likely to be at least as advantageous to the individual subject as any alternative.

Guideline 7: Research involving prisoners

Prisoners with serious illness or at risk of serious illness should not arbitrarily be denied access to investigational drugs, vaccines or other agents that show promise of therapeutic or preventive benefit.

Guideline 8: Research involving subjects in underdeveloped communities

Before undertaking research involving subjects in underdeveloped communities, whether in developed or developing countries, the investigator must ensure that:

— persons in underdeveloped communities will not ordinarily be involved in research that could be carried out reasonably well in developed communities;
— the research is responsive to the health needs and the priorities of the community in which it is to be carried out;
— every effort will be made to secure the ethical imperative that the consent of individual subjects be informed; and
— the proposals for the research have been reviewed and approved by an ethical review committee that has among its members or consultants persons who are thoroughly familiar with the customs and traditions of the community.

Guideline 9: Informed consent in epidemiological studies

For several types of epidemiological research individual informed consent is either impracticable or inadvisable. In such cases the ethical review committee should determine whether it is ethically acceptable to proceed without individual informed consent and whether the investigator's plans to protect the safety and respect the privacy of research subjects and to maintain the confidentiality of the data are adequate.

Selection of Research Subjects

Guideline 10: Equitable distribution of burdens and benefits

Individuals or communities to be invited to be subjects of research should be selected in such a way that the burdens and benefits of the research will be equitably distributed. Special justification is required for inviting vulnerable individuals and, if they are selected, the means of protecting their rights and welfare must be particularly strictly applied.

Guideline 11: Selection of pregnant or nursing (breastfeeding) women as research subjects

Pregnant or nursing women should in no circumstances be the subjects of non-clinical research unless the research carries no more than minimal risk to the fetus or nursing infant and the object of the research is to obtain new knowledge about pregnancy or lactation. As a general rule, pregnant or nursing women should not be subjects of any clinical trials except such trials as are designed to protect or advance the health of pregnant or nursing women or fetuses or nursing infants, and for which women who are not pregnant or nursing would not be suitable subjects.

Confidentiality of Data

Guideline 12: Safeguarding confidentiality

The investigator must establish secure safeguards of the confidentiality of research data. Subjects should be told of the limits to the investigators' ability to safeguard confidentiality and of the anticipated consequences of breaches of confidentiality.

Compensation of Research Subjects for Accidental Injury

Guideline 13: Right of subjects to compensation

Research subjects who suffer physical injury as a result of their participation are entitled to such financial or other assistance as would compensate them equitably for any temporary or permanent impairment or disability. In the case of death, their dependents are entitled to material compensation. The right to compensation may not be waived.

Review Procedures

Guideline 14: Constitution and responsibilities of ethical review committees

All proposals to conduct research involving human subjects must be submitted for review and approval to one or more independent ethical and scientific review committees. The investigator must obtain such approval of the proposal to conduct research before the research is begun.

Externally Sponsored Research

Guideline 15: Obligations of sponsoring and host countries

Externally sponsored research entails two ethical obligations:

  • An external sponsoring agency should submit the research protocol to ethical and scientific review according to the standards of the country of the sponsoring agency, and the ethical standards applied should be no less exacting than they would be in the case of ethical standards applied should be no less exacting than they would be in the case of research carried out in that country.
  • After scientific and ethical approval in the country of the sponsoring agency, the appropriate authorities of the host country, including a national or local ethical review committee or its equivalent, should satisfy themselves that the proposed research meets their own ethical requirements.

•   •   •

Appendix 2
EUROPEAN TRANSNATIONAL RESEARCH
ETHICS POLICIES

Appendix 2.1   Council of the European Communities, Directive on the Protection of Animals used for Experimental and other Scientific Purposes (1986)

European Community Council (now European Union) Council Directive on the Approximation of Laws, Regulations and Administrative Provisions of the Member States Regarding the Protection of Animals Used for Experimental and Other Scientific Purposes.

Article 1

The aim of this Directive is to ensure that where animals are used for experimental or other scientific purposes the provisions laid down by law, regulation or administrative provisions in the Member States for their protection are approximated so as to avoid affecting the establishment and functioning of the common market, in particular by distorsions of competition or barriers to trade.

Article 2

For the purposes of this Directive the following definitions shall apply:

(a) "animal" unless otherwise qualified, means any live non-human vertebrate, including free-living larval and/or reproducing larval forms, but excluding foetal or embryonic forms;

(b) "experimental animals" means animals used or to be used in experiments;

(c) "bred animals" means animals specially bred for use in experiments in facilities approved by, or registered with, the authority;

(d) "experiment" means any use of an animal for experimental or other scientific purposes which may cause it pain, suffering, distress or lasting harm, including any course of action intended, or liable, to result in the birth of an animal in any such condition, but excluding the least painful methods accepted in modern practice (i.e., "humane" methods) of killing or marking an animal; an experiment starts when an animal is first prepared for use and ends when no further observations are to be made for that experiment; the elimination of pain, suffering, distress or lasting harm by the successful use of anaesthesia or analgesia or other methods does not place the use of an animal outside the scope of this definition. Non experimental, agricultural or clinical veterinary practices are excluded;

(e) "authority" means the authority or authorities designated by each Member State as being responsible for supervising the experiments within the meaning of this Directive;

(f) "competent person" means any person who is considered by a Member State to be competent to perform the relevant function described in this Directive;

(g) "establishment" means any installation, building, group of buildings or other premises and may include a place which is not wholly enclosed or covered and mobile facilities;

(h) "breeding establishment" means any establishment where animals are bred with a view to their use in experiments;

(i) "supplying establishment" means any establishment, other than a breeding establishment, from which animals are supplied with a view to their use in experiments;

(j) "user establishment" means any establishment where animals are used for experiments;

(k) "properly anaesthetized" means deprived of sensation by methods of anaesthesia (whether local or general) as effective as those used in good veterinary practice;

(l) "humane method of killing" means the killing of an animal with a minimum of physical and mental suffering, depending on the species.

Article 3

This Directive applies to the use of animals in experiments which are undertaken for one of the following purposes:

(a) the development, manufacture, quality, effectiveness and safety testing of drugs, foodstuffs and other substances or products:

(i) for the avoidance, prevention, diagnosis or treatment of disease, ill-health or other abnormality or their effects in man, animals or plants;

(ii) for the assessment, detection, regulation or modification of physiological conditions in man, animals or plants;

(b) the protection of the natural environment in the interests of the health or welfare of man or animal.

Article 4

Each Member State shall ensure that experiments using animals considered as endangered under Appendix I of the Convention on International Trade in Endangered Species of Fauna and Flora and Annex C.I. of Regulation (EEC) No. 3626/82 are prohibited unless they are in conformity with the above Regulation and the objects of the experiment are:

— research aimed at preservation of the species in question, or
— essential biomedical purposes where the species in question exceptionally proves to be the only one suitable for those purposes.

Article 5

Member States shall ensure that, as far as the general care and accommodations of animals is concerned:

(a) all experimental animals shall be provided with housing, an environment, at least some freedom of movement, food, water and care which are appropriate to their health and well-being;

(b) any restriction on the extent to which an experimental animal can satisfy its physiological and ethnological needs shall be limited to the absolute minimum;

(c) the environmental conditions in which experimental animals are bred, kept or used must be checked daily;

(d) the well-being and state of health of experimental animals shall be observed by a competent person to prevent pain or avoidable suffering, distress or lasting harm;

(e) arrangements are made to ensure that any defect or suffering discovered is eliminated as quickly as possible.

For the implementation of the provisions of paragraphs (a) and (b), Member States shall pay regard to the guidelines set out in Annex II.

Article 6

1. Each Member State shall designate the authority or authorities responsible for verifying that the provisions of this Directive are properly carried out.

2. In the framework of the implementation of this Directive, Member States shall adopt the necessary measures in order that the designated authority mentioned in paragraph 1 above may have the advice of experts competent for the matters in question.

Article 7

1. Experiments shall be performed solely by competent authorized persons, or under the direct responsibility of such a person, or if the experimental or other scientific project concerned is authorized in accordance with the provisions of national legislation.
2. An experiment shall not be performed if another scientifically satisfactory method of obtaining the result sought, not entailing the use of an animal, is reasonably and practicably available.
3. When an experiment has to be performed, the choice of species shall be carefully considered and, where necessary, explained to the authority. In a choice between experiments, those which use the minimum number of animals, involve animals with the lowest degree of neurophysiological sensitivity, cause the least pain, suffering, distress or lasting harm and which are most likely to provide satisfactory results shall be selected.

Experiments on animals taken from the wild may not be carried out unless experiments on other animals would not suffice for the aims of the experiment.
4. All experiments shall be designed to avoid distress and unnecessary pain and suffering to the experimental animals. They shall be subject to the provisions laid down in Article 8. The measures set out in Article 9 shall be taken in all cases.

Article 8

1. All experiments shall be carried out under general or local anaesthesia.
2. Paragraph 1 above does not apply when:
    (a) anaesthesia is judged to be more traumatic to the animal than the experiment itself;
    (b) anaesthesia is incompatible with the object of the experiment. In such cases appropriate legislative and/or administrative measures shall be taken to ensure that no such experiment is carried out unnecessarily.
Anaesthesia should be used in the case of serious injuries which may cause severe pain.
3. If anaesthesia is not possible, analgesics or other appropriate methods should be used in order to ensure as far as possible that pain, suffering, distress or harm are limited and that in any event the animal is not subject to severe pain, distress or suffering.
4. Provided such action is compatible with the object of the experiment, an anaesthetized animal, which suffers considerable pain once anaesthesia has worn off, shall be treated in good time with pain-relieving means or, if this is not possible, shall be immediately killed by a humane method.

Article 9

1. At the end of any experiment, it shall be decided whether the animal shall be kept alive or killed by a humane method, subject to the condition that it shall not be kept alive if, even though it has been restored to normal health in all other respects, it is likely to remain in lasting pain or distress.
2. The decisions referred to in paragraph 1 shall be taken by a competent person, preferably a veterinarian.
3. Where, at the end of an experiment:
(a) an animal is to be kept alive, it shall receive the care appropriate to its state of health, be placed under the supervision of a veterinarian or other competent person and shall be kept

under conditions conforming to the requirements of Article 5. The conditions laid down in this subparagraph may, however, be waived where, in the opinion of a veterinarian, the animal would not suffer as a consequence of such exemption;

(b) an animal is not to be kept alive or cannot benefit from the provisions of Article 5 concerning its well-being, it shall be killed by a humane method as soon as possible.

Article 10

Member States shall ensure that any re-use of animals in experiments shall be compatible with the provisions of this Directive.

In particular, an animal shall not be used more than once in experiments entailing severe pain, distress or equivalent suffering.

Article 11

Notwithstanding the other provisions of this Directive, where it is necessary for the legitimate purposes of the experiment, the authority may allow the animal concerned to be set free, provided that it is satisfied that the maximum possible care has been taken to safeguard the animal's well-being, as long as its state of health allows this to be done and there is no danger for public health and the environment.

Article 12

1. Member States shall establish procedures whereby experiments themselves or the details of persons conducting such experiments shall be notified in advance to the authority.

2. Where it is planned to subject an animal to an experiment in which it will, or may, experience severe pain which is likely to be prolonged, that experiment must be specifically declared and justified to, or specifically authorized by, the authority. The authority shall take appropriate judicial or administrative action if it is not satisfied that the experiment is of sufficient importance for meeting the essential needs of man or animal.

• • •

Article 23

1. The Commission and Member States should encourage research into the development and validation of alternative techniques which could provide the same level of information as that obtained in experiments using animals but which involve fewer animals or which entail less painful procedures, and shall take such other steps as they consider appropriate to encourage research in this field. The Commission and Member States shall monitor trends in experimental methods.

2. The Commission shall report before the end of 1987 on the possibility of modifying tests and guidelines laid down in existing Community legislation taking into account the objectives referred to in paragraph 1.

Appendix 2.2   Council of Europe, Recommendation Concerning Medical Research on Human Beings (1990)

Principles Concerning Medical Research on Human Beings

Scope and Definition

For the purpose of application of these principles, medical research means any trial and experimentation carried out on human beings, the purpose of which or one of the purposes of which is to increase medical knowledge.

Principle 1

Any medical research must be carried out within the framework of a scientific plan and in accordance with the following principles.

Principle 2

1. In medical research the interests and well-being of the person under-going medical research must always prevail over the interests of science and society.
2. The risks incurred by a person undergoing medical research must be kept to a minimum. The risks should not be disproportionate to the benefits to that person or the importance of the aims pursued by the research.

Principle 3

1. No medical research may be carried out without the informed, free, express and specific consent of the person undergoing it. Such consent may be freely withdrawn at any phase of the research and the person undergoing the research should be informed, before being included in it, of his right to withdraw his consent.
2. The person who is to undergo medical research should be given information on the purpose of the research and the methodology of the experimentation. He should also be informed of the foreseeable risks and inconveniences to him of the proposed research. This information should be sufficiently clear and suitably adapted to enable consent to be given or refused in full knowledge of the relevant facts.
3. The provisions of this principle should apply also to a legal representative and to a legally incapacitated person having the capacity of understanding, in the situations described in Principles 4 and 5.

Principle 4

A legally incapacitated person may only undergo medical research where authorised by Principle 5 and if his legal representative, or an authority or an individual authorised or designated under his national law, consents. If the legally incapacitated person is capable of understanding, his consent is also required and no research may be undertaken if he does not give his consent.

Principle 5

1. A legally incapacitated person may not undergo medical research unless it is expected to produce a direct and significant benefit to his health.
2. However, by way of exception, national law may authorise research involving a legally

incapacitated person which is not a direct benefit to his health when that person offers no objection, provided that the research is to the benefit of persons in the same category and that the same scientific results cannot be obtained by research on persons who do not belong to this category.

Principle 6

Pregnant or nursing women may not undergo medical research where their health and/or that of the child would not benefit directly unless this research is aimed at benefiting other women and children who are in the same position and the same scientific results cannot be obtained by research on women who are not pregnant or nursing.

Principle 7

Persons deprived of liberty may not undergo medical research unless it is expected to produce a direct and significant benefit to their health.

Principle 8

In an emergency situation, notwithstanding Principle 3, where a patient is unable to give a prior consent, medical research can be carried out only when the following conditions are fulfilled:

— the research must have been planned to be carried out in the emergency in question;
— the systematic research plan must have been approved by an ethics committee;
— the research must be intended for the direct health benefit of the patient.

Principle 9

Any information of a personal nature obtained during medical research should be treated as confidential.

Principle 10

Medical research may not be carried out unless satisfactory evidence as to its safety for the person undergoing research is furnished.

Principle 11

Medical research that is not in accordance with scientific criteria in its design and cannot answer the questions posed is unacceptable even if the way it is to be carried out poses no risk to the person undergoing research.

Principle 12

1. Medical research must be carried out under the responsibility of a doctor or a person who exercises full clinical responsibility and who possesses appropriate knowledge and qualifications to meet any clinical contingency.
2. The responsible doctor or other person referred to in the preceding paragraph should enjoy full professional independence and should have the power to stop the research at any time.

Principle 13

1. Potential subjects of medical research should not be offered any inducement which compromises free consent. Persons undergoing medical research should not gain any financial

benefit. However, expenses and any financial loss may be refunded and in appropriate cases a modest allowance may be given for any inconvenience inherent in the medical research.

2. If the person undergoing research is legally incapacitated, his legal representatives should not receive any form of remuneration whatever, except for the refund of their expenses.

Principle 14

1. Persons undergoing medical research and/or their dependants should be compensated for injury and loss caused by the medical research.

2. Where there is no existing system providing compensation for the persons concerned, states should ensure that sufficient guarantees for such compensation are provided.

3. Terms and conditions which exclude or limit, in advance, compensation to the victim should be considered to be null and void.

Principle 15

All proposed medical research plans should be the subject of an ethical examination by an independent and multidisciplinary committee.

Principle 16

Any medical research which is:

— unplanned, or
— contrary to any of the preceding principles, or
— in any other way contrary to ethics or law, or
— not in accordance with scientific methods in its design and cannot answer the questions posed

should be prohibited or, if it has already begun, stopped or revised, even if it poses no risk to the person(s) undergoing the research.

Explanatory Memorandum to Recommendation R(90) 3 (1990)

Principle 1

17. Trials and experimentation on humans must be carried out in the framework of a scientific plan. However, these terms should not be interpreted in a narrow sense but should include any planned research even in cases where it is conducted on a single individual at a given stage of this research.

18. As the Principles concern medical research on human beings carried out in the framework of a plan, it is clear that in the case of comparative trials they also apply to persons belonging to a control group including a placebo group.

19. Subject to the specific situation in Principle 6, these Principles cover medical research on humans from birth.

20. It should be noted that the experts wished to prepare rules which would apply to medical research on human beings, the aim of which is essentially diagnostic or therapeutic for a patient as well as to medical research, the essential object of which is scientific. Principles 2, 5, 6, 7 and 8 take account of the existing differences between research where a direct health benefit can be expected for the person undergoing such research and other research, in particular with regard to the degree of risk which can be accepted.

21. Observational studies which do not involve any direct medical intervention on human beings as well as epidemiological research based on personal data without the participation of the persons

involved were considered but it was decided that they would not be covered by the scope of these Principles.

22. According to Principle 1, experiments which are not planned should not be regarded as medical research. Such experiments are without scientific value and therefore not acceptable.

Principle 2

23. The first element in this Principle establishes the precedence of the individual over science and society. Consequently, in conformity with the Helsinki Declaration, the interests of society and science, no matter how important and serious they may be, cannot be promoted without taking into account the dignity and the well-being of the person undergoing research. The interests of this person are the touchstone where there is a conflict with the interests of society or science.

24. Paragraph 2 provides that risks of the medical research must be kept to a minimum for the person undergoing it. In some medical research there will inevitably be some degree of risk to the person undergoing it. This is acceptable provided that the risk is not to be of a serious nature and should not have irreversible harmful consequences.

25. The Principle also provides that the risks taken by the person undergoing medical research should not be disproportionate to the benefits to that person or to the importance of the aim pursued by such research. A risk which is considered to be too high with regard to the aim of the research is not acceptable.

When medical research is intended to be of direct benefit to the health of the person undergoing it, a higher degree of risk may be acceptable provided that it is in proportion with the person's disease. A direct benefit of a person's health means not only treatment to cure the patient but also treatment which may alleviate his suffering thus improving his quality of life. However, it should be emphasized that even in the latter case the Principle set out in Paragraph 1 must be respected. That is to say, if the research that incurs risk is more for the benefit of science and society than for the patient, that research is not acceptable under the Principles.

26. The Committee of experts wished to emphasize that the ''importance of the aim pursued by medical research'' refers to the importance to the patient who undergoes research for the direct benefit to his health and to the scientific and medical importance for mankind but not to the financial importance and cost of the research to the promoter.

Principle 3

27. This Principle deals with the problem of consent and contains a fundamental legal principle that no research may be imposed on anyone without his consent. This consent should be free, informed, express and specific. Principle 3 is based on the aforementioned Helsinki declaration and goes beyond it.

28. In order to give his informed consent, the person concerned must have knowledge of the pertinent facts concerning the research he is to undergo. To make this requirement clear, Paragraph 2 of the Principle lists the minimum information to be given to the person concerned:

— the purpose of the medical research;
— the methodology of the experimentation;
— the foreseeable risks of the research;
— the inconveniences to be suffered.

29. This information should be sufficiently clear and suitably adapted to the person who is to undergo the research. The requirement that the information should be ''suitably adapted'' means that it should be given in a way to make it understandable taking into account of level of knowledge and education and psychological state of the person undergoing the medical research, be this person a sick patient or a healthy volunteer.

30. In addition, the Principle requires that the person must always consent clearly and specifically for each separate research study for which he is the subject. A general consent is not acceptable

and in some research studies the research subject's consent may additionally be required by the ethical committee (see Principle 15) for each successive stage of research study, particularly when a study is very prolonged.

31. While the Principle does not impose a formal requirement of written consent, it is evident that such form of consent may be desirable in certain circumstances not only to establish proof of the consent given but to make the person who is to undergo medical research think more seriously about his own decision. This Principle presents no obstacle for member States requiring written consent either for all medical research or for certain medical research under conditions determined by national law.

32. The giving of consent does not prevent a person from deciding at any stage in the research not to participate in it any more. In any event he cannot be held liable for any consequences in particular of a financial nature. Any obligation arising out of the mere fact of withdrawing would be contrary to the right to withdraw from research.

In any case if either before or during the medical research there is any doubt concerning free and informed consent it should be concluded that there is no such consent. Subject to circumstances described in Principle 8, the consent must be given expressly and its existence can never be implied or presumed.

33. Paragraph 3 of this Principle extends the application of these provisions to legal representatives where a legally incapacitated person is to undergo research and consequently the consent of his legal representatives is required. In these particular cases the legal representatives as well as legally incapacitated persons having the capacity of understanding (see paragraph 36 below) should give their consent according to the conditions set out in paragraphs 1, 2 and 3 of this Principle.

Principle 4

34. This Principle deals with the consent of legally incapacitated persons as defined by national law. As the medical research they undergo is restricted to that which is of direct and significant benefit to their health and to exceptional cases which are mentioned in paragraph 2 of Principle 5, Principle 4 makes a cross reference to Principle 5 in order to show clearly that the problem of the consent of these persons may arise only in cases where they are allowed to undergo medical research under the Principles. The persons referred to as "legally incapacitated persons" are minors and those who are legally incapacitated because of their mental disorder. It is specifically not intended to include here other persons who are legally incapacitated for reasons other than minority or mental disorder (eg prodigality, imprisonment, etc) which exist in the legal system in some member States.

35. In these Principles, the phrase "legal representatives" means those with legal responsibility for taking decisions on behalf of persons who do not have the legal capacity to take such decisions concerning themselves.

In addition to the legal representative "an authority or an individual authorised or designated under his national law" is also mentioned in this Principle. This addition intends to cover the possibility under the law of some States of appointing a person or authority empowered to give such consent but who without being guardian would have general representative power.

36. If the legally incapacitated person is capable of understanding, his consent is also required. Owing to the fact that the research concerns the person himself, the experts considered that it was necessary to take account of the view of the incapacitated person when he is able to express such views. No medical research may be carried out on that person if he refuses to undergo medical research, regardless of whether consent has already been given by his legal representative(s).

In order to protect the legally incapacitated person capable of understanding, his consent is not sufficient to authorise medical research. The consent of the legal representative or representatives is always required. The aim of the Committee of experts in adopting such a rule was twofold: on the one hand it did not wish to force a person capable of understanding to undergo medical research merely because consent had been given by his legal representative. On the other hand, recognising the mechanism protecting legally incapacitated persons, the Committee wished the refusal of the legal representative(s) to be respected.

Principle 5

37. Principles 5 to 7 list the prohibitions and restrictions concerning the possibility of carrying out medical research on certain categories of persons. Principle 5 deals with legally incapacitated persons.

38. Paragraph 1 of Principle 5 sets out the general principle concerning medical research on legally incapacitated persons and states that this should be restricted to research which is of direct and significant benefit to their health.

39. The second paragraph of this Principle emphasises that a person who is unable to understand or consent to research, but who by his behaviour clearly objects to what is involved in the research, must not be forced to be the subject of any research.

Paragraph 2 allows national law, where appropriate, to authorise medical research on these persons which will not bring them a direct benefit to their health when the research is aimed at benefiting persons belonging to the same category as the legally incapacitated person and analogous scientific results cannot be obtained on persons not belonging to this category. These include, in particular, research in paediatrics which requires specific trials on children and which cannot be replaced by identical research on adults. This provision also applies to certain adult persons suffering from given mental disorders where the research specifically concerns this category of persons and it is not possible to obtain analogous results by research on persons who do not suffer from such disorders.

Those persons who have given their consent in full legal capacity but who subsequently become legally incapacitated will thereafter be treated as legally incapacitated persons pursuant to Principles 4 and 5.

It should be underlined that even in the exceptional cases mentioned in Paragraph 2, the requirements of Principle 2 should be respected (eg medical research which is not of direct benefit should never involve any risk more than minimum).

Principle 6

40. Medical research on pregnant or nursing (breast-feeding) women presents a particular problem because of the potential harmful effect or danger of this research to the embryo, the foetus or to the newborn baby. This Principle aims at preventing medical research on these women unless the research is carried out in the interest of these women or their children (for example, to improve delivery conditions, to improve the health of the foetus). Naturally the term ''child'' employed in this Principle includes also child to be born. However the research may be carried out when the health of the persons concerned will not benefit directly, providing that it cannot be carried out on other categories.

Even in these cases the persons concerned may not undergo research where the tests would constitute more than a minimal risk to their own health or that of the embryo, foetus or newborn baby or where Principle 2 would be contravened in some other respect.

Principle 7

41. This Principle completely excludes the possibility of carrying out medical research on persons deprived of liberty unless they can gain a direct and significant benefit to their health. The Committee of experts, when drawing up this rule, felt that the particular condition of these persons justified this exclusion as the free nature of their consent may be doubtful.

42. Without directly referring to the European Convention on Human Rights, the experts included the different situations mentioned in its Article 5 (eg detention by order of a court; detention by the police; detention of persons suffering from mental disorders; putting in quarantine of persons to prevent the spread of infectious diseases, etc). This Principle does not deal with the lawful and correct nature of these detentions. Therefore, any detained person comes automatically within the

application of Principle 7 even if the decision was not lawfully made. Medical research on these persons will be forbidden until they regain their freedom.

43. This Principle, by its clear wording, revises Articles 5 of Recommendation R (83) 2 on the legal protection of persons suffering from mental disorders placed as involuntary patients and renders invalid the second sentence of Paragraph 3 (ie "clinical trials having psychiatric therapeutic purposes are a matter for national legal provisions"). These trials are no longer left to the national law but are simply excluded in the case of persons suffering from mental disorder placed as involuntary patients unless such trials are in the direct interest of the person concerned.

44. Finally Principle 7 also clarifies the rather general wording of Principle 27 of the European Prison Rules [Recommendation No R (87) 3] which states" "Prisoners may not be submitted to any experiments which may result in physical or moral injury". Principle 7 certainly prevents prisoners' undergoing medical research on a voluntary basis as mentioned in the Explanatory Memorandum (pages 44 to 45, paragraph 27) to the European Prison Rules. Voluntary participation of prisoners in medical research is not allowed unless it is to produce a direct and significant benefit to their health.

Principle 8

45. While Principle 3 requires that consent should always be given prior to medical research, there are emergency situations where a person is unable to give consent because of the nature of the emergency situation (for example, coma following an accident).

If such a patient has a legal representative and his opinion can be obtained without undue delay his consent should of course be sought.

If no legal representative can be reached the doctor may carry out medical research in accordance with Principle 8 without prior consent. However, the doctor must not carry out any medical research in an emergency when he knows or has reasons to believe that the research subject would object for reasons of his own convictions.

The experts also considered that a person close to the research subject who is present should be informed and his opinion sought but this opinion is not mandatory. It is for the doctor to decide on the treatment necessary for the medical care of an individual person undergoing research.

46. If and when the research subject recovers his full understanding while he is still undergoing research, he must be asked for his consent to its continuation. It must be a matter for the doctor's judgment to decide on the appropriate time during the patient's recovery to ask for consent. It will not always be in the research subject's best interest to insist that consent is asked as soon as the patient shows signs of recovering his full understanding.

Principle 9

47. This Principle is intended to protect confidentiality of data of a personal nature concerning the research subject. Taking into account Article 8 of the European Convention on human rights and Article 7 of the United Nations Covenant on civil and political rights the Principle states that information of a personal nature obtained during medical research must be treated as confidential. This rule applies to all persons having access to personal information obtained during medical research.

There should be full compliance with the Council of Europe's corpus of law relating to data protection which inter alia applies to personal data obtained during or as a result of medical research.

The Convention of 28 January 1981 for the protection of individuals with regard to automatic processing of personal data (ETS No. 108), to which nine member States were Parties at the time of preparation of the present Recommendation and which had been signed by eight other States, ranks medical data in the category of sensitive data for which reinforced protection standards are required. The general data protection rules have been amplified in a series of Recommendations of the Committee of Ministers to the member States, several of which deal with problems concerning medical data files and their use.

Principle 10

48. Before starting medical research on human subjects, appropriate proof should be furnished as to its safety. This means that the question of safety must be addressed and satisfactory evidence produced to demonstrate the nature and extent of any risk to the person undergoing the research in question.

The experts did not wish to prescribe a specific kind of proof (eg results of tests of a pharmaceutical drug on several mammalian species) as different types of medical research inevitably require different types of proof. The nature, the relevance and the degree of proof to be furnished will be determined in the light of scientific knowledge.

The notion of safety mentioned here only concerns the effect of research on the person undergoing it.

The experts emphasized that before any research is carried out on human beings it is necessary for all appropriate research to have been undertaken through other means.

Principle 11

49. Having regard to the fact that these principles not only aim at protecting persons undergoing medical research from risks and dangers, but also at respecting human dignity, the experts wished to exclude by this Principle medical research which has no scientific value (eg research which in its design or method cannot answer the hypothesis posed). Such research, being contrary to principles established in "Scope and Definition" and Principle 1, cannot be considered as "medical research" because it contributes nothing to medical knowledge. It should also be noted that in all member States unnecessary duplication of research is always considered unethical.

Principle 12

50. Paragraph 1 provides that medical research should be conducted under the supervision of a doctor or a person who exercises full clinical responsibility and possesses appropriate knowledge, resources and qualifications. The experts considered that medical research should be carried out under the direct clinical supervision of either the doctor or such a person. The words "appropriate knowledge and qualifications" have been included in this Paragraph in order to underline the fact that specific knowledge resources and skill, related to the type of medical research in question are required as well as the qualification to meet any foreseeable clinical contingency which may occur.

By "full clinical responsibility" the experts referred to persons having clinical responsibility for patients' care.

The experts noted that in certain States clinical control may be entrusted not only to doctors but also to dentists or nurses when the research concerns dentistry or care to be given by nurses.

51. Under Paragraph 2 of Principle 12 the supervising doctor or other person exercising clinical responsibility must be able to exercise independent judgment in the conduct of research and should be empowered to stop the research at any time. Such professional independence should exist even if the doctor, or the mentioned person, is paid by the promoter of the research.

The supervising doctor or the person exercising clinical responsibility is expected to intervene if the research no longer complies with the rules contained in the Principles. He may therefore have to stop medical research on certain persons (eg a woman becoming pregnant after the research started; an experiment where the risks have become unacceptable because of the abnormal reaction of the person undergoing it) but he may continue the research on other persons who do not have the same problems. If medical research which originally seemed without risk turns out to present more than a minimal risk (see Principle 2) the supervising doctor or the person referred to in Paragraph 1 should have the power to stop that medical research on all persons.

52. In some member States dentists supervise research within their expertise. Where a dentist is to exercise such supervision he will do so under the same conditions as apply to doctors and other

persons mentioned in Paragraph 1 (in particular with regard to qualifications, full professional independence and the power to stop the research at any time).

Principle 13

53. In this Principle the experts formulated the rule that no one should undergo medical research
for profit. In fact for several reasons the experts considered that medical research should not give
rise to any financial or equivalent benefit for the person undergoing such research: a person cannot
be subject to a commercial transaction; free consent should be ensured; the creation of a category
of persons who could be described as "professional guinea pigs" for medical research should be
avoided.

54. The experts agreed that, although any profit is excluded, expenses and financial loss may be
refunded. Medical research should not result in expenses or any loss for the person undergoing
research. The nature and the extent of these expenses and financial loss is to be determined in each
particular case.

55. The majority of experts considered that payment of a modest allowance may be allowed to
persons undergoing medical research where there are particular inconveniences (eg several daily
attendances which restrict the freedom of movement of the person undergoing that research, etc).
Such modest allowance must never compromise or prejudice the free nature of consent and never
be so large as to encourage persons undergoing research. A practice contrary to this would constitute,
inter alia, a violation of Principle 3 which requires "free consent".

56. In those cases where legally incapacitated persons may, under the Principles, be allowed to
undergo medical research, Paragraph 2 of this Principle prohibits their legal representatives from
receiving payment in their own name. The experts believed that it would be completely unethical
to allow someone to receive allowances for inconvenience suffered by someone else. In order to
avoid abuses the experts thought that legal representative(s) should only receive their expenses but
should not be paid for any losses which they incur.

Principle 14

57. The experts observed that in most member States social security schemes or doctor's malpractice insurance would give insufficient cover for persons undergoing research; in addition the
remedies available to persons harmed may often seem insufficient, uncertain, long and costly. Such
absence of protection occurs in particular in cases of injury and loss caused by unforeseen risks of
medical research. The resulting damage cannot be considered to be a consequence of malpractice.
Even most life insurance policies taken out by persons undergoing medical research exclude from
their cover injury and loss sustained as a result of an incident in medical research. Being aware of
the fact that undergoing medical research is, particularly for healthy volunteers, a highly com-
mendable act for the benefit of humanity and science for whose good the research will be employed,
the Committee wished to establish a rule that, where injury and loss are sustained as a result of
medical research, persons undergoing that research or their dependants must be compensated irrespective of social security rules or the promoter's or doctor's fault or malpractice.

The experts emphasised that it is not the purpose of the present Recommendation to deal with
the substantive law governing liability and compensation for damage. This matter is governed by
the domestic laws of the member States as well as by several international instruments.

58. After stating this general Principle, Paragraph 2 calls upon States, where there is no existing
system providing such compensation, to ensure that sufficient guarantees for compensation are
provided. The experts preferred this general wording, which does not specify any particular kind
of guarantee, owing to the differing administrative structures and practices in member States. The
Principle, which does not intend to harmonise existing administrative structures and practices, seeks
to ensure that sufficient guarantees in fact exist to give the person undergoing medical research the
compensation mentioned in Paragraph 1. The words "where there is no existing system providing

compensation'' have been added to the text to take account of the fact that in some States medical research is allowed to take place only in State establishments. Social security schemes would cover all treatment necessary in cases of accidents in some of these States. In order to provide a solution where no such systems exist or where existing systems provide inadequate cover, the experts discussed the possibility of obtaining insurance to provide cover for accidents which do not come within the doctor's malpractice insurance.

59. However, the experts did not make a specific reference to insurance as, in certain States, other types of guarantees could provide similar cover.

60. The person undergoing medical research must not be required to pay the costs of any guarantee (eg insurance premiums). A practice to the contrary would be against the spirit of the Principles. It should be recalled that Principle 13 provides that the expenses of persons undergoing research may be refunded.

This paragraph does not prevent a ceiling for the amount of compensation to be fixed provided that it is a reasonable one.

61. The third paragraph of the Principle was added to deal with a particular problem existing in certain States. In many member States a waiver of the right to compensation would be without legal effect. However, the experts, having noted that in some countries such terms and conditions might be valid, agreed to state in the Principles clearly that they should be considered null and void as otherwise such terms and conditions would render paragraphs 1 and 2 of the Principle meaningless.

Principle 15

62. The most important requirement of this Principle is that the committee which carries out the ethical examination of proposed research should be independent and multidisciplinary. "Independent" means being independent both of the promoter and the research teams. The ethics committee should not follow any orders or instructions of any other body or person. "Multidisciplinary" does not refer merely to a body composed of doctors and scientists of different specialisations, but also refers to other professions (lawyers, nurses, social workers, philosophers, theologians, etc) and the general public. The role of the ethics committee is to examine the proposed research from an ethical point of view. However, the ethical examination may require a detailed study of scientific aspects of the research project.

The experts believed that not all research projects would have to be submitted to an ethics committee. The manner in which ethics committees assess research projects submitted to them and publicity given to their conclusions should be governed by national or by committees' own rules of procedure (for example committees may decide to delegate certain matters to their chairman or to sub-committees).

The words "proposed medical research" imply that the examination should necessarily be made before the beginning of the research. It should be possible to continue or resume this examination at any time during the research.

Although this ethical examination is required to precede a medical research, the opinion of the ethics committee is, in most States, of an advisory nature and obtaining a favourable opinion would by no means do away with the liability of persons involved in doing medical research (eg promoter, supervising physician etc).

Principle 16

63. This Principle makes it clear that medical research which contravenes the rules established by the Principles or is in any other way contrary to ethics, law or scientific data should be prohibited; if it has already started it should be stopped. An experiment which is to be started again should be modified in accordance with the above-mentioned concepts.

Appendix 2.3   Council of Europe, Convention for the Protection of Human Rights and Dignity of the Human Being with Regard to the Application of Biology and Medicine: Convention on Human Rights and Biomedicine (1996)

· · ·

Chapter IV, Human Genome

Article 11. (Non-discrimination)

Any form of discrimination against a person on grounds of his or her genetic heritage is prohibited.

Article 12. (Predictive genetic tests)

Tests which are predictive of genetic diseases or which serve either to identify the subject as a carrier of a gene responsible for a disease or to detect a genetic predisposition or susceptibility to a disease may be performed only for health purposes or for scientific research linked to health purposes, and subject to appropriate genetic counseling.

Article 13. (Interventions on the human genome)

An intervention seeking to modify the human genome may only be undertaken for preventive, diagnostic or therapeutic purposes and only if its aim is not to introduce any modification in the genome of any descendants.

Article 14. (Non-selection of sex)

The use of techniques of medically assisted procreation shall not be allowed for the purpose of choosing a future child's sex, except where serious hereditary sex-related disease is to be avoided.

Chapter V, Scientific Research

Article 15. (General rule)

Scientific research in the field of biology and medicine shall be carried out freely, subject to the provisions of this Convention and the other legal provisions ensuring the protection of the human being.

Article 16. (Protection of persons undergoing research)

Research on a person may only be undertaken if all the following conditions are met:

i) there is no alternative of comparable effectiveness to research on humans,

ii) the risks which may be incurred by that person are not disproportionate to the potential benefits of the research,

iii) the research project has been approved by the competent body after independent examination of its scientific merit, including assessment of the importance of the aim of the research, and multidisciplinary review of its ethical acceptability,

iv) the persons undergoing research have been informed of their rights and the safeguards prescribed by law for their protection,

v) the necessary consent as provided for under Article 5 has been given expressly, specifically and is documented. Such consent may be freely withdrawn at any time.

Article 17. (Protection of persons not able to consent to research)

1. Research on a person without the capacity to consent as stipulated in Article 5 may be undertaken only if all the following conditions are met:

i. the conditions laid down in Article 16, sub-paragraphs (i) to (iv), are fulfilled;
ii. the results of the research have the potential to produce real and direct benefit to his or her health;
iii. research of comparable effectiveness cannot be carried out on individuals capable of giving consent;
iv. the necessary authorisation provided for under Article 6 has been given specifically and in writing, and
v. the person concerned does not object.

2. Exceptionally and under the protective conditions prescribed by law, where the research has not the potential to produce results of direct benefit to the health of the person concerned, such research may be authorised subject to the conditions laid down in paragraph 1, sub-paragraphs (i), (iii), (iv) and (v) above, and to the following additional conditions:

i. the research has the aim of contributing, through significant improvement in the scientific understanding of the individual's condition, disease or disorder, to the ultimate attainment of results capable of conferring benefit to the person concerned or to other persons in the same age category or afflicted with the same disease or disorder or having the same condition.
ii. the research entails only minimal risk and minimal burden for the individual concerned.

Article 18. (Research on embryos in vitro)

1. Where the law allows research on embryos in vitro, it shall ensure adequate protection of the embryo.
2. The creation of human embryos for research purposes is prohibited.

• • •

Appendix 2.4   Council of Europe, Scientific Research and/or Experimentation on Human Gametes, Embryos and Foetuses and Donation of Such Human Material (1989)

A. On Gametes

1. Gametes may be used independently for purposes of basic or experimental investigation, subject to the provisions of the following paragraphs;
2. Investigations shall be permitted:

— on fertility, sterility and contraception;
— on phenomena of histocompatibility or immunity related to procreation;
— on the process of gametogenesis and embryonic development, for the prevention or treatment of genetic diseases;

3. The human gametes employed for investigation or experimentation shall not be used to create zygotes or embryos *in vitro* for the purpose of procreation.

B. On Live Pre-Implantation Embryos

4. In accordance with Recommendations 934 (1982) and 1046 (1986), investigations of viable embryos *in vitro* shall only be permitted:

— for applied purposes of a diagnostic nature or for preventive or therapeutic purposes;
— if their non-pathological genetic heritage is not interfered with.

5. In accordance with paragraph 14.A.iv, eleventh sub-paragraph, of Recommendation 1046, research on living embryos must be prohibited, particularly:

— if the embryo is viable;
— if it is possible to use an animal model;
— if not foreseen within the framework of projects duly presented to and authorised by the appropriate public health or scientific authority or, by delegation, to and by the relevant national multidisciplinary committee;
—if not within the time-limits laid down by the authorities mentioned above.

6. Moreover, any proposed investigation which meets the above conditions for authorisation must be excluded:

— unless it is accompanied by all the required details on the embryonic material to be used, its source, foreseen time-limits of implementation and the aims pursued;
— unless, on completion of the investigation, those responsible agree to inform the authorising body of its outcome.

7. Embryos at the pre-implantation stage which have been expelled spontaneously from the uterus shall in no circumstances be retransferred back.

C. On Dead Pre-Implantation Embryos

8. Investigation of and experimentation on dead embryos for scientific, diagnostic, therapeutic or other purposes shall be permitted subject to prior authorisation.

D. On Post-Implantation Embryos or Live Foetuses in Utero

9. The removal of cells, tissues or embryonic or foetal organs, or of the placenta or the membranes, if live, for investigations other than of a diagnostic character and for preventive or therapeutic purposes shall be prohibited.

10. The pregnant woman and her husband or partner must be provided beforehand with as full information as necessary: i. on the technical operations to be performed for the removal of cells, and/ or embryonic or foetal tissues, or for the removal of the membranes, the placenta and/or the amniotic fluid, ii. on the intended purposes, and iii. on the risks involved.

11. Persons removing embryos or foetuses or parts thereof from the uterus without clinical or legal justification or without the prior consent of the pregnant woman and, where appropriate, of her husband or partner in a stable relationship, and persons using such embryological materials in breach of the relevant legislation or regulations shall be duly penalised.

E. On Post-Implantation Embryos or Live Foetuses Outside the Uterus

12. Foetuses shed prematurely and spontaneously and considered to be biologically viable may be the subject of clinical operations solely in order to promote their development and autonomous existence.

13. The performance of any operation on or the removal of cells, tissues or organs from embryos or foetuses outside the uterus shall be subject to, among other things, the parents' prior written consent.

14. Experiments on living embryos or foetuses, whether viable or not, shall be prohibited. None the less, where a state authorises certain experiments on non-viable foetuses or embryos only, these experiments may be undertaken in accordance with the terms of this recommendation and subject to prior authorisation from the health or scientific authorities or, where applicable, the national multidisciplinary body.

F. On Dead Embryos or Foetuses

15. Before proceeding to any intervention on dead embryos or foetuses, centres and clinics shall ascertain whether death is partial (when the embryo is clinically dead, its cells, tissues or organs may still remain alive for several hours) or total (when clinical death is matched by death of the cells).

16. The use of biological matter from dead embryos or foetuses for scientific, preventive, diagnostic, therapeutic, pharmaceutical, clinical or surgical purposes shall be permitted within the framework of the rules governing investigation, experimentation, diagnosis and therapy, in accordance with the terms of this recommendation.

G. Applications of Scientific Research to the Human Being in the Fields of Health and Heredity

17. Genetic technology shall only be used for investigations on or with human or recombinant genetic material if appropriate authorisation has been obtained. Such authorisation shall be granted by the competent authorities or, by delegation, by the national multidisciplinary body.

18. Scientific research projects on genetic engineering using genetic or recombinant genetic material shall be permitted, subject to approval:

— for diagnostic purposes, as in the case of prenatal diagnosis *in vitro or in utero* of genetic or hereditary diseases, in order to study the biological materials obtained with a

view to the treatment where possible of specific diseases or the prevention of their transmission, provided that the techniques used do not harm the embryo or the mother;
— for industrial purposes of a preventive, diagnostic or therapeutic nature, such as the
pharmaceutical manufacture (by molecular or gene cloning) of substances or products for
health or clinical purposes in suitable quantities, when they cannot be produced by any
other method, natural or otherwise, such as hormones, blood proteins which control the
immune responses, antiviral, antibacterial or anticarcinogenic agents, or the manufacture
of vaccines without any extra risk of a biological, immunological or infectious nature:
— for therapeutic purposes, in particular for the selection of sex in the case of diseases
linked to the sex chromosomes (particularly the X female chromosome), with a view to
preventing transmission; also for the creation by surgical means of beneficial gene mo-
saics, by transplanting genetically and biologically healthy cells, tissues or organs from
other persons to replace the diseased, damaged or defective counterparts in the person
being treated. In this connection, the approval of the use of healthy recombinant DNA to
replace pathological DNA causing a specific disease shall depend on the degree of scientific and technical safety which, in the opinion of the scientific and public authorities,
can be achieved in the human being with the type of molecular recombination envisaged.
Any form of therapy on the human germinal line shall be forbidden;
— for purposes of scientific investigation, for studying DNA sequences in the human
genome—their location, functions, dynamics, interrelationships and pathology; for studying recombinant DNA within human cells (as well as in the cells of simpler organisms
such as viruses and bacteria) with a view to obtaining a better understanding of the
mechanisms of molecular recombination, of expression of the genetic message, of the
development of cells and their components and their functional organisation; for studying
the ageing processes of cells, tissues and organs; and, more particularly, for studying the
general or specific mechanisms governing the development of diseases;
— for any other purpose considered useful and beneficial to the individual and to humanity, and incorporated in projects already approved.

19. Investigations or acts involving genetic technology shall only be authorised at centres and
establishments which have been registered, approved and authorised for such purposes, and
which have the requisite specialised personnel and technical resources.

H. Donation of Human Embryological Material

20. The donation of human embryological material shall be authorised solely for scientific
research on diagnostic, prevention or therapeutic purposes. Its sale shall be prohibited.
21. The intentional creation and/or keeping alive of embryos or foetuses whether *in vitro or
in utero* for any scientific research purpose, for instance to obtain genetic material, cells, tissues
or organs therefrom, shall be prohibited.
22. The donation and use of human embryological material shall be conditional on the freely
given written consent of the donor parents.
23. The donation of organs shall be devoid of any commercial aspect. The purchase or sale
of embryos or foetuses or parts thereof by their donor parents or other parties, and their
importation or exportation, shall also be prohibited.
24. The donation and use of human embryological material for the manufacture of dangerous
and exterminatory biological weapons shall be forbidden.
25. For the whole of this recommendation, "viable" embryos shall be understood to mean
embryos which are free of biological characteristics likely to prevent their development; however, the non-viability of human embryos and foetuses shall be determined solely by objective
biological criteria based on the embryo's intrinsic defects.

Appendix 2.5   Council of Europe, Recommendation on Genetic Testing and Screening for Health Care Purposes (1992)

Principle 1—Informing the Public

a. Plans for the introduction of genetic testing and screening should be brought to the notice of individuals, families and the public.

b. The public should be informed about genetic testing and screening, in particular their availability, purpose and implications—medical, legal, social and ethical—as well as the centres where they are carried out. Such information should start within the school system and be continued by the media.

Principle 2—Quality of Genetic Services

a. Proper education should be provided regarding human genetics and genetic disorders, particularly for health professionals and the paramedical professions, but also for any other profession concerned.

b. Genetic tests may only be carried out under the responsibility of a duly qualified physician.

c. It is desirable for centres where laboratory tests are performed to be approved by the state or by a competent authority in the state, and to participate in an external quality assurance.

Principle 3—Counselling and Support

a. Any genetic testing and screening procedure should be accompanied by appropriate counselling, both before and after the procedure.

Such counselling must be non-directive. The information to be given should include the pertinent medical facts, the results of tests, as well as the consequences and choices. It should explain the purpose and the nature of the tests and point out possible risks. It must be adapted to the circumstances in which individuals and families receive genetic information.

b. Everything should be done to provide, where necessary, continuing support for the tested persons.

Principle 4—Equality of Access—Non-discrimination

a. There should be equality of access to genetic testing, without financial considerations and without preconditions concerning eventual personal choices.

b. No condition should be attached to the acceptance or the undergoing of genetic tests.

c. The sale to the public of tests for diagnosing genetic disease or a predisposition for such diseases, or for the identification of carriers of such diseases, should only be allowed subject to strict licensing conditions laid down by national legislation.

Principle 5—Self-determination

a. The provision of genetic services should be based on respect for the principle of self-determination of the persons concerned. For this reason, any genetic testing, even when offered systematically, should be subject to their express, free and informed consent.

b. The testing of the following categories of persons should be subject to special safeguards:

— minors;

— persons suffering from mental disorders;

— adults placed under limited guardianship. Testing of these persons for diagnostic purposes should be permitted only when this is necessary for their own health or if the information is imperatively needed to diagnose the existence of a genetic disease in family members.

The consent of the person to be tested is required, except where national law provides otherwise.

Principle 6—Non-compulsory Nature of Tests

a. Health service benefits, family allowances, marriage requirements or other similar formalities, as well as the admission to, or the continued exercise of, certain activities, especially employment, should not be made dependent on the undergoing of genetics tests or screening.

Exceptions to this principle must be justified by reasons of direct protection of the person concerned or of a third party and be directly related to the specific conditions of the activity.

b. Only if expressly allowed by law may tests be made compulsory for the protection of individuals or the public.

Principle 7—Insurance

Insurers should not have the right to require genetic testing or to enquire about results of previously performed tests, as a pre-condition for the conclusion or modification of an insurance contract.

Principle 8—Data Protection

a. The collection and storage of substances and of samples, and the processing of information derived therefrom, must be in conformity with the Council of Europe's basic principles of data protection and data security laid down in the Convention for the Protection of Individuals with regard to Automatic Processing of Personal Data, European Treaty Series No. 108 of 28 January 1981 and the relevant recommendations of the Committee of Ministers in this field.

In particular in genetic screening and testing or associated genetic counselling personal data may be collected, processed and stored only for the purposes of health care, diagnosis and disease prevention, and for research closely related to these matters, as outlined in Principle 5.

b. Nominative genetic data may be stored as part of medical records and may also be stored in disease-related or test-related registers. The establishment and maintenance of such registers should be subject to national legislation.

Principle 9—Professional Secrecy

Persons handling genetic information should be bound by professional rules of conduct and rules laid down by national legislation aimed at preventing the misuse of such information and, in particular, by the duty to observe strict confidentiality. Personal information obtained by genetic testing is protected on the same basis as other medical data by the rules of medical data protection.

However, in the case of a severe genetic risk for other family members, consideration should be given, in accordance with national legislation and professional rules of conduct, to informing family members about matters relevant to their health or that of their future children.

Principle 10—Separate Storage of Genetic Information

Genetic data collected for health care purposes, as for all medical data, should as a general rule be kept separate from other personal records.

Principle 11—Unexpected Findings

In conformity with national legislation, unexpected findings may be communicated to the person tested only if they are of direct importance to the person or the family.

Communication of unexpected findings to family members of the person tested should only be authorised by national law if the person tested refuses expressly to inform them even though their lives are in danger.

Principle 12—Supervision

Research projects involving medical genetic data have to be carried out, in conformity with the standards of medical ethics, under the direct supervision of a responsible physician or, in exceptional circumstances, of a responsible scientist.

Principle 13—Handling of Data

a. Samples collected for a specific medical or scientific purpose may not, without permission of the persons concerned or the persons legally entitled to give permission on their behalf, be used in ways which could be harmful to the persons concerned.

b. The use of genetic data for population and similar studies has to respect rules governing data protection, and in particular concerning anonymity and confidentiality. The same applies to the publishing of such data.

Appendix 2.6   European Medical Research Councils Gene Therapy in Man (1988)

Over the past decade there have been major advances in the understanding at the molecular level of the structure and organisation of the genetic material of living organisms, including man. These advances have been driven by the application of recombinant DNA technology which, despite early concerns, has been used safely in laboratories throughout the world under the regulation of simple guidelines. Animal and human genes have been isolated and characterised; and the appropriate gene products, such as proteins or hormones, have been expressed following the introduction of genes into cultured cells in the laboratory. A further advance—the expression of specific genes after their introduction into laboratory animals—has raised the possibility that certain genetic defects in man might be corrected by applying similar techniques. Discussion of this possibility is well advanced in the USA, and the European Medical Research Councils (EMRC) consider it timely to formulate guidelines for the conduct of research on gene therapy in man and member countries.

General Considerations

Scope of Gene Therapy

The central consideration in this document is the correction of specific genetic defects in individual patients. This consideration should be distinguished from the application of gene therapy for the enhancement of general human characteristics such as physical appearance or intelligence, which raises profound ethical problems and should not be contemplated.

Distinction between Somatic and Germline Gene Therapy

Foreign genes may be inserted either into somatic cells (ie, any body cell except a germ cell) or into germ cells or cells that give rise to germ cells (eg, early embryonic cells). Insertion of genetic material into somatic cells and their subsequent transplantation is not fundamentally different from any form of organ transplantation or blood transfusion. The insertion of genes into fertilised eggs or very early embryos is fundamentally different because these genes would be passed on to the offspring in subsequent generations. Germline gene therapy should not be contemplated.

Experience with Experimental Systems

Somatic gene cell therapy in animals has given disappointing results and no successful "cures" can be claimed. This has been due mainly to the inefficiency of methods for inserting genes into somatic cells, such as marrow stem cells, and to the low level of expression after transfection. More encouraging results have been achieved in dogs, but further success in experimental systems will be necessary before trials in man can be justified.

Candidate Genetic Diseases and Target Tissues for Somatic Gene Therapy

Genetic diseases occur with an estimated frequency of 40–50 per 1000 population. They may be due to defects in single genes or to the interactions of a number of genes. Other diseases may have a genetic component but may also be influenced significantly by contributions from environmental factors. Single-gene defects, such as phenylketonuria (1 per 10 000 births) and muscular dystrophy (1 per 5 000 births) affect 1–2% of newborn babies.

For the foreseeable future, diseases which might be treated with gene therapy will be exclusively single-gene disorders. Diseases in which the affected gene has not been identified or in which regulation of the expression of the normal gene is very complex would not be appropriate for investigation in the near future. Candidates for gene therapy would be diseases which are invariably fatal or severely disabling and for which current possible therapies, such as bone marrow transplantation, are not always feasible or carry a high level of risk.

Bone marrow disorders are appropriate targets for early investigation because there is substantial experience of removal, treatment, and replacement of marrow cells in patients. Disorders such as adenosine deaminase deficiency and purine nucleoside phosphorylase deficiency, both of which result in immunodeficiency, would be suitable targets although they are rare. Although globin gene expression is tightly regulated, the haemoglobinopathies might also be suitable for study, since much is known about the mechanisms of regulation at the molecular level. The ability of transfected marrow cells to correct genetic defects in other tissues, such as the brain in Lesch-Nyhan disease, is less certain and should be accorded a lower priority. The possibility of implantation of modified fibroblasts or epidermal cells might also be considered in the future.

Technology and Safety of Introduction of Genes into Cells

In principle, genes may be introduced into human cells outside the body for later reimplantation, or cells may be treated in situ. There are several possible techniques for the introduction of normal genes into human cells. Although direct transfection of DNA is currently an inefficient means of modifying the large numbers of cells required for therapy, improved techniques may be developed in the future. Techniques of site-directed recombination, involving the simple exchange of the defective gene with a normal copy, are also currently inefficient, and the production of mutations following application of this method has been reported. However, this method is attractive in principle, and advances during the next few years may increase its practical value for therapy in man.

Most attention has been focused on the viral vectors, retroviruses in particular, for the introduction of genes into cells. The vector virus must be disabled so that it does not subsequently replicate, and there must be no active "helper" virus (used to package the disabled vector) in the vector preparations. Both these dangers can be avoided with modern production techniques. Vectors specific for particular tissues and cells are being developed, and vectors that occur naturally in the species to be treated are likely to be the most useful.

Safety is a major consideration in the introduction of genes into cells. There must be no possibility of producing active, possibly cancer-inducing, helper or vector viruses through recombination between disabled vector and helper viruses. It is also possible that insertion of a gene into the genetic material of the treated cell might (through "promoter insertion") activate the expression of genes involved in the induction of cancer or cause other harmful disturbances of cell regulation or function. In addition, the insertion might lead to rearrangement or relocation of particular host genes known to be involved in the induction of cancer (oncogenes). It should be noted, however, that certain current medical treatments, such as cancer chemotherapy, immunosuppression, and radiation, also carry a risk of predisposition to cancer. Finally, it will be necessary to ensure that the expression of an introduced gene is stable and sufficient to achieve a therapeutic effect.

The techniques for the introduction of genes into the cells, whether inside or initially outside the body, should not allow the spread of such genes or of any vectors to other cells, in particular germ cells, within the body or to people in contact with the patient. In this respect, great caution should be exercised with methods designed to target the introduction of genes into specific tissues within the body.

Manipulations in vitro must ensure that normal gene is introduced into a high proportion of stem cells and that such cells are given a proliferative advantage by procedures that specifically select for cells containing the gene. It seems that cells in the division cycle are more susceptible to the successful introduction of genes in retroviral vectors, and special methods, such as the use of growth factors, may be required to ensure that all the cells to be treated are in cycle. Techniques to select for, and therefore ensure the survival of, treated cells after transplantation into the patient will need investigation and may require the use of toxic drugs, with the possible complication of drug resistance, particularly if the selective therapies have to be applied for long periods.

Ethical Considerations

Somatic gene cell therapy by reimplantation of the patient's own cells is in principle similar to current routine therapies such as organ transplantation and therefore raises no new ethical issues. Judgments on the ethics of gene therapy in man will initially apply to individual cases and will require assessment of factors such as safety, efficacy, alternative treatments, and prognosis—in other words, the balance of risk and benefit for the patient. In the near future treatment by gene therapy might be justified in cases of invariably fatal or life-threatening diseases for which no alternative treatment is available. The patient should understand the issues involved and normally be asked to give informed consent to the treatment, although legal issues associated with "consent" by parents on behalf of a child may present difficulties. If damage caused by the genetic disorder in a particular patient is irreversible, then there may be no case for intervention through gene therapy. In the future, consideration might be given in particular disorders to treatment of the fetus before birth in order to prevent damage caused by early expression of the defect.

Regulation

National guidelines for the conduct of human gene therapy are essential. There should therefore be an expert national body to consider and approve proposals for such therapy in order to ensure public confidence in the introduction of a new and sophisticated treatment. In addition local ethical committees should subsequently consider and approve proposals. The assessment of early trials of human gene therapy should be monitored by a central body.

Summary

1. The purpose of gene therapy currently under consideration is the correction of genetic defects; attempts to enhance general human characteristics should not be contemplated. Only somatic cell gene therapy, resulting in non-heritable changes to particular body tissues, should be contemplated. Germline therapy, for introduction of heritable genetic modifications, is not acceptable. Further technical improvements in the expression of transferred genes in somatic cells will be necessary before successful gene therapy can be achieved even in animal models; in the meantime trials in man are not justified.

2. The most appropriate ''candidate'' genetic diseases for early investigation of treatment by gene therapy are single-gene disorders for which the affected gene and its regulation have been characterised.

3. In the near future, it is likely that success in the introduction of normal genes into human cells will be achieved through the use of disabled retrovirus vectors, although other techniques may advance rapidly. Much further work is required in the development of safe species-specific and tissue-specific retrovirus vectors. The methods of gene introduction should not result in the spread of gene or vector to other tissues within the body or to people in contact with the patient. The possibility of a significant increase in the predisposition of the patient to cancer should be evaluated in considering the risks and benefits of the treatment. In addition, the expression and regulation of the gene inserted should be stable and sufficient to ensure a therapeutic effect.

4. General ethical considerations applicable to any new clinical treatment apply to human gene therapy and, in the first instance, will require assessment in individual cases. In the near future it is likely that such therapy will be clinically justified in particular patients with invariably fatal or life-threatening diseases, provided informed consent is obtained and no alternative treatment is available.

5. A national body should consider all proposals for human gene therapy and ensure the application of agreed national guidelines. Early trials should be monitored by a central body.

Appendix 3
U.S. RESEARCH ETHICS POLICIES

Appendix 3.1 Department of Health and Human Services, Regulations for the Protection of Human Subjects (45 CFR 46)

Subpart A—Federal Policy for the Protection of Human Subjects (1991)

§46.101 To What Does This Policy Apply?

(a) Except as provided in paragraph (b) of this section, this policy applies to all research involving human subjects conducted, supported or otherwise subject to regulation by any Federal Department or Agency which takes appropriate administrative action to make the policy applicable to such research. This includes research conducted by Federal civilian employees or military personnel, except that each Department or Agency head may adopt such procedural modifications as may be appropriate from an administrative standpoint. It also includes research conducted, supported, or otherwise subject to regulation by the Federal Government outside the United States.

(1) Research that is conducted or supported by a Federal Department or Agency, whether or not it is regulated as defined in §46.102(e) must comply with all sections of this policy.

(2) Research that is neither conducted nor supported by a Federal Department or Agency but is subject to regulation as defined in §46.102(e) must be reviewed and approved, in compliance with §46.101, §46.102, and §46.107 through §46.117 of this policy, by an Institutional Review Board (IRB) that operates in accordance with the pertinent requirements of this policy.

(b) Unless otherwise required by Department or Agency heads, research activities in which the only involvement of human subjects will be in one or more of the following categories are exempt from this policy:

(1) Research conducted in established or commonly accepted educational settings, involving normal educational practices, such as

(i) research on regular and special education instructional strategies, or

(ii) research on the effectiveness of or the comparison among instructional techniques, curricula, or classroom management methods.

(2) Research involving the use of educational tests (cognitive, diagnostic, aptitude, achievement), survey procedures, interview procedures or observation of public behavior, unless:

(i) information obtained is recorded in such a manner that human subjects can be identified, directly or through identifiers linked to the subjects; and

(ii) any disclosure of the human subjects' responses outside the research could reasonably place the subjects at risk of criminal or civil liability or be damaging to the subjects' financial standing, employability, or reputation.

(3) Research involving the use of educational tests (cognitive, diagnostic, aptitude, achievement), survey procedures, interview procedures, or observation of public behavior that is not exempt under paragraph (b)(2) of this section, if:

(i) the human subjects are elected or appointed public officials or candidates for public office; or

(ii) Federal statute(s) require(s) without exception that the confidentiality of the personally identifiable information will be maintained throughout the research and thereafter.

(4) Research involving the collection or study of existing data, documents, records, pathological specimens, or diagnostic specimens, if these sources are publicly available or if

the information is recorded by the investigator in such a manner that subjects cannot be identified, directly or through identifiers linked to the subjects.

(5) Research and demonstration projects which are conducted by or subject to the approval of Department or Agency heads, and which are designed to study, evaluate, or otherwise examine:

(i) Public benefit or service programs;

(ii) procedures for obtaining benefits or services under those programs;

(iii) possible changes in or alternatives to those programs or procedures; or

(iv) possible changes in methods or levels of payment for benefits or services under those programs.

(6) Taste and food quality evaluation and consumer acceptance studies,

(i) if wholesome foods without additives are consumed or

(ii) if a food is consumed that contains a food ingredient at or below the level and for a use found to be safe, or agricultural chemical or environmental contaminant at or below the level found to be safe, by the Food and Drug Administration or approved by the Environmental Protection Agency or the Food Safety and Inspection Service of the U.S. Department of Agriculture.

(c) Department or Agency heads retain final judgment as to whether a particular activity is covered by this policy.

(d) Department or Agency heads may require that specific research activities or classes of research activities conducted, supported, or otherwise subject to regulation by the Department or Agency but not otherwise covered by this policy, comply with some or all of the requirements of this policy.

(e) Compliance with this policy requires compliance with pertinent Federal laws or regulations which provide additional protection for human subjects.

(f) This policy does not affect any state or local laws or regulations which may otherwise be applicable and which provide additional protections for human subjects.

(g) This policy does not affect any foreign laws or regulations which may otherwise be applicable and which provide additional protections to human subjects of research.

(h) When research covered by this policy takes place in foreign countries, procedures normally followed in the foreign countries to protect human subjects may differ from those set forth in this policy. [An example is a foreign institution which complies with guidelines consistent with the World Medical Assembly Declaration (Declaration of Helsinki amended 1989) issued either by sovereign states or by an organization whose function for the protection of human research subjects is internationally recognized.] In these circumstances, if a Department or Agency head determines that the procedures prescribed by the institution afford protections that are least equivalent to those provided in this policy, the Department or Agency head may approve the substitution of the foreign procedures in lieu of the procedural requirements provided in this policy. Except when otherwise required by statute, Executive Order, or the Department or Agency head, notices of these actions as they occur will be published in the Federal Register or will be otherwise published as provided in Department or Agency procedures.

(i) Unless otherwise required by law, Department or Agency heads may waive the applicability of some or all of the provisions of this policy to specific research activities or classes of research activities otherwise covered by this policy. Except when otherwise required by statute or Executive Order, the Department or Agency head shall forward advance notices of these actions to the Office for Protection from Research Risks, National Institutes of Health, Department of Health and Human services (DHHS), and shall also publish them in the Federal Register or in such other manner as provided in Department or Agency procedures.

§46.102 Definitions

(a) *Department or Agency head* means the head of any Federal Department or Agency and any other officer or employee of any Department or Agency to whom authority has been delegated.

(b) *Institution* means any public or private entity or Agency (including Federal, State, and other agencies).

(c) *Legally authorized representative* means an individual or judicial or other body authorized under applicable law to consent on behalf of a prospective subject to the subject's participation in the procedure(s) involved in the research.

(d) *Research* means a systematic investigation, including research development, testing and evaluation, designed to develop or contribute to generalizable knowledge. Activities which meet this definition constitute research for purposes of this policy, whether or not they are conducted or supported under a program which is considered research for other purposes. For example, some demonstration and service programs may include research activities.

(e) *Research subject to regulation,* and similar terms are intended to encompass those research activities for which a Federal Department or Agency has specific responsibility for regulating as a research activity, (for example, Investigational New Drug requirements administered by the Food and Drug Administration). It does not include research activities which are incidentally regulated by a Federal Department or Agency solely as part of the Department's or Agency's broader responsibility to regulate certain types of activities whether research or non-research in nature (for example, Wage and Hour requirements administered by the Department of Labor).

(f) *Human subject* means a living individual about whom an investigator (whether professional or student) conducting research obtains.

(1) data through intervention or interaction with the individual, or

(2) identifiable private information. *Intervention* includes both physical procedures by which data are gathered (for example, venipuncture) and manipulations of the subject or the subject's environment that are performed for research purposes. Interaction includes communication or interpersonal contact between investigator and subject. *Private information* includes information about behavior that occurs in a context in which an individual can reasonably expect that no observation or recording is taking place, and information which has been provided for specific purposes by an individual and which the individual can reasonably expect will not be made public (for example, a medical record). Private information must be individually identifiable (i.e., the identity of the subject is or may readily be ascertained by the investigator or associated with the information) in order for obtaining the information to constitute research involving human subjects.

(g) *IRB* means an Institutional Review Board established in accord with and for the purposes expressed in this policy.

(h) *IRB approval* means the determination of the IRB that the research has been reviewed and may be conducted at an institution within the constraints set forth by the IRB and by other institutional and Federal requirements.

(i) *Minimal risk* means that the probability and magnitude of harm or discomfort anticipated in the research are not greater in and of themselves than those ordinarily encountered in daily life or during the performance of routine physical or psychological examinations or tests.

(j) *Certification* means the official notification by the institution to the supporting Department or Agency, in accordance with the requirements of this policy, that a research project or activity involving human subjects has been reviewed and approved by an IRB in accordance with an approved assurance.

§46.103 Assuring Compliance With This Policy—Research Conducted or Supported By Any Federal Department or Agency

(a) Each institution engaged in research which is covered by this policy and which is conducted or supported by a Federal Department or Agency shall provide written assurance satisfactory to the Department or Agency head that it will comply with the requirements set forth in this policy. In lieu of requiring submission of an assurance, individual Department or Agency heads shall accept the existence of a current assurance, appropriate for the research in question, on file with the Office for Protection from Research Risks, National Institutes Health, DHHS, and approved for Federalwide use by that office. When the existence of an DHHS-approved assurance is accepted in lieu of requiring submission of an assurance, reports (except certification) required by this policy to be made to Department and Agency heads shall also be made to the Office for Protection from Research Risks, National Institutes of Health, DHHS.

(b) Department and agencies will conduct or support research covered by this policy only if the institution has an assurance approved as provided in this section, and only if the institution has certified to the Department or Agency head that the research has been reviewed and approved by an IRB provided for in the assurance, and will be subject to continuing review by the IRB. Assurances applicable to federally supported or conducted research shall at a minimum include:

(1) A statement of principles governing the institution in the discharge of its responsibilities for protecting the rights and welfare of human subjects of research conducted at or sponsored by the institution, regardless of whether the research is subject to Federal regulation. This may include an appropriate existing code, declaration, or statement of ethical principles, or a statement formulated by the institution itself. This requirement does not preempt provisions of this policy applicable to Department-or Agency-supported or regulated research and need not be applicable to any research exempted or waived under §46.101 (b) or (i).

(2) Designation of one or more IRBs established in accordance with the requirements of this policy, and for which provisions are made for meeting space and sufficient staff to support the IRB's review and recordkeeping duties.

(3) A list of IRB members identified by name; earned degrees; representative capacity; indications of experience such as board certifications, licenses, etc., sufficient to describe each member's chief anticipated contributions to IRB deliberations; and any employment or other relationship between each member and the institution; for example: full-time employee, part-time employee, member of governing panel or board, stockholder, paid or unpaid consultant. Changes in IRB membership shall be reported to the Department or Agency head, unless in accord with §46.103(a) of this policy, the existence of a DHHS-approved assurance is accepted. In this case, change in IRB membership shall be reported to the Office for Protection from Research Risks, National Institutes of Health, DHHS.

(4) Written procedures which the IRB will follow

(i) for conducting its initial and continuing review of research and for reporting its findings and actions to the investigator and the institution;

(ii) for determining which projects require review more often than annually and which projects need verification from sources other than the investigators that no material changes have occurred since previous IRB review; and

(iii) for ensuring prompt reporting to the IRB of proposed changes in a research activity, and for ensuring that such changes in approved research, during the period for which IRB approval has already been given, may not be initiated without IRB review and approval except when necessary to eliminate apparent immediate hazards to the subject.

(5) Written procedures for ensuring prompt reporting to the IRB, appropriate institutional officials, and the Department or Agency head of

(i) any unanticipated problems involving risks to subjects or others or any serious or continuing noncompliance with this policy or the requirements or determinations of the IRB: and

(ii) any suspension or termination of IRB approval.

(c) The assurance shall be executed by an individual authorized to act for the institution and to assume on behalf of the institution the obligations imposed by this policy and shall be filed in such form and manner as the Department or Agency head prescribes.

(d) The Department or Agency head will evaluate all assurances submitted in accordance with this policy through such officers and employees of the Department or Agency and such experts or consultants engaged for this purpose as the Department or Agency head determines to be appropriate. The Department or Agency head's evaluation will take into consideration the adequacy of the proposed IRB in light of the anticipated scope of the institution's research activities and the types of subject populations likely to be involved, the appropriateness of the proposed initial and continuing review procedures in light of the probable risks, and the size and complexity of the institution.

(e) On the basis of this evaluation, the Department or Agency head may approve or disapprove the assurance, or enter into negotiations to develop an approvable one. The Department or Agency head may limit the period during which any particular approved assurance or class of approved assurances shall remain effective or otherwise condition or restrict approval.

(f) Certification is required when the research is supported by a Federal Department or Agency and not otherwise exempted or waived under §46.101 (b) or (i). An institution with an approved assurance shall certify that each application or proposal for research covered by the assurance and by §46.103 of this policy has been reviewed and approved by the IRB. Such certification must be submitted with the application or proposal or by such later date as may be prescribed by the Department or Agency to which the application or proposal is submitted. Under no condition shall research covered by §46.103 of the policy be supported prior to receipt of the certification that the research has been reviewed and approved by the IRB. Institutions without an approved assurance covering the research shall certify within 30 days after receipt of a request for such a certification from the Department or Agency, that the application or proposal has been approved by the IRB. If the certification is not submitted within these time limits, the application or proposal may be returned to the institution.

§§46.104–46.106 [Reserved]

§46.107 IRB Membership

(a) Each IRB shall have at least five members, with varying backgrounds to promote complete and adequate review of research activities commonly conducted by the institution. The IRB shall be sufficiently qualified through the experience and expertise of its members, and the diversity of the members, including consideration of race, gender, and cultural backgrounds and sensitivity to such issues as community attitudes, to promote respect for its advice and counsel in safeguarding the rights and welfare of human subjects. In addition to possessing the professional competence necessary to review specific research activities, the IRB shall be able to ascertain the acceptability of proposed research in terms of institutional commitments and regulations, applicable law, and standards of professional conduct and practice. The IRB shall therefore include persons knowledgeable in these areas. If an IRB regularly reviews research that involves a vulnerable category of subjects, such as children, prisoners, pregnant women, or handicapped or mentally disabled persons, consideration shall be given to the inclusion of one or more individuals who are knowledgeable about and experienced in working with these subjects.

(b) Every nondiscriminatory effort will be made to ensure that no IRB consists entirely of men or entirely of women, including the institution's consideration of qualified persons of both sexes, so long as no selection is made to the IRB on the basis of gender. No IRB may consist entirely of members of one profession.

(c) Each IRB shall include at least one member whose primary concerns are in scientific areas and at least one member whose primary concerns are in nonscientific areas.

(d) Each IRB shall include at least one member who is not otherwise affiliated with the institution and who is not part of the immediate family of a person who is affiliated with the institution.

(e) No IRB may have a member participate in the IRB's initial or continuing review of any project in which the member has a conflicting interest, except to provide information requested by the IRB.

(f) An IRB may, in its discretion, invite individuals with competence in special areas to assist in the review of issues which require expertise beyond or in addition to that available on the IRB. These individuals may not vote with the IRB.

§46.108 IRB Functions and Operations

In order to fulfill the requirements of this policy each IRB shall:

(a) Follow written procedures in the same detail as described in §46.103(b)(4) and to the extent required by §46.103(b)(5).

(b) Except when an expedited review procedure is used (see §46.110), review proposed research at convened meetings at which a majority of the members of the IRB are present, including at least one member whose primary concerns are in nonscientific areas. In order for the research to be approved, it shall receive the approval of a majority of those members present at the meeting.

§46.109 IRB Review of Research

(a) An IRB shall review and have authority to approve, require modifications in (to secure approval), or disapprove all research activities covered by this policy.

(b) An IRB shall require that information given to subjects as part of informed consent is in accordance with §46.116. The IRB may require that information, in addition to that specifically mentioned in §46.116, be given to the subjects when in the IRB's judgment the information would meaningfully add to the protection of the rights and welfare of subjects.

(c) An IRB shall require documentation of informed consent or may waive documentation in accordance with §46.117.

(d) An IRB shall notify investigators and the institution in writing of its decision to approve or disapprove the proposed research activity, or of modifications required to secure IRB approval of the research activity. If the IRB decides to disapprove a research activity, it shall include in its written notification a statement of the reasons for its decision and give the investigator an opportunity to respond in person or in writing.

(e) An IRB shall conduct continuing review of research covered by this policy at intervals appropriate to the degree of risk, but not less than once per year, and shall have authority to observe or have a third party observe the consent process and the research.

§46.110 Expedited Review Procedures For Certain Kinds of Research Involving No More Than Minimal Risk, and For Minor Changes in Approved Research

(a) The Secretary, HHS, has established, and published as a Notice in the Federal Register, a list of categories of research that may be reviewed by the IRB through an expedited review procedure. The list will be amended, as appropriate, after consultation with other departments and agencies, through periodic republication by the Secretary, HHS, in the Federal Register. A copy of the list is available from the Office for Protection from Research Risks, National Institutes of Health, DHHS, Bethesda, Maryland 20892.

(b) An IRB may use the expedited review procedure to review either or both of the following:

(1) some or all of the research appearing on the list and found by the reviewer(s) to involve no more than minimal risk,

(2) minor changes in previously approved research during the period (of one year or less) for which approval is authorized.

Under an expedited review procedure, the review may be carried out by the IRB chairperson or by one or more experienced reviewers designated by the chairperson from among members of the IRB. In reviewing the research, the reviewers may exercise all of the authorities of the IRB except that the reviewers may not disapprove the research. A research activity may be disapproved only after review in accordance with the non-expedited procedure set forth in §46.108(b).

(c) Each IRB which uses an expedited review procedure shall adopt a method for keeping all members advised of research proposals which have been approved under the procedure.

(d) The Department or Agency head may restrict, suspend, terminate, or choose not to authorize an institution's or IRB's use of the expedited review procedure.

§46.111 Criteria for IRB Approval of Research

(a) In order to approve research covered by this policy the IRB shall determine that all of the following requirements are satisfied::

    (1) Risks to subjects are minimized:

        (i) by using procedures which are consistent with sound research design and which do not unnecessarily expose subjects to risk, and

        (ii) whenever appropriate, by using procedures already being performed on the subjects for diagnostic or treatment purposes.

    (2) Risks to subjects are reasonable in relation to anticipated benefits, if any, to subjects, and the importance of the knowledge that may reasonably be expected to result. In evaluating risks and benefits, the IRB should consider only those risks and benefits that may result from the research (as distinguished from risks and benefits of therapies subjects would receive even if not participating in the research). The IRB should not consider possible long-range effects of applying knowledge gained in the research (for example, the possible effects of the research on public policy) as among those research risks that fall within the purview of its responsibility.

    (3) Selection of subjects is equitable. In making this assessment the IRB should take into account the purposes of the research and the setting in which the research will be conducted and should be particularly cognizant of the special problems of research involving vulnerable populations, such as children, prisoners, pregnant women, mentally disabled persons, or economically or educationally disadvantaged persons.

    (4) Informed consent will be sought from each prospective subject or the subject's legally authorized representative, in accordance with, and to the extent required by §46.116.

    (5) Informed consent will be appropriately documented, in accordance with, and to the extent required by §46.117.

    (6) When appropriate, the research plan makes adequate provision for monitoring the data collected to ensure the safety of subjects.

    (7) When appropriate, there are adequate provisions to protect the privacy of subjects and to maintain the confidentiality of data.

(b) When some or all of the subjects are likely to be vulnerable to coercion or undue influence, such as children, prisoners, pregnant women, mentally disabled persons, or economically or educationally disadvantaged persons, additional safeguards have been included in the study to protect the rights and welfare of these subjects.

§46.112 Review by Institution

Research covered by this policy that has been approved by an IRB may be subject to further appropriate review and approval or disapproval by officials of the institution. However, those officials may not approve the research if it has not been approved by an IRB.

§46.113 Suspension or Termination of IRB Approval of Research

An IRB shall have authority to suspend or terminate approval of research that is not being conducted in accordance with the IRB's requirements or that has been associated with unexpected serious harm to subjects. Any suspension or termination of approval shall include a statement of the reasons for the IRB's action and shall be reported promptly to the investigator, appropriate institutional officials, and the Department or Agency head.

§46.114 Cooperative Research

Cooperative research projects are those projects covered by this policy which involve more than one institution. In the conduct of cooperative research projects, each institution is responsible for safeguarding the rights and welfare of human subjects and for complying with this policy. With the approval of the Department or Agency head, an institution participating in a cooperative project may enter into a joint review arrangement, rely upon the review of another qualified IRB, or make similar arrangements for avoiding duplication of effort.

§46.115 IRB Records

(a) An institution, or when appropriate an IRB, shall prepare and maintain adequate documentation of IRB activities, including the following:

(1) Copies of all research proposals reviewed, scientific evaluations, if any, that accompany the proposals, approved sample consent documents, progress reports submitted by investigators, and reports of injuries to subjects.

(2) Minutes of IRB meetings which shall be in sufficient detail to show attendance at the meetings; actions taken by the IRB; the vote on these actions including the number of members voting for, against, and abstaining; the basis for requiring changes in or disapproving research; and a written summary of the discussion of controverted issues and their resolution.

(3) Records of continuing review activities.

(4) Copies of all correspondence between the IRB and the investigators.

(5) A list of IRB members in the same detail as described in §46.103(b)(3).

(6) Written procedures for the IRB in the same detail as described in §46.103(b)(4) and §46.103(b)(5).

(7) Statements of significant new findings provided to subjects, as required by §46.116(b)(5).

(b) The records required by this policy shall be retained for at least 3 years, and records relating to research which is conducted shall be retained for at least 3 years after completion of the research. All records shall be accessible for inspection and copying by authorized representatives of the Department or Agency at reasonable times and in a reasonable manner.

§46.116 General Requirements for Informed Consent

Except as provided elsewhere in this policy, no investigator may involve a human being as a subject in research covered by this policy unless the investigator has obtained the legally effective informed consent of the subject or the subject's legally authorized representative. An investigator shall seek such consent only under circumstances that provide the prospective subject or the representative sufficient opportunity to consider whether or not to participate and that minimize the possibility of coercion or undue influence. The information that is given to the subject or the representative shall be in language understandable to the subject or the representative. No informed consent, whether oral or written, may include any exculpatory language through which the subject or the representative is made to waive or appear to waive any of the subject's legal rights, or releases or appears to release the investigator, the sponsor, the institution or its agents from liability for negligence.

(a) Basic elements of informed consent. Except as provided in paragraph (c) or (d) of this section, in seeking informed consent the following information shall be provided to each subject:

(1) a statement that the study involves research, an explanation of the purposes of the research and the expected duration of the subject's participation, a description of the procedures to be followed, and identification of any procedures which are experimental;

(2) a description of any reasonably foreseeable risks or discomforts to the subject;

(3) a description of any benefits to the subject or to others which may reasonably be expected from the research;

(4) a disclosure of appropriate alternative procedures or courses of treatment, if any, that might be advantageous to the subject;

(5) a statement describing the extent, if any, to which confidentiality of records identifying the subject will be maintained;

(6) for research involving more than minimal risk, an explanation as to whether any compensation and an explanation as to whether any medical treatments are available if injury occurs and, if so, what they consist of, or where further information may be obtained;

(7) an explanation of whom to contact for answers to pertinent questions about the research and research subjects' rights, and whom to contact in the event of a research-related injury to the subject; and

(8) a statement that participation is voluntary, refusal to participate will involve no penalty or loss of benefits to which the subject is otherwise entitled, and the subject may discontinue participation at any time without penalty or loss of benefits to which the subject is otherwise entitled.

(b) additional elements of informed consent. When appropriate, one or more of the following elements of information shall also be provided to each subject:

(1) a statement that the particular treatment or procedure may involve risks to the subject (or to the embryo or fetus, if the subject is or may become pregnant) which are currently unforeseeable;

(2) anticipated circumstances under which the subject's participation may be terminated by the investigator without regard to the subject's consent;

(3) any additional costs to the subject that may result from participation in the research;

(4) the consequences of a subject's decision to withdraw from the research and procedures for orderly termination of participation in the research;

(5) a statement that significant new findings developed during the course of the research which may relate to the subject's willingness to continue participation will be provided to the subject; and

(6) the approximate number of subjects involved in the study.

(c) An IRB may approve a consent procedure which does not include, or which alters, some or all of the elements of informed consent set forth above, or waive the requirement to obtain informed consent provided the IRB finds and documents that:

(1) the research or demonstration project is to be conducted by or subject to the approval of state or local government officials and is designed to study, evaluate, or otherwise examine: (i) public benefit or service programs; (ii) procedures for obtaining benefits or services under those programs; (iii) possible changes in or alternatives to those programs or procedures; or (iv) possible changes in methods or levels of payment for benefits or services under those programs; and

(2) the research could not practicably be carried out without the waiver or alteration.

(d) An IRB may approve a consent procedure which does not include, or which alters, some or all of the elements of informed consent set forth in this section, or waive the requirement to obtain informed consent provided the IRB finds and documents that:

(1) the research involves no more than minimal risk to the subjects;

(2) the waiver or alteration will not adversely affect the rights and welfare of the subjects;

(3) the research could not practicably be carried out without the waiver or alteration; and

(4) whenever appropriate, the subjects will be provided with additional pertinent information after participation.

(e) The informed consent requirements in this policy are not intended to preempt any applicable Federal, State, or local laws which require additional information to be disclosed in order for informed consent to be legally effective.

(f) Nothing in this policy is intended to limit the authority of a physician to provide emergency medical care, to the extent the physician is permitted to do so under applicable Federal, State, or local law.

§46.117 Documentation of Informed Consent

(a) Except as provided in paragraph (c) of this section, informed consent shall be documented by the use of a written consent form approved by the IRB and signed by the subject or the subject's legally authorized representative. A copy shall be given to the person signing the form.

(b) Except as provided in paragraph (c) of this section, the consent form may be either of the following:

(1) A written consent document that embodies the elements of informed consent required by §46.116. This form may be read to the subject or the subject's legally authorized representative, but in any event, the investigator shall give either the subject or the representative adequate opportunity to read it before it is signed; or

(2) A short form written consent document stating that the elements of informed consent required by §46.116 have been presented orally to the subject or the subject's legally authorized representative. When this method is used, there shall be a witness to the oral presentation. Also, the IRB shall approve a written summary of what is to be said to the subject or the representative. Only the short form itself is to be signed by the subject or the representative. However, the witness shall sign both the short form and a copy of the summary, and the person actually obtaining consent shall sign a copy of the summary. A copy of the summary shall be given to the subject or the representative, in addition to a copy of the short form.

(c) An IRB may waive the requirement for the investigator to obtain a signed consent form for some or all subjects if it finds either:

(1) That the only record linking the subject and the research would be the consent document and the principal risk would be potential harm resulting from a breach of confidentiality. Each subject will be asked whether the subject wants documentation linking the subject with the research, and the subject's wishes will govern; or

(2) That the research presents no more than minimal risk of harm to subjects and involves no procedures for which written consent is normally required outside of the research context.

In cases in which the documentation requirement is waived, the IRB may require the investigator to provide subjects with a written statement regarding the research.

§46.118 Applications and Proposals Lacking Definite Plans for Involvement of Human Subjects

Certain types of applications for grants, cooperative agreements, or contracts are submitted to departments or agencies with the knowledge that subjects may be involved within the period of support, but definite plans would not normally be set forth in the application or proposal. These include activities such as institutional type grants when selection of specific projects is the institution's responsibility; research training grants in which the activities involving subjects remain to be selected; and projects in which human subjects' involvement will depend upon completion of instruments, prior animal studies, or purification of compounds. These applications need not be reviewed by an IRB before an award may be made. However, except for research exempted or waived under §46.101 (b) or (i), no human subjects may be involved in any project supported by these awards until the project has been reviewed and approved by the IRB, as provided in this policy, and certification submitted, by the institution, to the Department or Agency.

§46.119 Research Undertaken Without the Intention of Involving Human Subjects

In the event research is undertaken without the intention of involving human subjects, but it is later proposed to involve human subjects in the research, the research shall first be reviewed and approved by an IRB, as provided in this policy, a certification submitted, by the institution, to the Department or Agency, and final approval given to the proposed change by the Department or Agency.

§46.120 Evaluation and Disposition of Applications and Proposals for Research to be Conducted or Supported by a Federal Department or Agency

(a) The Department or Agency head will evaluate all applications and proposals involving human subjects submitted to the Department or Agency through such officers and employees of the Department or Agency and such experts and consultants as the Department or Agency head determines to be appropriate. This evaluation will take into consideration the risks to the subjects, the adequacy of protection against these risks, the potential benefits of the research to the subjects and others, and the importance of the knowledge gained or to be gained.

(b) On the basis of this evaluation, the Department or Agency head may approve or disapprove the application or proposal, or enter into negotiations to develop an approvable one.

§46.121 [Reserved]

§46.122 Use of Federal Funds

Federal funds administered by a Department or Agency may not be expended for research involving human subjects unless the requirements of this policy have been satisfied.

§46.123 Early Termination of Research Support: Evaluation of Applications and Proposals

(a) The Department or Agency head may require that Department or Agency support for any project be terminated or suspended in the manner prescribed in applicable program requirements, when the Department or Agency head finds an institution has materially failed to comply with the terms of this policy.

(b) In making decisions about supporting or approving applications or proposals covered by this policy the Department or Agency head may take into account, in addition to all other eligibility requirements and program criteria, factors such as whether the applicant has been subject to a termination or suspension under paragraph (a) of this section and whether the applicant or the person or persons who would direct or has/have directed the scientific and technical aspects of an activity has/have, in the judgment of the Department or Agency head, materially failed to discharge responsibility for the protection of the rights and welfare of human subjects (whether or not the research was subject to Federal regulation).

§46.124 Conditions

With respect to any research project or any class of research projects the Department or Agency head may impose additional conditions prior to or at the time of approval when in the judgment of the Department or Agency head additional conditions are necessary for the protection of human subjects.

Subpart B—Additional DHHS Protections Pertaining to Research, Development, and Related Activities Involving Fetuses, Pregnant Women, and Human In Vitro Fertilization (1981)

§46.201 Applicability

(a) The regulations in this subpart are applicable to all Department of Health and Human Services grants and contracts supporting research, development, and related activities involving:
  (1) the fetus,
  (2) pregnant women, and
  (3) human *in vitro* fertilization.

(b) Nothing in this subpart shall be construed as indicating that compliance with the procedures set forth herein will in any way render inapplicable pertinent State or local laws bearing upon activities covered by this subpart.

(c) The requirements of this subpart are in addition to those imposed under the other subparts of this part.

§46.202 Purpose

It is the purpose of this subpart to provide additional safeguards in reviewing activities to which this subpart is applicable to assure that they conform to appropriate ethical standards and relate to important societal needs.

§46.203 Definitions

As used in this subpart:

(a) "Secretary" means the Secretary of Health and Human Services and any other officer or employee of the Department of Health and Human Services (DHHS) to whom authority has been delegated.

(b) "Pregnancy" encompasses the period of time from confirmation of implantation (through any of the presumptive signs of pregnancy, such as missed menses, or by a medically acceptable pregnancy test), until expulsion or extraction of the fetus.

(c) "Fetus" means the product of conception from the time of implantation (as evidenced by any of the presumptive signs of pregnancy, such as missed menses, or a medically acceptable pregnancy test), until a determination is made, following expulsion or extraction of the fetus, that it is viable.

(d) "Viable" as it pertains to the fetus means being able, after either spontaneous or induced delivery, to survive (given the benefit of available medical therapy) to the point of independently maintaining heart beat and respiration. The Secretary may from time to time, taking into account medical advances, publish in the **Federal Register** guidelines to assist in determining whether a fetus is viable for purposes of this subpart. If a fetus is viable after delivery, it is a premature infant.

(e) "Nonviable fetus" means a fetus *ex utero* which, although living, is not viable.

(f) "Dead fetus" means a fetus *ex utero* which exhibits neither heartbeat, spontaneous respiratory activity, spontaneous movement of voluntary muscles, nor pulsation of the umbilical cord (if still attached).

(g) "*In vitro* fertilization" means any fertilization of human ova which occurs outside the body of a female, either through admixture of donor human sperm and ova or by any other means.

§46.204 Ethical Advisory Boards

(a) One or more Ethical Advisory Boards shall be established by the Secretary. Members of these Board(s) shall be so selected that the Board(s) will be competent to deal with medical, legal, social, ethical, and related issues and may include, for example, research scientists, physicians, psychologists, sociologists, educators, lawyers, and ethicists, as well as representatives of the general public. No Board member may be a regular, full-time employee of the Department of Health and Human Services.

(b) At the request of the Secretary, the Ethical Advisory Board shall render advice consistent with the policies and requirements of this part as to ethical issues, involving activities covered by this subpart, raised by individual applications or proposals. In addition, upon request by the Secretary, the Board shall render advice as to classes of applications or proposals and general policies, guidelines, and procedures.

(c) A Board may establish, with the approval of the Secretary, classes of applications or proposals which: (1) must be submitted to the Board, or (2) need not be submitted to the Board. Where the Board so establishes a class of applications or proposals which must be submitted, no application or proposal within the class may be funded by the Department or any component thereof until the application or proposal has been reviewed by the Board and the Board has rendered advice as to its acceptability from an ethical standpoint.

(d) No application or proposal involving human *in vitro* fertilization may be funded by the Department or any component thereof until the application or proposal has been reviewed by the Ethical Advisory Board and the Board has rendered advice as to its acceptability from an ethical standpoint.

§46.205 Additional Duties of the Institutional Review Boards in Connection with Activities Involving Fetuses, Pregnant Women, or Human In Vitro Fertilization

(a) In addition to the responsibilities prescribed for Institutional Review Boards under Subpart A of this part, the applicant's or offeror's Board shall, with respect to activities covered by this subpart, carry out the following additional duties:

(1) determine that all aspects of the activity meet the requirements of this subpart;

(2) determine that adequate consideration has been given to the manner in which potential subjects will be selected, and adequate provision has been made by the applicant or offeror for monitoring the actual informed consent process (e.g., through such mechanisms, when appropriate, as participation by the Institutional Review Board or subject advocates in: (i) overseeing the actual process by which individual consents required by this subpart are secured either by approving induction of each individual into the activity or verifying, perhaps through sampling, that approved procedures for induction of individuals into the activity are being followed, and (ii) monitoring the progress of the activity and intervening as necessary through such steps as visits to the activity site and continuing evaluation to determine if any unanticipated risks have arisen);

(3) carry out such other responsibilities as may be assigned by the Secretary.

(b) No award may be issued until the applicant or offeror has certified to the Secretary that the Institutional Review Board has made the determinations required under paragraph (a) of this section and the Secretary has approved these determinations, as provided in §46.120 of Subpart A of this part.

(c) Applicants or offerors seeking support for activities covered by this subpart must provide for the designation of an Institutional Review Board, subject to approval by the Secretary, where no such Board has been established under Subpart A of this part.

§46.206 General Limitations

(a) No activity to which this subpart is applicable may be undertaken unless:

(1) appropriate studies on animals and nonpregnant individuals have been completed;

(2) except where the purpose of the activity is to meet the health needs of the mother or the particular fetus, the risk to the fetus is minimal and, in all cases, is the least possible risk for achieving the objectives of the activity;

(3) individuals engaged in the activity will have no part in: (i) any decisions as to the timing, method, and procedures used to terminate the pregnancy, and (ii) determining the viability of the fetus at the termination of the pregnancy; and

(4) no procedural changes which may cause greater than minimal risk to the fetus or the pregnant woman will be introduced into the procedure for terminating the pregnancy solely in the interest of the activity.

(b) No inducements, monetary or otherwise, may be offered to terminate pregnancy for purposes of the activity.

§46.207 Activities Directed Toward Pregnant Women as Subjects

(a) No pregnant woman may be involved as a subject in an activity covered by this subpart unless:

(1) the purpose of the activity is to meet the health needs of the mother and the fetus will be placed at risk only to the minimum extent necessary to meet such needs, or

(2) the risk to the fetus is minimal.

(b) An activity permitted under paragraph (a) of this section may be conducted only if the mother and father are legally competent and have given their informed consent after having been fully informed regarding possible impact on the fetus, except that the father's informed consent need not be secured if:

(1) the purpose of the activity is to meet the health needs of the mother;

(2) his identity or whereabouts cannot reasonably be ascertained;

(3) he is not reasonably available; or

(4) the pregnancy resulted from rape.

§46.208 Activities Directed Toward Fetuses In Utero as Subjects

(a) No fetus *in utero* may be involved as a subject in any activity covered by this subpart unless:

(1) the purpose of the activity is to meet the health needs of the particular fetus and the fetus will be placed at risk only to the minimum extent necessary to meet such needs, or

(2) the risk to the fetus imposed by the research is minimal and the purpose of the activity is the development of important biomedical knowledge which cannot be obtained by other means.

(b) An activity permitted under paragraph (a) of this section may be conducted only if the mother and father are legally competent and have given their informed consent, except that the father's consent need not be secured if:

(1) his identity or whereabouts cannot reasonably be ascertained

(2) he is not reasonably available, or

(3) the pregnancy resulted from rape.

§46.209 Activities Directed Toward Fetuses Ex Utero, Including Nonviable Fetuses, as Subjects

(a) Until it has been ascertained whether or not a fetus *ex utero* is viable, a fetus *ex utero* may not be involved as a subject in an activity covered by this subpart unless:

(1) there will be no added risk to the fetus resulting from the activity, and the purpose of the activity is the development of important biomedical knowledge which cannot be obtained by other means, or

(2) the purpose of the activity is to enhance the possibility of survival of the particular fetus to the point of viability.

(b) No nonviable fetus may be involved as a subject in an activity covered by this subpart unless:

(1) vital functions of the fetus will not be artificially maintained,

(2) experimental activities which of themselves would terminate the heartbeat or respiration of the fetus will not be employed, and

(3) the purpose of the activity is the development of important biomedical knowledge which cannot be obtained by other means.

(c) In the event the fetus *ex utero* is found to be viable, it may be included as a subject in the activity only to the extent permitted by and in accordance with the requirements of other subparts of this part.

(d) An activity permitted under paragraph (a) or (b) of this section may be conducted only if the mother and father are legally competent and have given their informed consent, except that the father's informed consent need not be secured if:

(1) his identity or whereabouts cannot reasonably be ascertained,

(2) he is not reasonably available, or

(3) the pregnancy resulted from rape.

§46.210 Activities Involving the Dead Fetus, Fetal Material, or the Placenta

Activities involving the dead fetus, mascerated fetal material, or cells, tissue, or organs excised from a dead fetus shall be conducted only in accordance with any applicable State or local laws regarding such activities.

§46.211 Modification or Waiver of Specific Requirements

Upon the request of an applicant or offeror (with the approval of its Institutional Review Board), the Secretary may modify or waive specific requirements of this subpart, with the approval of the Ethical Advisory Board after such opportunity for public comment as the Ethical Advisory Board considers appropriate in the particular instance. In making such decisions, the Secretary will consider whether the risks to the subject are so outweighed by the sum of the benefit to the subject and the importance of the knowledge to be gained as to warrant such modification or waiver and that such benefits cannot be gained except through a modification or waiver. Any such modifications or waivers will be published as notices in the Federal Register.

Subpart C—Additional DHHS Protections Pertaining to Biomedical and Behavioral Research Involving Prisoners as Subjects (1981)

§46.301 Applicability

(a) The regulations in this subpart are applicable to all biomedical and behavioral research conducted or supported by the Department of Health and Human Services involving prisoners as subjects.

(b) Nothing in this subpart shall be construed as indicating that compliance with the procedures set forth herein will authorize research involving prisoners as subjects, to the extent such research is limited or barred by applicable State or local law.

(c) The requirements of this subpart are in addition to those imposed under the other subparts of this part.

§46.302 Purpose

Inasmuch as prisoners may be under constraints because of their incarceration which could affect their ability to make a truly voluntary and uncoerced decision whether or not to participate as subjects in research, it is the purpose of this subpart to provide additional safeguards for the protection of prisoners involved in activities to which this subpart is applicable.

§46.303 Definitions

As used in this subpart:

(a) "Secretary" means the Secretary of Health and Human Services and any other officer or employee of the Department of Health and Human Services to whom authority has been delegated.

(b) "DHHS" means the Department of Health and Human Services.

(c) "Prisoner" means any individual involuntarily confined or detained in a penal institution.

The term is intended to encompass individuals sentenced to such an institution under a criminal or civil statute, individuals detained in other facilities by virtue of statutes or commitment procedures which provide alternatives to criminal prosecution or incarceration in a penal institution, and individuals detained pending arraignment, trial, or sentencing.

(d) "Minimal risk" is the probability and magnitude of physical or psychological harm that is normally encountered in the daily lives, or in the routine medical, dental, or psychological examination of healthy persons.

§46.304 Composition of Institutional Review Boards Where Prisoners are Involved

In addition to satisfying the requirements in §46.107 of this part, an Institutional Review Board, carrying out responsibilities under this part with respect to research covered by this subpart, shall also meet the following specific requirements:

(a) A majority of the Board (exclusive of prisoner members) shall have no association with the prison(s) involved, apart from their membership on the Board.

(b) At least one member of the Board shall be a prisoner, or a prisoner representative with appropriate background and experience to serve in that capacity, except that where a particular research project is reviewed by more than one Board only one Board need satisfy this requirement.

§46.305 Additional Duties of the Institutional Review Boards Where Prisoners are Involved

(a) In addition to all other responsibilities prescribed for Institutional Review Boards under this part, the Board shall review research covered by this subpart and approve such research only if it finds that:

(1) the research under review represents one of the categories of research permissible under §46.306(a)(2);

(2) any possible advantages accruing to the prisoner through his or her participation in the research, when compared to the general living conditions, medical care, quality of food, amenities and opportunity for earnings in the prison, are not of such a magnitude that his or her ability to weigh the risks of the research against the value of such advantages in the limited choice environment of the prison is impaired;

(3) the risks involved in the research are commensurate with risks that would be accepted by nonprisoner volunteers;

(4) procedures for the selection of subjects within the prison are fair to all prisoners and immune from arbitrary intervention by prison authorities or prisoners. Unless the principal investigator provides to the Board justification in writing for following some other procedures, control subjects must be selected randomly from the group of available prisoners who meet the characteristics needed for that particular research project;

(5) the information is presented in language which is understandable to the subject population;

(6) adequate assurance exists that parole boards will not take into account a prisoner's participation in the research in making decisions regarding parole, and each prisoner is clearly informed in advance that participation in the research will have no effect on his or her parole; and

(7) where the Board finds there may be a need for follow-up examination or care of participants after the end of their participation, adequate provision has been made for such examination or care, taking into account the varying lengths of individual prisoners' sentences, and for informing participants of this fact.

(b) The Board shall carry out such other duties as may be assigned by the Secretary.

(c) The institution shall certify to the Secretary, in such form and manner as the Secretary may require, that the duties of the Board under this section have been fulfilled.

§46.306 Permitted Research Involving Prisoners

(a) Biomedical or behavioral research conducted or supported by DHHS may involve prisoners as subjects only if:

(1) the institution responsible for the conduct of the research has certified to the Secretary that the Institutional Review Board has approved the research under §46.305 of this subpart; and

(2) in the judgment of the Secretary the proposed research involves solely the following:

(A) study of the possible causes, effects, and processes of incarceration, and of criminal behavior, provided that the study presents no more than minimal risk and no more than inconvenience to the subjects;

(B) study of prisons as institutional structures or of prisoners as incarcerated persons, provided that the study presents no more than minimal risk and no more than inconvenience to the subjects;

(C) research on conditions particularly affecting prisoners as a class (for example, vaccine trials and other research on hepatitis which is much more prevalent in prisons than elsewhere; and research on social and psychological problems such as alcoholism, drug addiction, and sexual assaults) provided that the study may proceed only after the Secretary has consulted with appropriate experts including experts in penology, medicine, and ethics, and published notice, in the Federal Register, of his intent to approve such research; or

(D) research on practices, both innovative and accepted, which have the intent and reasonable probability of improving the health or well-being of the subject. In cases in which those studies require the assignment of prisoners in a manner consistent with protocols approved by the IRB to control groups which may not benefit from the research, the study may proceed only after the Secretary has consulted with appropriate experts, including experts in penology, medicine, and ethics, and published notice, in the Federal Register, of the intent to approve such research.

(b) Except as provided in paragraph (a) of this section, biomedical or behavioral research conducted or supported by DHHS shall not involve prisoners as subjects.

Subpart D—Additional DHHS Protections for Children Involved as Subjects in Research (1983)

§46.401 To What Do These Regulations Apply?

(a) This subpart applies to all research involving children as subjects, conducted or supported by the Department of Health and Human Services.

(1) This includes research conducted by Department employees, except that each head of an Operating Division of the Department may adopt such nonsubstantive, procedural modifications as may be appropriate from an administrative standpoint.

(2) It also includes research conducted or supported by the Department of Health and Human Services outside the United States, but in appropriate circumstances, the Secretary may, under paragraph (e) of §46.101 of Subpart A, waive the applicability of some or all of the requirements of these regulations for research of this type.

(b) Exemptions at §46.101(b)(1) and (b)(3) through (b)(6) are applicable to this subpart. The exemption at §46.101(b)(2) regarding educational tests is also applicable to this subpart. However, the exemption at §46.101(b)(2) for research involving survey or interview procedures or observations of public behavior does not apply to research covered by this subpart, except for research involving observation of public behavior when the investigator(s) do not participate in the activities being observed.

(c) The exceptions, additions, and provisions for waiver as they appear in paragraphs (c) through (i) of §46.101 of Subpart A are applicable to this subpart.

§46.402 Definitions

The definitions in §46.102 of Subpart A shall be applicable to this subpart as well. In addition, as used in this subpart:

(a) "Children" are persons who have not attained the legal age for consent to treatments or procedures involved in the research, under the applicable law of the jurisdiction in which the research will be conducted.

(b) "Assent" means a child's affirmative agreement to participate in research. Mere failure to object should not, absent affirmative agreement, be construed as assent.

(c) "Permission" means the agreement of parent(s) or guardian to the participation of their child or ward in research.

(d) "Parent" means a child's biological or adoptive parent.

(e) "Guardian" means an individual who is authorized under applicable State or local law to consent on behalf of a child to general medical care.

§46.403 IRB Duties

In addition to other responsibilities assigned to IRBs under this part, each IRB shall review research covered by this subpart and approve only research which satisfies the conditions of all applicable sections of this subpart.

§46.404 Research Not Involving Greater Than Minimal Risk

DHHS will conduct or fund research in which the IRB finds that no greater than minimal risk to children is presented, only if the IRB finds that adequate provisions are made for soliciting the assent of the children and the permission of their parents or guardians, as set forth in §46.408.

§46.405 Research Involving Greater Than Minimal Risk But Presenting the Prospect of Direct Benefit to the Individual Subjects

DHHS will conduct or fund research in which the IRB finds that more than minimal risk to children is presented by an intervention or procedure that holds out the prospect of direct benefit for the individual subject, or by a monitoring procedure that is likely to contribute to the subject's well-being, only if the IRB finds that:

(a) the risk is justified by the anticipated benefit to the subjects;

(b) the relation of the anticipated benefit to risk is at least as favorable to the subjects as that presented by available alternative approaches; and

(c) adequate provisions are made for soliciting the assent of the children and permission of their parents or guardians, as set forth in §46.408.

§46.406 Research Involving Greater Than Minimal Risk and No Prospect of Direct Benefit to Individual Subjects, But Likely to Yield Generalizable Knowledge About the Subject's Disorder or Condition

DHHS will conduct or fund research in which the IRB finds that more than minimal risk to children is presented by an intervention or procedure that does not hold out the prospect of direct benefit for the individual subject, or by a monitoring procedure which is not likely to contribute to the well-being of the subject, only if the IRB finds that:

(a) the risk represents a minor increase over minimal risk;

(b) the intervention or procedure presents experiences to subjects that are reasonably commensurate with those inherent in their actual or expected medical, dental, psychological, social, or educational situations;

(c) the intervention or procedure is likely to yield generalizable knowledge about the subjects' disorder or condition which is of vital importance for the understanding or amelioration of the subjects' disorder or condition; and

(d) adequate provisions are made for soliciting assent of the children and permission of their parents or guardians, as set forth in §46.408.

§46.407 Research Not Otherwise Approvable Which Presents an Opportunity to Understand, Prevent, or Alleviate a Serious Problem Affecting the Health or Welfare of Children

DHHS will conduct or fund research that the IRB does not believe meets the requirements of §46.404, §46.405, or §46.406 only if:

(a) the IRB finds that the research presents a reasonable opportunity to further the understanding, prevention, or alleviation of a serious problem affecting the health or welfare of children; and

(b) the Secretary, after consultation with a panel of experts in pertinent disciplines (for example: science, medicine, education, ethics, law) and following opportunity for public review and comment, has determined either:

(1) that the research in fact satisfies the conditions of §46.404, §46.405, or §46.406, as applicable, or

(2) the following:

(i) the research presents a reasonable opportunity to further the understanding, prevention, or alleviation of a serious problem affecting the health or welfare of children;

(ii) the research will be conducted in accordance with sound ethical principles;

(iii) adequate provisions are made for soliciting the assent of children and the permission of their parents or guardians, as set forth in §46.408.

§46.408 Requirements for Permission by Parents or Guardians and for Assent by Children

(a) In addition to the determinations required under other applicable sections of this subpart, the IRB shall determine that adequate provisions are made for soliciting the assent of the children, when in the judgment of the IRB the children are capable of providing assent. In determining whether children are capable of assenting, the IRB shall take into account the ages, maturity, and psychological state of the children involved. This judgment may be made for all children to be involved in research under a particular protocol, or for each child, as the IRB deems appropriate. If the IRB determines that the capability of some or all of the children is so limited that they cannot reasonably be consulted or that the intervention or procedure involved in the research holds out a prospect of direct benefit that is important to the health or well-being of the children and is available only in the context of the research, the assent of the children is not a necessary condition for proceeding with the research. Even where the IRB determines that the subjects are capable of assenting, the IRB may still waive the assent requirement under circumstances in which consent may be waived in accord with §46.116 of Subpart A.

(b) In addition to the determinations required under other applicable sections of this subpart, the IRB shall determine, in accordance with and to the extent that consent is required by §46.116 of Subpart A, that adequate provisions are made for soliciting the permission of each child's parents or guardian. Where parental permission is to be obtained, the IRB may find that the permission of one parent is sufficient for research to be conducted under §46.404 or

§46.405. Where research is covered by §46.406 and §46.407 and permission is to be obtained from parents, both parents must give their permission unless one parent is deceased, unknown, incompetent, or not reasonably available, or when only one parent has legal responsibility for the care and custody of the child.

(c) In addition to the provisions for waiver contained in §46.116 of Subpart A, if the IRB determines that a research protocol is designed for conditions or for a subject population for which parental or guardian permission is not a reasonable requirement to protect the subjects (for example, neglected or abused children), it may waive the consent requirements in Subpart A of this part and paragraph (b) of this section, provided an appropriate mechanism for protecting the children who will participate as subjects in the research is substituted, and provided further that the waiver is not inconsistent with Federal, State, or local law. The choice of an appropriate mechanism would depend upon the nature and purpose of the activities described in the protocol, the risk and anticipated benefit to the research subjects, and their age, maturity, status, and condition.

(d) Permission by parents or guardians shall be documented in accordance with and to the extent required by §46.117 of Subpart A.

(e) When the IRB determines that assent is required, it shall also determine whether and how assent must be documented.

§46.409 Wards

(a) Children who are wards of the State or any other agency, institution, or entity can be included in research approved under §46.406 or §46.407 only if such research is:

(1) related to their status as wards; or

(2) conducted in schools, camps, hospitals, institutions, or similar settings in which the majority of children involved as subjects are not wards.

(b) If the research is approved under paragraph (a) of this section, the IRB shall require appointment of an advocate for each child who is a ward, in addition to any other individual acting on behalf of the child as guardian or in loco parentis. One individual may serve as advocate for more than one child. The advocate shall be an individual who has the background and experience to act in, and agrees to act in, the best interests of the child for the duration of the child's participation in the research and who is not associated in any way (except in the role as advocate or member of the IRB) with the research, the investigator(s), or the guardian organization.

Appendix 3.2 National Commission, The Belmont Report (1979)

Ethical Principles and Guidelines for Research Involving Human Subjects

Scientific research has produced substantial social benefits. It has also posed some troubling ethical questions. Public attention was drawn to these questions by reported abuses of human subjects in biomedical experiments, especially during the Second World War. During the Nuremberg War Crime Trials, the Nuremberg code was drafted as a set of standards for judging physicians and scientists who had conducted biomedical experiments on concentration camp prisoners. This code became the prototype of many later codes intended to assure that research involving human subjects would be carried out in an ethical manner.

The codes consist of rules, some general, others specific, that guide the investigators or the reviewers of research in their work. Such rules often are inadequate to cover complex situations; at times they come into conflict, and they are frequently difficult to interpret or apply. Broader ethical principles will provide a basis on which specific rules may be formulated, criticized and interpreted.

Three principles, or general prescriptive judgments, that are relevant to research involving human subjects are identified in this statement. Other principles may also be relevant. These three are comprehensive, however, and are stated at a level of generalization that should assist scientists, subjects, reviewers and interested citizens to understand the ethical issues inherent in research involving human subjects. These principles cannot always be applied so as to resolve beyond dispute particular ethical problems. The objective is to provide an analytical framework that will guide the resolution of ethical problems arising from research involving human subjects.

This statement consists of a distinction between research and practice, a discussion of the three basic ethical principles, and remarks about the application of these principles.

A. Boundaries Between Practice and Research

It is important to distinguish between biomedical and behavioral research, on the one hand, and the practice of accepted therapy on the *other*, in order to know what activities ought to undergo review for the protection of human subjects of research. The distinction between research and practice is blurred partly because both often occur together (as in research designed to evaluate a therapy) and partly because notable departures from standard practice are often called "experimental" when the terms "experimental" and "research" are not carefully defined.

For the most part, the term "practice" refers to interventions that are designed solely to enhance the well-being of an individual patient or client and that have a reasonable expectation of success. The purpose of medical or behavioral practice is to provide diagnosis, preventive treatment or therapy to particular individuals. By contrast, the term "research" designates an activity designed to test an hypothesis, permit conclusions to be drawn, and thereby to develop or contribute to generalizable knowledge (expressed, for example, in theories, principles, and statements of relationships). Research is usually described in a formal protocol that sets forth an objective and a set of procedures designed to reach that objective.

When a clinician departs in a significant way from standard or accepted practice, the innovation does not, in and of itself, constitute research. The fact that a procedure is "experimental," in the sense of new, untested or different, does not automatically place it in the category of research. Radically new procedures of this description should, however, be made the object of formal research at an early stage in order to determine whether they are safe and effective. Thus, it is the responsibility of medical practice committees, for example, to insist that a major innovation be incorporated into a formal research project.

Research and practice may be carried on together when research is designed to evaluate the safety and efficacy of a therapy. This need not cause any confusion regarding whether or not the activity requires review; the general rule is that if there is any element of research in an activity, that activity should undergo review for the protection of human subjects.

B. Basic Ethical Principles

The expression "basic ethical principles" refers to those general judgments that serve as a basic justification for the many particular ethical prescriptions and evaluations of human actions. Three basic principles, among those generally accepted in our cultural tradition, are particularly relevant to the ethics of research involving human subjects: the principles of respect for persons, beneficence and justice.

1. *Respect for Persons.*—Respect for persons incorporates at least two ethical convictions: first, that individuals should be treated as autonomous agents, and second, that persons with diminished autonomy are entitled to protection. The principle of respect for persons thus divides into two separate moral requirements: the requirement to acknowledge autonomy and the requirement to protect those with diminished autonomy.

An autonomous person is an individual capable of deliberation about personal goals and of acting under the direction of such deliberation. To respect autonomy is to give weight to autonomous persons' considered opinions and choices while refraining from obstructing their actions unless they are clearly detrimental to others. To show lack of respect for an autonomous agent is to repudiate that person's considered judgments, to deny an individual the freedom to act on those considered judgments, or to withhold information necessary to make a considered judgment, when there are no compelling reasons to do so.

However, not every human being is capable of self-determination. The capacity for self-determination matures during an individual's life, and some individuals lose this capacity wholly or in part because of illness, mental disability, or circumstances that severely restrict liberty. Respect for the immature and the incapacitated may require protecting them as they mature or while they are incapacitated.

Some persons are in need of extensive protection, even to the point of excluding them from activities which may harm them; other persons require little protection beyond making sure they undertake activities freely and with awareness of possible adverse consequences. The extent of protection afforded should depend upon the risk of harm and the likelihood of benefit. The judgment that any individual lacks autonomy should be periodically reevaluated and will vary in different situations.

In most cases of research involving human subjects, respect for persons demands that subjects enter into the research voluntarily and with adequate information. In some situations, however, application of the principle is not obvious. The involvement of prisoners as subjects of research provides an instructive example. On the one hand, it would seem that the principle of respect for persons requires that prisoners not be deprived of the opportunity to volunteer for research. On the other hand, under prison conditions they may be subtly coerced or unduly influenced to engage in research activities for which they would not otherwise volunteer. Respect for persons would then dictate that prisoners be protected. Whether to allow prisoners to "volunteer" or to "protect" them presents a dilemma. Respecting persons, in most hard cases, is often a matter of balancing competing claims urged by the principle of respect itself.

2. *Beneficence.*—Persons are treated in an ethical manner not only by respecting their decisions and protecting them from harm, but also by making efforts to secure their well-being. Such treatment falls under the principle of beneficence. The term "beneficence" is often understood to cover acts of kindness or charity that go beyond strict obligation. In this document, beneficence is understood in a stronger sense, as an obligation. Two general rules have been formulated as complementary expressions of beneficent actions in this sense: (1) do not harm and (2) maximize possible benefits and minimize possible harms.

The Hippocratic maxim "do no harm" has long been a fundamental principle of medical ethics. Claude Bernard extended it to the realm of research, saying that one should not injure one person regardless of the benefits that might come to others. However, even avoiding harm requires learning what is harmful; and, in the process of obtaining this information, persons may be exposed to risk of harm. Further, the Hippocratic Oath requires physicians to benefit their patients "according to their best judgment." Learning what will in fact benefit may require exposing persons to risk. The problem posed by these imperatives is to decide when it is justifiable to seek certain benefits despite the risks involved, and when the benefits should be foregone because of the risks.

The obligations of beneficence affect both individual investigators and society at large, because they extend both to particular research projects and to the entire enterprise of research. In the case of particular projects, investigators and members of their institutions are obliged to give forethought to the maximization of benefits and the reduction of risk that might occur from the research investigation. In the case of scientific research in general, members of the larger society are obliged to recognize the longer term benefits and risks that may result from the improvement of knowledge and from the development of novel medical, psychotherapeutic, and social procedures.

The principle of beneficence often occupies a well-defined justifying role in many areas of research involving human subjects. An example is found in research involving children. Effective ways of treating childhood diseases and fostering healthy development are benefits that serve to justify research involving children—even when individual research subjects are not direct benefi-ciaries. Research also makes is possible to avoid the harm that may result from the application of previously accepted routine practices that on closer investigation turn out to be dangerous. But the role of the principle of beneficence is not always so unambiguous. A difficult ethical problem remains, for example, about research that presents more than minimal risk without immediate pros-pect of direct benefit to the children involved. Some have argued that such research is inadmissible, while others have pointed out that this limit would rule out much research promising great benefit to children in the future. Here again, as with all hard cases, the different claims covered by the principle of beneficence may come into conflict and force difficult choices.

3. *Justice.*—Who ought to receive the benefits of research and bear its burdens? This is a question of justice, in the sense of "fairness in distribution" or "what is deserved." An injustice occurs when some benefit to which a person is entitled is denied without good reason or when some burden is imposed unduly. Another way of conceiving the principle of justice is that equals ought to be treated equally. However, this statement requires explication. Who is equal and who is unequal? What considerations justify departure from equal distribution? Almost all commentators allow that distinctions based on experience, age, deprivation, competence, merit and position do sometimes constitute criteria justifying differential treatment for certain purposes. It is necessary, then, to explain in what respects people should be treated equally. There are several widely accepted for-mulations of just ways to distribute burdens and benefits. Each formulation mentions some relevant property on the basis of which burdens and benefits should be distributed. These formulations are (1) to each person an equal share, (2) to each person according to individual need, (3) to each person according to individual effort, (4) to each person according to societal contribution, and (5) to each person according to merit.

Questions of justice have long been associated with social practices such as punishment, taxation and political representation. Until recently these questions have not generally been associated with scientific research. However, they are foreshadowed even in the earliest reflections on the ethics of research involving human subjects. For example, during the 19th and early 20th centuries the bur-dens of serving as research subjects fell largely upon poor ward patients, while the benefits of improved medical care flowed primarily to private patients. Subsequently, the exploitation of un-willing prisoners as research subjects in Nazi concentration camps was condemned as a particularly flagrant injustice. In this country, in the 1940's, the Tuskegee syphilis study used disadvantaged, rural black men to study the untreated course of a disease that is by no means confined to that population. These subjects were deprived of demonstrably effective treatment in order not to inter-rupt the project, long after such treatment became generally available.

Against this historical background, it can be seen how conceptions of justice are relevant to research involving human subjects. For example, the selection of research subjects needs to be scrutinized in order to determine whether some classes (e.g., welfare patients, particular racial and ethnic minorities, or persons confined to institutions) are being systematically selected simply be-cause of their easy availability, their compromised position, or their manipulability, rather than for reasons directly related to the problem being studied. Finally, whenever research supported by public funds leads to the development of therapeutic devices and procedures, justice demands both that these not provide advantages only to those who can afford them and that such research should not unduly involve persons from groups unlikely to be among the beneficiaries of subsequent applica-tions of the research.

C. Applications

Applications of the general principles to the conduct of research leads to consideration of the following requirements: informed consent, risk/benefit assessment, and the selection of subjects of research.

1. *Informed Consent.*—Respect for persons requires that subjects, to the degree that they are capable, be given the opportunity to choose what shall or shall not happen to them. This opportunity is provided when adequate standards for informed consent are satisfied.

While the importance of informed consent is unquestioned, controversy prevails over the nature and possibility of an informed consent. Nonetheless, there is widespread agreement that the consent process can be analyzed as containing three elements: information, comprehension and voluntariness.

Information. Most codes of research establish specific items for disclosure intended to assure that subjects are given sufficient information. These items generally include: the research procedure, their purposes, risks and anticipated benefits, alternative procedures (where therapy is involved), and a statement offering the subject the opportunity to ask questions and to withdraw at any time from the research. Additional items have been proposed, including how subjects are selected, the person responsible for the research, etc.

However, a simple listing of items does not answer the question of what the standard should be for judging how much and what sort of information should be provided. One standard frequently invoked in medical practice, namely the information commonly provided by practitioners in the field or in the locale, is inadequate since research takes place precisely when a common understanding does not exist. Another standard, currently popular in malpractice law, requires the practitioner to reveal the information that reasonable persons would wish to know in order to make a decision regarding their care. This, too, seems insufficient since the research subject, being in essence a volunteer, may wish to know considerably more about risks gratuitously undertaken than do patients who deliver themselves into the hand of a clinician for needed care. It may be that a standard of "the reasonable volunteer" should be proposed: the extent and nature of the information should be such that persons, knowing that the procedure is neither necessary for their care nor perhaps fully understood, can decide whether they wish to participate in the furthering of knowledge. Even when some direct benefit to them is anticipated, the subjects should understand clearly the range of risk and the voluntary nature of participation.

A special problem of consent arises where informing subjects of some pertinent aspect of the research is likely to impair the validity of the research. In many cases, it is sufficient to indicate to subjects that they are being invited to participate in research of which some features will not be revealed until the research is concluded. In all cases of research involving incomplete disclosure, such research is justified only if it is clear that (1) incomplete disclosure is truly necessary to accomplish the goals of the research, (2) there are no undisclosed risks to subjects that are more than minimal, and (3) there is an adequate plan for debriefing subjects, when appropriate, and for dissemination of research results to them. Information about risks should never be withheld for the purpose of eliciting the cooperation of subjects, and truthful answers should always be given to direct questions about the research. Care should be taken to distinguish cases in which disclosure would destroy or invalidate the research from cases in which disclosure would simply inconvenience the investigator.

Comprehension. The manner and context in which information is conveyed is as important as the information itself. For example, presenting information in a disorganized and rapid fashion, allowing too little time for consideration or curtailing opportunities for questioning, all may adversely affect a subject's ability to make an informed choice.

Because the subject's ability to understand is a function of intelligence, rationality, maturity and language, it is necessary to adapt the presentation of the information to the subject's capacities. Investigators are responsible for ascertaining that the subject has comprehended the information. While there is always an obligation to ascertain that the information about risk to subjects is complete and adequately comprehended, when the risks are more serious, that obligation increases. On occasion, it may be suitable to give some oral or written tests of comprehension.

Special provision may need to be made when comprehension is severely limited—for example, by conditions of immaturity or mental disability. Each class of subjects that one might consider as incompetent (e.g., infants and young children, mentally disabled patients, the terminally ill and the comatose) should be considered on its own terms. Even for these persons, however, respect requires giving them the opportunity to choose to the extent they are able, whether or not to participate in research. The objections of these subjects to involvement should be honored, unless the research entails providing them a therapy unavailable elsewhere. Respect for persons also requires seeking the permission of other parties in order to protect the subjects from harm. Such persons are thus respected both by acknowledging their own wishes and by the use of third parties to protect them from harm.

The third parties chosen should be those who are most likely to understand the incompetent subject's situation and to act in that person's best interest. The person authorized to act on behalf of the subject should be given an opportunity to observe the research as it proceeds in order to be able to withdraw the subject from the research, if such action appears in the subject's best interest.

Voluntariness. An agreement to participate in research constitutes a valid consent only if voluntarily given. This element of informed consent requires conditions free of coercion and undue influence. Coercion occurs when an overt threat of harm is intentionally presented by one person to another in order to obtain compliance. Undue influence, by contrast, occurs through an offer of an excessive, unwarranted, inappropriate or improper reward or other overture in order to obtain compliance. Also, inducements that would ordinarily be acceptable may become undue influences if the subject is especially vulnerable.

Unjustifiable pressures usually occur when persons in positions of authority or commanding influence—especially where possible sanctions are involved—urge a course of action for a subject. A continuum of such influencing factors exists, however, and it is impossible to state precisely where justifiable persuasion ends and undue influence begins. But undue influence would include actions such as manipulating a person's choice through the controlling influence of a close relative and threatening to withdraw health services to which an individual would otherwise be entitled.

2. *Assessment of Risks and Benefits.*—The assessment of risks and benefits requires a careful arrayal of relevant data, including, in some cases, alternative ways of obtaining the benefits sought in the research. Thus, the assessment presents both an opportunity and a responsibility to gather systematic and comprehensive information about proposed research. For the investigator, it is a means of examine whether the proposed research is properly designed. For a review committee, it is a method for determining whether the risks that will be presented to subjects are justified. For prospective subjects, the assessment will assist the determination whether or not to participate.

The Nature and Scope of Risks and Benefits. The requirement that research be justified on the basis of a favorable risk/benefit assessment bears a close relation to the principle of beneficence, just as the moral requirement that informed consent be obtained is derived primarily from the principle of respect for persons. The term "risk" refers to a possibility that harm may occur. However, when expressions such as "small risk" or "high risk" are used, they usually refer (often ambiguously) both to the chance (probability) of experiencing a harm and the severity (magnitude) of the envisioned harm.

The term "benefit" is used in the research context to refer to something of positive value related to health or welfare. Unlike "risk," "benefit" is not a term that expresses probabilities. Risk is properly contrasted to probability of benefits, and benefits are properly contrasted with harms rather than risks of harm. Accordingly, so-called risk/benefit assessments are concerned with the probabilities and magnitudes of possible harms and anticipated benefits. Many kinds of possible harms and benefits need to be taken into account. There are, for example, risks of psychological harm, physical harm, legal harm, social harm and economic harm and the corresponding benefits. While the most likely types of harms to research subjects are those of psychological or physical pain or injury, other possible kinds should not be overlooked.

Risks and benefits of research may affect the individual subjects, the families of the individual subjects, and society at large (or special groups of subjects in society). Previous codes and Federal regulations have required that risks to subjects be outweighed by the sum of both the anticipated benefit to the subject, if any, and the anticipated benefit to society in the form of knowledge to be gained from the research. In balancing these different elements, the risks and benefits affecting the immediate research subject will normally carry special weight. On the other hand, interests other than those of the subject may on some occasions be sufficient by themselves to justify the risks involved in the research, so long as the subjects' rights have been protected. Beneficence thus requires that we protect against risk of harm to subjects and also that we be concerned about the loss of the substantial benefits that might be gained from research.

The Systematic Assessment of Risks and Benefits. It is commonly said that benefits and risks must be "balanced" and shown to be "in a favorable ratio." The metaphorical character of these terms draws attention to the difficulty of making precise judgments. Only on rare occasions will quantitative techniques be available for the scrutiny of research protocols. However, the idea of systematic, nonarbitrary analysis of risks and benefits should be emulated insofar as possible. This ideal requires those making decisions about the justifiability of research to be thorough in the accumulation and assessment of information about all aspects of the research, and to consider alternatives systematically. This procedure renders the assessment of research more rigorous and precise, while making communication between review board members and investigators less subject to misinterpretation, misinformation and conflicting judgments. Thus, there should first be a determination of the validity of the presuppositions of the research; then the nature, probability and magnitude of risk should be distinguished with as much clarity as possible. The method of ascertaining risks should be explicit, especially where there is no alternative to the use of such vague categories as small or slight risk. It should also be determined whether an investigator's estimates of the probability of harm or benefits are reasonable, as judged by known facts or other available studies.

Finally, assessment of the justifiability of research should reflect at least the following considerations: (i) Brutal or inhumane treatment of human subjects is never morally justified. (ii) Risks should be reduced to those necessary to achieve the research objective. It should be determined whether it is in fact necessary to use human subjects at all. Risk can perhaps never be entirely eliminated, but it can often be reduced by careful attention to alternative procedures. (iii) When research involves significant risk of serious impairment, review committees should be extraordinarily insistent on the justification of the risk (looking usually to the likelihood of benefit to the subject—or, in some rare cases, to the manifest voluntariness of the participation). (iv) When vulnerable populations are involved in research, the appropriateness of involving them should itself be demonstrated. A number of variables go into such judgments, including the nature and degree of risk, the condition of the particular population involved, and the nature and level of the anticipated benefits. (v) Relevant risks and benefits must be thoroughly arrayed in documents and procedures used in the informed consent process.

3. *Selection of Subjects.*—Just as the principle of respect for persons finds expression in the requirements for consent, and the principle of beneficence in risk/benefit assessment, the principle of justice gives rise to moral requirements that there be fair procedures and outcomes in the selection of research subjects.

Justice is relevant to the selection of subjects of research at two levels: the social and the individual. Individual justice in the selection of subjects would require that researchers exhibit fairness: thus, they should not offer potentially beneficial research only to some patients who are in their favor or select only "undesirable" persons for risky research. Social justice requires that distinction be drawn between classes of subjects that ought, and ought not, to participate in any particular kind of research, based on the ability of members of that class to bear burdens and on the appropriateness of placing further burdens on already burdened persons. Thus, it can be considered a matter of social justice that there is an order of preference in the selection of classes of subjects (e.g., adults before children) and that some classes of potential subjects (e.g., the institutionalized mentally infirm or prisoners) may be involved as research subjects, if at all, only on certain conditions.

Injustice may appear in the selection of subjects, even if individual subjects are selected fairly by investigators and treated fairly in the course of research. Thus injustice arises from social, racial, sexual and cultural biases institutionalized in society. Thus, even if individual researchers are treating their research subjects fairly, and even if IRBs are taking care to assure that subjects are selected fairly within a particular institution, unjust social patterns may nevertheless appear in the overall distribution of the burdens and benefits of research. Although individual institutions or investigators may not be able to resolve a problem that is pervasive in their social setting, they can consider distributive justice in selecting research subjects.

Some populations, especially institutionalized ones, are already burdened in many ways by their infirmities and environments. When research is proposed that involves risks and does not include a therapeutic component, other less burdened classes of persons should be called upon first to accept these risks of research, except where the research is directly related to the specific conditions of the class involved. Also, even though public funds for research may often flow in the same directions as public funds for health care, it seems unfair that populations dependent on public health care constitute a pool of preferred research subjects if more advantaged populations are likely to be the recipients of the benefits.

One special instance of injustice results from the involvement of vulnerable subjects. Certain groups, such as racial minorities, the economically disadvantaged, the very sick, and the institutionalized may continually be sought as research subjects, owing to their ready availability in settings where research is conducted. Given their dependent status and their frequently compromised capacity for free consent, they should be protected against the danger of being involved in research solely for administrative convenience, or because they are easy to manipulate as a result of their illness or socioeconomic condition.

Appendix 3.3   Public Health Service, U.S. Government Principles for the Utilization and Care of Vertebrate Animals Used in Testing, Research, and Training (1986)

The development of knowledge necessary for the improvement of the health and well-being of humans as well as other animals requires *in vivo* experimentation with a wide variety of animal species. Whenever U.S. Government agencies develop requirements for testing, research, or training procedures involving the use of vertebrate animals, the following principles shall be considered; and whenever these agencies actually perform or sponsor such procedures, the responsible Institutional Official shall ensure that these principles are adhered to:

I. The transportation, care, and use of animals should be in accordance with the Animal Welfare Act (7 U.S.C. 2131 et. seq.) and other applicable Federal laws, guidelines, and policies.

II. Procedures involving animals should be designed and performed with due consideration of their relevance to human or animal health, the advancement of knowledge, or the good of society.

III. The animals selected for a procedure should be of an appropriate species and quality and the minimum number required to obtain valid results. Methods such as mathematical models, computer simulation, and *in vitro* biological systems should be considered.

IV. Proper use of animals, including the avoidance or minimization of discomfort, distress, and pain when consistent with sound scientific practices, is imperative. Unless the contrary is established, investigators should consider that procedures that cause pain or distress in human beings may cause pain or distress in other animals.

V. Procedures with animals that may cause more than momentary or slight pain or distress should be performed with appropriate sedation, analgesia, or anethesia. Surgical or other painful procedures should not be performed on unanesthetized animals paralyzed by chemical agents.

VI. Animals that would otherwise suffer severe or chronic pain or distress that cannot be relieved should be painlessly killed at the end of the procedure or, if appropriate, during the procedure.

VII. The living conditions of animals should be appropriate for their species and contribute to their health and comfort. Normally, the housing, feeding, and care of all animals used for biomedical purposes must be directed by a veterinarian or other scientist trained and experienced in the proper care, handling, and use of the species being maintained or studied. In any case, veterinary care shall be provided as indicated.

VIII. Investigators and other personnel shall be appropriately qualified and experienced for conducting procedures on living animals. Adequate arrangements shall be made for their in-service training, including the proper and humane care and use of laboratory animals.

IX. Where exceptions are required in relation to the provisions of these Principles, the decisions should not rest with the investigators directly concerned but should be made, with due regard to Principle II, by an appropriate review group such as an institutional animal care and use committee. Such exceptions should not be made solely for the purposes of teaching or demonstration.

Appendix 3.4   Food and Drug Administration, (21 CFR 314.126) Adequate and Well-Controlled Studies (1985)

(a) The purpose of conducting clinical investigations of a drug is to distinguish the effect of a drug from other influences, such as spontaneous change in the course of the disease, placebo effect, or biased observation. The characteristics described in paragraph (b) of this section have been developed over a period of years and are recognized by the scientific community as the essentials of an adequate and well-controlled clinical investigation. The Food and Drug Administration considers these characteristics in determining whether an investigation is adequate and well-controlled for purposes of sections 505 and 507 of the act. Reports of adequate and well-controlled investigations provide the primary basis for determining whether there is "substantial evidence" to support the claims of effectiveness for new drugs and antibiotics. Therefore, the study report should provide sufficient details of study design, conduct, and analysis to allow critical evaluation and a determination of whether the characteristics of an adequate and well-controlled study are present.

(b) An adequate and well-controlled study has the following characteristics:

(1) There is a clear statement of the objectives of the investigation and a summary of the proposed or actual methods of analysis in the protocol for the study and in the report of its results. In addition, the protocol should contain a description of the proposed methods of analysis, and the study report should contain a description of the methods of analysis actually used. If the protocol does not contain a description of the proposed methods of analysis, the study report should describe how the methods used were selected.

(2) The study uses a design that permits a valid comparison with a control to provide a quantitative assessment of drug effect. The protocol for the study and report of results should describe the study design precisely; for example, duration of treatment periods, whether treatments are parallel, sequential, or crossover, and whether the sample size is predetermined or based upon some interim analysis. Generally, the following types of control are recognized:

(i) *Placebo concurrent control.* The test drug is compared with an inactive preparation designed to resemble the test drug as far as possible. A placebo-controlled study may include additional treatment groups, such as an active treatment control or a dose-comparison control, and usually includes randomization and blinding of patients or investigators, or both.

(ii) *Dose-comparison concurrent control.* At least two doses of the drug are compared. A dose-comparison study may include additional treatment groups, such as placebo control or active control. Dose-comparison trials usually include randomization and blinding of patients or investigators, or both.

(iii) *No treatment concurrent control.* Where objective measurements of effectiveness are available and placebo effect is negligible, the test drug is compared with no treatment. No treatment concurrent control trials usually include randomization.

(iv) *Active treatment concurrent control.* The test drug is compared with known effective therapy; for example, where the condition treated is such that administration of placebo or no treatment would be contrary to the interest of the patient. An active treatment study may include additional treatment groups, however, such as a placebo control or a dose-comparison control. Active treatment trials usually include randomization and blinding of patients or investigators, or both. If the intent of the trial is to show similarity of the test and control drugs, the report of the study should assess the ability of the study to have detected a difference between treatments. Similarity of test drug and active control can mean either that both drugs were effective or that neither was effective. The analysis of the study should explain why the drugs should be considered effective in the study, for example, by reference to results in previous placebo-controlled studies of the active control drug.

(v) *Historical control.* The results of treatment with the test drug are compared with experience historically derived from the adequately documented natural history of the disease or condition, or from the results of active treatment, in comparable patients or populations. Because historical control populations usually cannot be as well assessed with respect to pertinent variables as can concurrent control populations, historical control designs are usually reserved for special circumstances. Examples include studies of diseases with high and predictable mortality (for example, certain malignancies) and studies in which the effect of the drug is self-evident (general anesthetics, drug metabolism).

(3) The method of selection of subjects provides adequate assurance that they have the disease or condition being studied, or evidence of susceptibility and exposure to the condition against which prophylaxis is directed.

(4) The method of assigning patients to treatment and control groups minimizes bias and is intended to assure comparability of the groups with respect to pertinent variables such as age, sex, severity of disease, duration of disease, and use of drugs or therapy other than the test drug. The protocol for the study and the report of its results should describe how subjects were assigned to groups. Ordinarily, in a concurrently controlled study, assignment is by randomization, with or without stratification.

(5) Adequate measures are taken to minimize bias on the part of the subjects, observers, and analysts of the data. The protocol and report of the study should describe the procedures used to accomplish this, such as blinding.

(6) The methods of assessment of subjects' response are well-defined and reliable. The protocol for the study and the report of results should explain the variables measured, the methods of observation, and criteria used to assess response.

(7) There is an analysis of the results of the study adequate to assess the effects of the drug. The report of the study should describe the results and the analytic methods used to evaluate them, including any appropriate statistical methods. The analysis should assess, among other things, the comparability of test and control groups with respect to pertinent variables, and the effects of any interim data analyses performed.

(c) The Director of the Center for Drug Evaluation and Research may, on the Director's own initiative or on the petition of an interested person, waive in whole or in part any of the criteria in paragraph (b) of this section with respect to a specific clinical investigation, either prior to the investigation or in the evaluation of a completed study. A petition for a waiver is required to set forth clearly and concisely the specific criteria from which waiver is sought, why the criteria are not reasonably applicable to the particular clinical investigation, what alternative procedures, if any, are to be, or have been employed, and what results have been obtained. The petition is also required to state why the clinical investigations so conducted will yield, or have yielded, substantial evidence of effectiveness, notwithstanding nonconformance with the criteria for which waiver is requested.

(d) For an investigation to be considered adequate for approval of a new drug, it is required that the test drug be standardized as to identity, strength, quality, purity, and dosage form to give significance to the results of the investigation.

(e) Uncontrolled studies or partially controlled studies are not acceptable as the sole basis for the approval of claims of effectiveness. Such studies carefully conducted and documented, may provide corroborative support of well-controlled studies regarding efficacy and may yield valuable data regarding safety of the test drug. Such studies will be considered on their merits in the light of the principles listed here, with the exception of the requirement for the comparison of the treated subjects with controls. Isolated case reports, random experience, and reportslacking the details which permit scientific evaluation will not be considered.

Supplementary Advisory:
Placebo-Controlled and Active Controlled Drug Study Designs (1989)

Before a new drug can be marketed, its sponsor must show, through adequate and well-controlled clinical studies, that the drug is effective. A well-controlled study permits a comparison of patients treated with the new agent with a suitable control population, so that the effect of the new agent can be determined and distinguished from other influences, such as spontaneous change, "placebo" effects, concomitant therapy, or observer expectations. Regulations (Attachment 1) cite five different kinds of controls [(1) placebo concurrent control, (2) dose comparison concurrent control (3) no treatment concurrent control, (4) active treatment concurrent control, and (5) historical control] that can be useful in particular circumstances. No general preference is expressed for any one type, but the study design chosen must be adequate to the task. Thus, in discussing historical controls, the regulation notes that because it is relatively difficult to be sure that historical control groups are comparable to the treated patients with respect to variables that could affect outcome, use of historical control studies has been reserved for special circumstances, notably cases where the disease treated has high and predictable mortality (a large difference from this usual course would be easy to detect) and those in which the effect is self-evident (e.g., a general anesthetic).

Placebo control, no treatment control (suitable where objective measurements are felt to make blinding unnecessary), and dose-comparison control studies are all study designs in which a *difference* is intended to be shown between the new drug and some control. The alternative study design generally proposed to these kinds of studies is an active treatment concurrent control in which a finding of *no difference* between the new drug and the recognized effective agent (active control) would be considered evidence of effectiveness of the new agent. There are circumstances in which this is a fully valid design. Active controls are usually used in antibiotic trials, for example, because it is easy to tell the difference between antibiotics that have the expected effect on specific infections and those that do not. In many cases, however, the active control design may be simply incapable of allowing any conclusion as to whether or not a drug is having an effect.

Three principal difficulties in interpreting active control trials have been described in two publications (Attachments 2 & 3). First, active-control trials are often too small to provide assurance that a clinically meaningful difference between the two treatments, if present, could have been detected with reasonable assurance; i.e., the trials have a high beta-error. In part this can be overcome by increasing sample size, but two other problems remain even if studies are large. One problem is that there are numerous ways of conducting a study that can obscure differences between treatments, such as poor diagnostic criteria, poor methods of measurement, poor compliance, medication errors, or poor training of observers. As a general statement, sloppiness of all kinds will tend to obscure differences between treatments. Where the objective of a study is to show a difference, investigators have powerful stimuli toward assuring study excellence. Active control studies, however, which are intended to show *no significant difference* between treatments, do not provide the same incentives toward study excellence, and it is difficult to detect or assess the kinds of poor study quality that can arise. The second additional problem is that a finding of no difference between a new drug and an effective treatment may not be meaningful, even in an excellent study. Even where all the incentives toward study excellence are present, i.e., in placebo-controlled trials, effective drugs are not necessarily demonstrably effective (i.e., superior to placebo) every time they are studied. In the absence of a placebo group, a finding of no difference in an active control study therefore can mean *either* that both agents are effective, that neither drug was effective in that study, or that the study was simply unable to tell effective from ineffective drugs. In other words, to draw the conclusion that the new drug was effective, one has to know with assurance that the active control would have shown superior results to a placebo, had a placebo group been included in the study.

For certain drug classes, such as analgesics, antidepressants or antianxiety drugs, failure to show superiority to placebo in a given study is common. It is also seen reasonably often with antihypertensives, antiangina drugs, anti-heart failure treatments, antihistamines, and drugs for asthma prophylaxis. In those situations active control trials showing no difference between the new drug and control are of little value as primary evidence of effectiveness and the active control design, the study design most often proposed as an alternative to use of a placebo, is not credible.

In many situations, deciding whether an active control design is likely to be a useful basis for providing data for marketing approval is a matter of judgment influenced by available evidence. If, for example, examination of prior studies of a proposed active control reveals that the drug can very regularly (almost always) be distinguished from placebo in a particular setting (patient population, dose, etc.), an active control design may be reasonable if it reproduces the setting in which the active control has been regularly effective.

It may also be possible to design a successful placebo-controlled trial that does not cause investigator discomfort and raise ethical issues. Treatment periods can be kept short; early "escape" mechanisms can be built into the study so that patients will not undergo prolonged placebo-treatment if they are not doing well. In some cases randomized placebo-controlled therapy withdrawal studies have been used to minimize exposure to placebo or unsuccessful therapy; in such studies apparent responders to a treatment in an open study are randomly assigned to continued treatment or to placebo. Patients who fail (blood pressure rises, angina worsens) can be removed promptly, with such failure representing a study endpoint.

Placebo-controlled trials, whatever their advantages in interpretability, are obviously not ethically acceptable where existing treatment is life-prolonging, but there are relatively few situations where this is the case. Although treatment of hypertension is clearly beneficial, for example, it would be difficult to argue that mild or moderate hypertensives (diastolic 95–115) would be placed at risk if given a placebo for 4–8 weeks with monitoring of blood pressure; a long-term study would of course be another matter. Although IRB's have expressed concern about placebo-controlled exercise-angina studies, there is no evidence that angina treatment enhances survival; an overview of all placebo controlled angina treatment trials in FDA files reveals no suggestion of a disadvantage (indeed there was a numerical advantage) in the placebo group with respect to adverse cardiovascular events.

Even where a placebo-controlled trial cannot be carried out on ethical grounds the active control trial may, unfortunately, not be informative. For example, a placebo-controlled trial of a beta-blocker in the post-infarction setting would appear unwarranted in view of available data showing improved survival in treated patients, yet only a few of the more than two dozen large placebo-controlled trials have shown a significant difference between the beta-blocker and placebo. A new trial showing no difference in mortality in patients treated with two different beta-blockers would thus prove nothing as only an occasional beta-blocker trial has been able to distinguish active drug from placebo.

IRB's may face difficult issues in deciding on the acceptability of placebo-controlled and active control trials. A placebo-controlled study that exposes patients to a documented serious risk will not be acceptable, but it is critical to review the evidence that harm would result from denial of active treatment, because alternative study designs, especially active control studies, may not be informative, exposing patients to risk but unable to collect useful information. It is often possible to design a study that, while using a placebo group to clearly delineate the efficacy of a proposed treatment, causes no unreasonable exposure of patients to no treatment; design features to consider include a dose-response study, early escape from ineffective treatment, randomized withdrawal from active-therapy, and minimizing study duration.

Appendix 3.5 Food and Drug Administration, Subpart H— Accelerated Approval of New Drugs for Serious or Life- Threatening Illnesses (1992)

21 CFR 314.500 Scope.

This subpart applies to certain new drug and antibiotic products that have been studied for their safety and effectiveness in treating serious or life-threatening illnesses and that provide meaningful therapeutic benefit to patients over existing treatments (e.g., ability to treat patients unresponsive to, or intolerant of, available therapy, or improved patient response over available therapy).

21 CFR 314.510 Approval Based on a Surrogate Endpoint or on an Effect on a Clinical Endpoint Other Than Survival or Irreversible Morbidity.

FDA may grant marketing approval for a new drug product on the basis of adequate and well- controlled clinical trials establishing that the drug product has an effect on a surrogate endpoint that is reasonably likely, based on epidemiologic, therapeutic, pathophysiologic, or other evidence, to predict clinical benefit or on the basis of an effect on a clinical endpoint other than survival or irreversible morbidity. Approval under this section will be subject to the requirement that the applicant study the drug further, to verify and describe its clinical benefit, where there is uncertainty as to the relation of the surrogate endpoint to clinical benefit, or of the observed clinical benefit to ultimate outcome. Postmarketing studies would usually be studies already underway. When required to be conducted, such studies must also be adequate and well-controlled. The applicant shall carry out any such studies with the due diligence.

21 CFR 314.520 Approval with Restrictions to Assure Safe Use.

(a) If FDA concludes that a drug product shown to be effective can be safely used only if distribution or use is restricted, FDA will require such postmarketing restrictions as are needed to assure safe use of the drug product, such as:
(1) Distribution restricted to certain facilities or physicians with special training or experience; or
(2) Distribution conditioned on the performance of specified medical procedures.
(3) The limitations imposed will be commensurate with the specific safety concerns presented by the drug product.

• • •

Appendix 3.6 Food and Drug Administration, Guideline for the Study and Evaluation of Gender Differences in the Clinical Evaluation of Drugs (1993)

I. Introduction

The Food and Drug Administration (FDA) advises that this guideline represents its current position on the clinical evaluation of drugs in humans. This guideline does not bind the agency, and it does not create or confer any rights, privileges, or benefits for or on any person.

The principles of inclusion of women in product development programs and analysis of subgroup differences outlined in this guideline also apply to the clinical development of biological products and medical devices.

A. Abstract

In general, drugs should be studied prior to approval in subjects representing the full range of patients likely to receive the drug once it is marketed. Although in most cases, drugs behave qualitatively similarly in demographic (age, gender, race) and other (concomitant illness, concomitant drugs) subsets of the population, there are many quantitative differences, for example, in dose-response, maximum size of effect, or in the risk of an adverse effect. Recognition of these differences can allow safer and more effective use of drugs. Rarely, there may be qualitative differences as well. It is very difficult to evaluate subsets of the overall population as thoroughly as the entire population, but sponsors are expected to include a full range of patients in their studies, carry out appropriate analyses to evaluate potential subset differences in the patients they have studied, study possible pharmacokinetic differences in patient subsets, and carry out targeted studies to look for subset pharmacodynamic differences that are especially probable, are suggested by existing data, or that would be particularly important if present. Study protocols are also expected to provide appropriate precautions against exposure of fetuses to potentially dangerous agents. Where animal data suggest possible effects on fertility, such as decreased sperm production, special studies in humans may be needed to evaluate this potential toxicity.

B. Underlying Observations

The following general observations and conclusions underlie the recommendations set forth in this guideline:

1. Variations in response to drugs, including gender-related differences, can arise from pharmacokinetic differences (that is, differences in the way a drug is absorbed, excreted, metabolized, or distributed) or pharmacodynamic differences (i.e., differences in the pharmacologic or clinical response to a given concentration of the drug in blood or other tissue).

2. Gender-related variations in drug effects may arise from a variety of sources. Some of these are specifically associated with gender, e.g., effects of endogenous and exogenous hormones. Gender-related differences could also arise, however, not because of gender itself, but because the frequency of a particular characteristic (for example, small size, concomitant hepatic disease or concomitant drug treatment, or habits such as smoking or alcohol use) is different in one gender, even if the characteristic could occur in either gender. Proper management of patients of both genders thus requires that physicians know all the factors that can influence the pharmacokinetics of a drug. An approach is needed that will identify, better than is done at present, all such factors. Understanding how various factors may influence pharmacokinetics will greatly enhance our ability to treat people of both genders appropriately.

3. For a number of practical and theoretical reasons, the evaluation of possible gender-related differences in response should focus initially on the evaluation of potential pharmacokinetic differences. Such differences are known to occur and have, at least to date, been documented much more commonly than documented pharmacodynamic differences. Moreover, pharmacokinetic differences are relatively easy to discover. Once reliable assays are developed for a drug and its metabolites (such assays are now almost always available early in the development of the drug), techniques exist for readily assessing gender-related or other subgroup-related pharmacokinetic differences.

Formal pharmacokinetic studies are one means of answering questions about specific subgroups. Another approach is use of a screening procedure, a "pharmacokinetic screen" (see "Guideline for the Study of Drugs Likely To Be Used in the Elderly"). Carried out in phase 2 and 3 study populations, the pharmacokinetic screen can greatly increase the ability to detect pharmacokinetic differences in subpopulations and individuals, even when these differences are not anticipated. By obtaining a small number of blood concentration determinations in most or all phase 2 and 3 patients, it is possible to detect markedly atypical pharmacokinetic behavior in individuals, such as that seen in slow metabolizers of debrisoquin, and pharmacokinetic differences in population subsets, such as patient populations of different gender, age, or race, or patients with particular underlying diseases or concomitant therapy. The screen may also detect interactions of two factors, e.g., gender and age. The relative ease with which pharmacokinetic differences among population subsets can be assessed contrasts with the difficulty of developing precise relationships of most clinical responses to drug dose or to the drug concentration in blood, which usually would be necessary when attempting to observe pharmacodynamic differences between two subgroups.

A final reason to emphasize pharmacokinetic evaluation is that it must be carried out to allow relevant assessment of pharmacodynamic differences or relationships. Assessing pharmacodynamic differences between groups or establishing blood concentration-response relationships is possible only when groups are reasonably well matched for blood concentrations. Enough pharmacokinetic data must therefore be available to permit the investigator to administer doses that will produce comparable blood concentrations in the subsets to be compared or, alternatively, to compare subsets that have been titrated to similar blood concentrations.

4. The number of documented gender-related pharmacodynamic differences of clinical consequence is at this time small, and conducting formal pharmacodynamic/effectiveness studies to detect them may be difficult, depending on the clinical endpoint. Such studies are therefore not routinely necessary. The by-gender analyses of clinical trials that include both men and women, however, which are specified in the 1988 guideline entitled ''Guideline for the Format and Content of the Clinical and Statistical Sections of New Drug Applications'' are not difficult to carry out. Particularly if these analyses are accompanied by blood concentration data for each patient, they can detect important pharmacodynamic/effectiveness differences related to gender.

C. Inclusion of Both Genders in Clinical Studies

The patients included in clinical studies should, in general, reflect the population that will receive the drug when it is marketed. For most drugs, therefore, representatives of both genders should be included in clinical trials in numbers adequate to allow detection of clinically significant gender-related differences in drug response. Although it may be reasonable to exclude certain patients at early stages because of characteristics that might make evaluation of therapy more difficult (e.g., patients on concomitant therapy), such exclusions should usually be abandoned as soon as possible in later development so that possible drug-drug and drug-disease interactions can be detected. Thus, for example, there is ordinarily no good reason to exclude women using oral contraceptives or estrogen replacement from trials. Rather, they should be included and differences in responses between them and patients not on such therapy examined. Pharmacokinetic interaction studies (or screening approaches) to look at the interactions resulting from concomitant treatment are also useful.

Ordinarily, patients of both genders should be included in the same trials. This permits direct comparisons of genders within the studies. In some cases, however, it may be appropriate to conduct studies in a single gender, e.g., to evaluate the effects of phases of the menstrual cycle on drug response.

Although clinical or pharmacokinetic data collected during phase 3 may provide evidence of gender-related differences, these data may become available too late to affect the design and dose-selection of the pivotal controlled trials. Inclusion of women in the earliest phases of clinical development, particularly in early pharmacokinetic studies, is, therefore, encouraged so that information on gender differences may be used to refine the design of later trials. Note that the strict limitation on the participation of women of childbearing potential in phase 1 and early phase 2 trials that was imposed by the 1977 guideline entitled, ''General Considerations for the Clinical Evaluation of Drugs,'' has been eliminated.

There is no regulatory or scientific basis for routine exclusion of women from bioequivalence trials. For certain drugs, however, it is possible that changes during the menstrual cycle may lead to increases in intra-subject variability. Such variability could be related to hormonally-mediated differences in metabolism or changes in fluid balance. Sponsors of bioequivalence trials are encouraged to examine available information on the pharmacokinetics and metabolism of the test drugs and related drugs to determine whether there is a basis for concern about variability in pharmacokinetics during the menstrual cycle. Where the available information does raise such concern, measures could be taken to reduce or adjust for variability, e.g., administration of each drug at the same phase of the menstrual cycle, or inclusion of larger numbers of subjects. Sponsors are encouraged to collect data that will contribute to the understanding of the relationship between hormonal variations and pharmacokinetics.

D. Analysis of Effectiveness and Adverse Effects by Gender

FDA's guideline on the clinical and statistical sections of NDA's calls for analyses of effectiveness, adverse effects, dose-response, and, if available, blood concentration-response, to look for the influence of: (1) Demographic features, such as age, gender, and race; and (2) other patient characteristics, such as body size (body weight, lean body mass, fat mass), renal, cardiac, and hepatic status, the presence of concomitant illness, and concomitant use of drugs, including ethanol and nicotine. Analyses to detect the influence of gender should be carried out both for individual studies and in the overall integrated analyses of effectiveness and safety. Such analyses of subsets with particular characteristics can be expected to detect only relatively large gender-related differences, but in general, small differences are not likely to be clinically important. The results of these analyses may suggest the need for more formal dose-response or blood concentration-response studies in men or women or in other patient subsets. Depending on the magnitude of the findings, or their potential importance (e.g., they would be more important for drugs with low therapeutic indices), these additional studies might be carried out before or after marketing.

E. Defining the Pharmacokinetics of the Drug in Both Genders

The factors most commonly having a major influence on pharmacokinetics are renal function, for drugs excreted by the kidney, and hepatic function, for drugs that are metabolized or excreted by the liver; these should be assessed directly as part of the ordinary development of drugs. The pharmacokinetic effects of other subgroup characteristics such as gender can be assessed either by a pharmacokinetic screening approach, described in the 1989 guideline entitled, "Guideline for the Study of Drugs Likely to Be Used in the Elderly," or by formal pharmacokinetic studies in specific gender or age groups.

Using either a specific pharmacokinetic study or a pharmacokinetic screen, the pharmacokinetics of a drug should be defined for both genders. In general, it is prudent to at least carry out pilot studies to look for major pharmacokinetic differences before conducting definitive controlled trials, so that differences that might lead to the need for different dosing regimens can be detected. Such studies are particularly important for drugs with low therapeutic indices, where the smaller average size of women alone might be sufficient to require modified dosing, and for drugs with nonlinear kinetics, where the somewhat higher milligram per kilogram dose caused by a woman's smaller size could lead to much larger differences in blood concentrations of drug. Gender may interact with other factors, such as age. The potential for such interactions should be explored.

Three pharmacokinetic issues related specifically to women that should be considered during drug development are: (1) The influence of menstrual status on the drug's pharmacokinetics, including both comparisons of premenopausal and postmenopausal patients and examination of within-cycle changes; (2) the influence of concomitant supplementary estrogen treatment or systemic contraceptives (oral contraceptives, long-acting progesterone) on the drug's pharmacokinetics; and (3) the influence of the drug on the pharmacokinetics of oral contraceptives. Which of these influences should be studied in a given case would depend on the drug's excretion, metabolism, and other pharmacokinetic properties, and on the steepness of the dose-response curve.

Hormonal status during the menstrual cycle may affect plasma volume and the volume of distribution (and thus clearance) of drugs. The activity of certain cytochrome P450 enzymes may be influenced by estrogen levels and, in addition, microsomal oxidation by these enzymes may decline in the elderly more in men than women. Oral contraceptives can cause decreased clearance of drugs (e.g., imipramine, diazepam, chlordiazepoxide, phenytoin, caffeine, and cyclosporine), apparently by inhibiting hepatic metabolism. They can also increase clearance by inducing drug metabolism (e.g., of acetaminophen, salicylic acid, morphine, lorazepam, temazepam, oxazepam, and clofibrate). Certain anticonvulsants (carbamazepine, phenytoin) and antibiotics (rifampin) can reduce the effectiveness of oral contraceptives. Many of the potential interactions of gender and gender-related characteristics (e.g., use of oral contraceptives) can be evaluated with the pharmacokinetic screen. In some cases, specific studies will be needed.

F. Gender-Specific Pharmacodynamic Studies

Because documented demographic differences in pharmacodynamics appear to be relatively uncommon, it is not necessary to carry out separate pharmacodynamic/effectiveness studies in each gender routinely. Evidence of such differences should be sought, however, in the data from clinical trials by carrying out the by-gender analyses suggested in the guideline on the clinical and statistical sections of NDA's. These analyses of controlled trials involving both genders are probably more likely to detect differences than studies carried out entirely in one gender. Experience has shown that gender differences can be detected with such approaches.

If the by-gender analyses suggest gender-related differences, or if such differences would be particularly important, e.g., because of a low therapeutic index, additional formal studies to seek such differences between the blood level-response curves of men and women should be conducted. Even in the absence of a particular concern based on the by-gender analyses, if there is a readily measured pharmacodynamic endpoint, such as blood pressure or rate of ventricular premature beats, and if there are good dose-response data for the overall population, it should be feasible to develop dose response data from population subsets (e.g., both genders) in the critical clinical trials.

G. Precautions in Clinical Trials Including Women of Childbearing Potential

Appropriate precautions should be taken in clinical studies to guard against inadvertent exposure of fetuses to potentially toxic agents and to inform subjects and patients of potential risk and the need for precautions. In all cases, the informed consent document and investigator's brochure should include all available information regarding the potential risk of fetal toxicity. If animal reproductive toxicity studies are complete, the results should be presented, with some explanation of their significance in humans. If these studies have not been completed, other pertinent information should be provided, such as a general assessment of fetal toxicity in drugs with related structures or pharmacologic effects. If no relevant information is available, the informed consent should explicitly note the potential for fetal risk.

In general, it is expected that reproductive toxicity studies will be completed before there is large-scale exposure of women of childbearing potential, i.e., usually by the end of phase 2 and before any expanded access program is implemented.

Except in the case of trials intended for the study of drug effects during pregnancy, clinical protocols should also include measures that will minimize the possibility of fetal exposure to the investigational drug. These would ordinarily include providing for the use of a reliable method of contraception (or abstinence) for the duration of drug exposure (which may exceed the length of the study), use of pregnancy testing (beta HOG) to detect unsuspected pregnancy prior to initiation of study treatment, and timing of studies (easier with studies of short duration) to coincide with, or immediately follow, menstruation. Female subjects should be referred to a study physician or other counselor knowledgeable in the selection and use of contraceptive approaches.

H. Potential Effects on Fertility

Where abnormalities of reproductive organs or their function (spermatogenesis or ovulation) have been observed in experimental animals, the decision to include patients of reproductive age in a clinical study should be based on a careful risk-benefit evaluation, taking into account the nature of the abnormalities, the dosage needed to induce them, the consistency of findings in different species, the severity of the illness being treated, the potential importance of the drug, the availability of alternative treatment, and the duration of therapy. Where patients of reproductive potential are included in studies of drugs showing reproductive toxicity in animals, the clinical studies should include appropriate monitoring and/or laboratory studies to allow detection of these effects. Long-term followup will usually be needed to evaluate the effects of such drugs in humans.

Appendix 3.7   Food and Drug Administration, (21 CFR 50.24) Exception from Informed Consent Requirements for Emergency Research (1996)

(a) The IRB responsible for the review, approval, and continuing review of the clinical investigation described in this section may approve that investigation without requiring that informed consent of all research subjects be obtained if the IRB (with the concurrence of a licensed physician who is a member of or consultant to the IRB and who is not otherwise participating in the clinical investigation) finds and documents each of the following:

(1) The human subjects are in a life-threatening situation, available treatments are unproven or unsatisfactory, and the collection of valid scientific evidence, which may include evidence obtained through randomized placebo-controlled investigations, is necessary to determine the safety and effectiveness of particular interventions.

(2) Obtaining informed consent is not feasible because:

(i) The subjects will not be able to give their informed consent as a result of their medical condition;

(ii) The intervention under investigation must be administered before consent from the subjects' legally authorized representatives is feasible; and

(iii) There is no reasonable way to identify prospectively the individuals likely to become eligible for participation in the clinical investigation.

(3) Participation in the research holds out the prospect of direct benefit to the subjects because:

(i) Subjects are facing a life-threatening situation that necessitates intervention;

(ii) Appropriate animal and other preclinical studies have been conducted, and the information derived from those studies and related evidence support the potential for the intervention to provide a direct benefit to the individual subjects; and

(iii) Risks associated with the investigation are reasonable in relation to what is known about the medical condition of the potential class of subjects, the risks and benefits of standard therapy, if any, and what is known about the risks and benefits of the proposed intervention or activity.

(4) The clinical investigation could not practicably be carried out without the waiver.

(5) The proposed investigational plan defines the length of the potential therapeutic window based on scientific evidence, and the investigator has committed to attempting to contact a legally authorized representative for each subject within that window of time and, if feasible, to asking the legally authorized representative contacted for consent within that window rather than proceeding without consent. The investigator will summarize efforts made to contact legally authorized representatives and make this information available to the IRB at the time of continuing review.

(6) The IRB has reviewed and approved informed consent procedures and an informed consent document consistent with Sec. 50.25. These procedures and the informed consent document are to be used with subjects or their legally authorized representatives in situations where use of such procedures and documents is feasible. The IRB has reviewed and approved procedures and information to be used when providing an opportunity for a family member to object to a subject's participation in the clinical investigation consistent with paragraph (a) (7) (v) of this section.

(7) Additional protections of the rights and welfare of the subjects will be provided, including, at least:

(i) Consultation (including, where appropriate, consultation carried out by the IRB) with representatives of the communities in which the clinical investigation will be conducted and from which the subjects will be drawn;

(ii) Public disclosure to the communities in which the clinical investigation will be conducted and from which the subjects will be drawn, prior to initiation of the clinical investigation, of plans for the investigation and its risks and expected benefits;

(iii) Public disclosure of sufficient information following completion of the clinical investigation to apprise the community and researchers of the study, including the demographic characteristics of the research population, and its results;

(iv) Establishment of an independent data monitoring committee to exercise oversight of the clinical investigation; and

(v) If obtaining informed consent is not feasible and a legally authorized representative is not reasonably available, the investigator has committed, if feasible, to attempting to contact within the therapeutic window the subject's family member who is not a legally authorized representative, and asking whether he or she objects to the subject's participation in the clinical investigation. The investigator will summarize efforts made to contact family members and make this information available to the IRB at the time of continuing review.

(b) The IRB is responsible for ensuring that procedures are in place to inform, at the earliest feasible opportunity, each subject, or if the subject remains incapacitated, a legally authorized representative of the subject, or if such a representative is not reasonably available, a family member, of the subject's inclusion in the clinical investigation, the details of the investigation and other information contained in the informed consent document. The IRB shall also ensure that there is a procedure to inform the subject, or if the subject remains incapacitated, a legally authorized representative of the subject, or if such a representative is not reasonably available, a family member, that he or she may discontinue the subject's participation at any time without penalty or loss of benefits to which the subject is otherwise entitled. If a legally authorized representative or family member is told about the clinical investigation and the subject's condition improves, the subject is also to be informed as soon as feasible. If a subject is entered into a clinical investigation with waived consent and the subject dies before a legally authorized representative or family member can be contacted, information about the clinical investigation is to be provided to the subject's legally authorized representative or family member, if feasible.

(c) The IRB determinations required by paragraph (a) of this section and the documentation required by paragraph (e) of this section are to be retained by the IRB for at least 3 years after completion of the clinical investigation, and the records shall be accessible for inspection and copying by FDA in accordance with Sec. 56.115 (b) of this chapter.

(d) Protocols involving an exception to the informed consent requirement under this section must be performed under a separate investigational new drug application (IND) or investigational device exemption (IDE) that clearly identifies such protocols as protocols that may include subjects who are unable to consent. The submission of those protocols in a separate IND/IDE is required even if an IND for the same drug product or an IDE for the same device already exists. Applications for investigations under this section may not be submitted as amendments under Secs. 312.30 or 812.35 of this chapter.

(e) If an IRB determines that it cannot approve a clinical investigation because the investigation does not meet the criteria in the exception provided under paragraph (a) of this section or because of other relevant ethical concerns, the IRB must document its findings and provide these findings promptly in writing to the clinical investigator and to the sponsor of the clinical investigation. The sponsor of the clinical investigation must promptly disclose this information to FDA and to the sponsor's clinical investigators who are participating or are asked to participate in this or a substantially equivalent clinical investigation of the sponsor, and to other IRB's that have been, or are, asked to review this or a substantially equivalent investigation by that sponsor.

Appendix 3.8   National Institutes of Health, Research Involving Impaired Human Subjects: Clinical Center Policy for the Consent Process (1986)

In September 1986, following a one year trial, the Medical Board of the Clinical Center (CC) approved a new policy for the consent process in clinical research with patients who are or will become cognitively impaired. The purposes of the policy are: 1) to protect the rights and welfare of such subjects, and 2) to encourage needed research in diseases which carry great cognitive deficits.

This document sets out the final policy and how it must be implemented by the Institute Clinical Review Subpanel (ICRS) and CC physicians and others who advise impaired patients and their families. The first section describes how the policy applies to the research review process. The second section sets out how the consent process must be administered by the subject's physician.

Section 1. Research Review of Studies Involving Impaired Human Subjects

The ICRS is authorized by Federal regulation to protect the rights and welfare of subjects of research who are temporarily or permanently impaired by including "appropriate additional safeguards". [45 CFR 46. 111 (b)] This policy specifies how the ICRS can approve "additional safeguards" for the consent process with impaired human subjects and their legally authorized representatives.

Investigators who plan research with human subjects who are or will become cognitively impaired must include a written section in the protocol which:

1) describes the risks of the proposed research,

2) describes the prospect of direct benefit(s) of the research to the subject, or if direct benefit to the subject is not expected, describes the importance of the knowledge sought by the research, and

3) describes the anticipated degree of clinical impairment of subjects during their participation, and

4) requests ICRS approval to use a Durable Power of Attorney (DPA) for the consent process, when appropriate.

The DPA is a legal document by which a prospective research subject appoints a surrogate to make decisions for the subject about his or her participation in research at the NIH.

In reviewing the research, the ICRS shall specify, in consultation with the principal investigator, the level of risk involved in the proposed research. The minutes of the ICRS shall record the assessment of risk level and approval of the planned use of the DPA.

Three levels of research risks are described in Federal regulations which are permitted in intramural research involving impaired subjects, provided that the consent process described in Section 2 is used.

Level 1. Research having minimal risk, e.g., non-invasive procedures; psychometric tests; medical record reviews; venipunctures; medical tests or procedures carried out in the routine medical care of patients with the diagnosis, etc.

Level 2. Research having greater than minimal risk but presenting the prospect of direct benefit to individual subjects, e.g., a drug trial with minimal side effects; tests involving minimal radiation but providing useful diagnostic information (CAT Scan), etc.

Level 3. Research having greater than minimal risk with no prospect of direct benefit to subjects, but likely to yield generalizable knowledge about the subject's disorder or condition, e.g., added lumber punctures or ionizing radiation done for research, etc.

Section 2. Consent Process with Impaired Human Subjects

CC policy is that consent of impaired subjects is necessary but is not sufficient to begin research. More must be done to provide the best substituted judgment that the subject would consent to the research if he or she were not impaired. When the subject is not seriously impaired, he or she shall be asked to appoint the surrogate decision maker. The patient may select the person of choice, not necessarily a relative. The DPA is the official record of the subject's choice. When the subject is so seriously impaired as to be incapable of understanding the intent or meaning of the DPA process, a next-of-kin surrogate may be chosen by the physician. However, a consultation is required from the Bioethics Program about the suitability and willingness of the prospective surrogate to serve in this role.

Further, the policy specifies that if higher levels of research risk and impairment are involved, a higher degree of monitoring will be required. Three levels of monitoring are embodied in the policy: 1) notification of Institute and CC officials of the use of the DPA, 2) required bioethics consultations in five of eight types of cases, and 3) family-initiated court appointment of a guardian in two types of cases.

Figure 1 describes eight case types, considerations of levels of research risk and impairment, and the action(s) required.

In Case 1 the subject is capable of understanding the DPA and the research risk is minimal. The DPA is executed, notification given, and research can proceed. Notification is done by sending copies of the signed and witnessed DPA forms to those designated on the carbons (Chair, ICRS; Institute Clinical Director; CC Bioethicist).

In Case 2 the subject is incapable of understanding the DPA and the research risk is minimal. The physician shall request an ethics consultation for the selection of a next-of-kin surrogate. Following a positive consultation report the substituted proxy consent of the relative can be obtained and research can proceed.

In Case 3 the subject is capable of understanding the DPA and the research risk is greater than minimal risk, but with a prospect of direct benefit to the subject. The physician shall request an ethics consultation to assure that the person appointed by the subject is capable of understanding the risks and benefits of the study. After the DPA is executed, notification shall occur, and research can proceed.

In Case 4 the subject is capable of understanding the DPA and the research risk is greater than minimal risk, but with no prospect of benefit to the subject. The physician shall request an ethics consultation to assure that the person appointed by the subject is capable of understanding the purpose and risks of the study. After the DPA is executed, notification shall occur, and research can proceed.

In Case 5, the subject is incapable of understanding the DPA and the research risk is greater than minimal, with a prospect of direct benefit to the subject. No court-appointed guardian exists, but family members desire the patient's participation in the research. The physician shall request an ethics consultation for the family members to assure their understanding of the risks and benefits and also of the CC's policy requiring court appointment of a guardian. Research shall not proceed until family members initiate court proceedings and a court-appointed guardian can give consent for the research.

In Case 6, the subject is incapable of understanding the DPA and the research risk is greater than minimal, with no prospect of benefit to the subject. No court-appointed guardian exists, but family members desire the subject's participation in the research. The physician shall request an ethics consultation for the family members to assure their understanding of the risks and lack of benefit in this case. Research shall not proceed until family members initiate court proceedings and a court-appointed guardian can give consent for the research.

In Case 7, the subject is incapable of understanding the DPA and the research risk is greater than minimal, with a prospect of direct benefit to the subject. The subject does not have an intact family; i.e., either no relatives are alive or able to act as surrogate decision makers. Research can proceed if the situation is a medical emergency, when a physician may give therapy, including experimental therapy, if in the physician's judgment it is necessary to protect the life or health of the patient.

In Case 8, the subject is incapable of understanding the DPA and the research risk is greater than minimal, with no benefit to the subject. The subject does not have an intact family or relatives. Research is prohibited in this case.

Patients with a valid DPA prepared elsewhere or with a court-appointed guardian need not execute a new DPA. Also, the DPA is valid for all research and clinical care involving the patient during his or her entire NIH stay.

The physician caring for the research subject is responsible for all phases of the DPA procedure: (1) securing consultation if needed, (2) explaining the DPA to the subject and the surrogate, (3) completing of the DPA and placing it in the chart, and (4) notifying designated officials by sending carbon copies as indicated.

DPA forms with instructions are available from all unit nursing stations and from the Bioethics Program.

Consultation on ethical problems in the consent process with impaired human subjects or answers to questions about the DPA policy can be obtained by calling the Bioethics Program, 496-2429, Building 10, Room 2C-202.

Appendix 3.9 National Institutes of Health, Report of the Human Embryo Research Panel (1994)

Charge to the Panel

The mandate of the National Institutes of Health (NIH) Human Embryo Research Panel (the Panel) was to consider various areas of research involving the ex utero preimplantation human embryo and to provide advice as to those areas that (1) are acceptable for Federal funding, (2) warrant additional review, and (3) are unacceptable for Federal support. For those areas of research considered acceptable for Federal funding, the Panel was asked to recommend specific guidelines for the review and conduct of this research.

The Panel's charge encompasses only research that involves extracorporeal human embryos produced by in vitro fertilization or from other sources, or parthenogenetically activated oocytes. Research involving in utero human embryos, or fetuses, is not part of the charge, since guidelines for such research are embodied in Federal laws and regulations governing human subjects research. Research involving human germ-line gene modification also is not within the Panel's scope. Therapeutic human fetal tissue transplantation research is also not part of the Panel's mandate; guidelines are already in place to govern such research.

Throughout this report, "ex utero preimplantation embryo" or "preimplantation embryo" refers to a fertilized ovum in vitro that has never been transferred to or implanted in a uterus. This includes a fertilized ovum that has been flushed from a woman before implantation in the uterus. This procedure, although infrequent and posing special risks, is included because it is one potential source of embryos.

Ethical Considerations

Throughout its deliberations, the Panel considered the wide range of views held by American citizens on the moral status of preimplantation embryos. In recommending public policy, the Panel was not called upon to decide which of these views is correct. Rather, its task was to propose guidelines for preimplantation human embryo research that would be acceptable public policy based on reasoning that takes account of generally held public views regarding the beginning and development of human life. The Panel weighed arguments for and against Federal funding of this research in light of the best available information and scientific knowledge and conducted its deliberations in terms that were independent of a particular religious or philosophical perspective.

The Panel received a considerable volume of public input, which it carefully considered. The

Panel heard from citizens who object to any research involving preimplantation embryos as well as those who support it and listened closely to the thinking underlying the various opinions expressed. In the process of receiving public input, the Panel realized that the scientific and policy issues involved in research on preimplantation embryos are complex and not easily comprehended. The Panel therefore recognizes that a special effort is required to enhance public understanding of the issues related to research involving the preimplantation embryo. It is the Panel's hope that this report will in some measure contribute to a process of increasing public awareness, discussion, and understanding of these issues.

From the perspective of public policy, the Panel concludes that sufficient arguments exist to support the permissibility of certain areas of research involving the preimplantation human embryo within a framework of stringent guidelines. This conclusion is based on an assessment of the moral status of the preimplantation embryo from various viewpoints and not solely on its location ex utero. In addition, the Panel weighed the important human benefits that might be achieved if preimplantation embryo research were federally funded under stringent guidelines.

The Panel believes that certain areas of research are permissible based on three primary considerations, which are listed below. Different members of the Panel may have accorded different weight to each of these considerations in reaching a conclusion about the permissibility of certain areas of research.

- The promise of human benefit from research is significant, carrying great potential benefit to infertile couples, families with genetic conditions, and individuals and families in need of effective therapies for a variety of diseases.
- Although the preimplantation human embryo warrants serious moral consideration as a developing form of human life, it does not have the same moral status as an infant or child. This is because of the absence of developmental individuation in the preimplantation embryo, the lack of even the possibility of sentience and most other qualities considered relevant to the moral status of persons, and the very high rate of natural mortality at this stage.
- In the continued absence of Federal funding and regulation in this area, preimplantation human embryo research that has been and is being conducted without Federal funding and regulation would continue, without consistent ethical and scientific review. It is in the public interest that the availability of Federal funding and regulation should provide consistent ethical and scientific review for this area of research. The Panel believes that because the preimplantation embryo possesses qualities requiring moral respect, research involving the ex utero preimplantation human embryo must be carefully regulated and consistently monitored.

Principles and Guidelines for Preimplantation Embryo Research

The Panel supports Federal funding of certain areas of preimplantation embryo research within the framework of the guidelines specified below. Any research conducted on the ex utero preimplantation human embryo or on gametes intended for fertilization should adhere to the following general principles as well as the more specific guidelines relevant to the nature of the particular research.

- The research must be conducted by scientifically qualified individuals in an appropriate research setting.
- The research must consist of a valid research design and promise significant scientific or clinical benefit.
- The research goals cannot be otherwise accomplished by using animals or unfertilized gametes. In addition, where applicable, adequate prior animal studies must have been conducted.
- The number of embryos required for the research must be kept to the minimum consistent with scientific criteria for validity.
- Donors of gametes or embryos must have given informed consent with regard to the nature and purpose of the specific research being undertaken.
- There must be no purchase or sale of gametes or embryos used in research. Reasonable compensation in clinical studies should be permissible to defray a subject's expenses, over

and above the costs of drugs and procedures required for standard treatment, provided that no compensation or financial inducements of any sort are offered in exchange for the donation of gametes or embryos, and so long as the level of compensation is in accordance with Federal regulations governing human subjects research and that it is consistent with general compensation practice for other federally funded experimental protocols.

• Research protocols and consent forms must be reviewed and approved by an appropriate institutional review board (IRB) and, for the immediate future, an ad hoc review process that extends beyond the existing review process to be established by NIH and operated for at least 3 years.

• There must be equitable selection of donors of gametes and embryos, and efforts must be made to ensure that benefits and risks are fairly distributed among subgroups of the population.

• Out of respect for the special character of the preimplantation human embryo, research involving preimplantation embryos should be limited to the shortest time period consistent with the goals of each research proposal and, for the present, research involving human embryos should not be permitted beyond the time of the usual appearance of the primitive streak in vivo (14 days). An exception to this is made for research protocols with the goal of reliably identifying in the laboratory the appearance of the primitive streak.

Fertilization of Oocytes Expressly for Research Purposes

One of the most difficult issues the Panel had to consider was whether it is ethically permissible to fertilize donated oocytes expressly for research purposes or whether researchers should be restricted to the use of embryos remaining from infertility treatments that are donated by women or couples. In developing its recommendation concerning this issue, the Panel considered both the deeply held moral concerns about the fertilization of oocytes for research as well as the potential clinical benefits to be gained from such research. The Panel concludes that studies that require the fertilization of oocytes are needed to answer crucial questions in reproductive medicine and that it would therefore not be wise to prohibit altogether the fertilization and study of oocytes for research purposes. The Panel had to balance important issues regarding the health and safety of women, children, and men against the moral respect due the preimplantation embryo. Given the conclusions the Panel reached about the moral status of the preimplantation embryo, it concludes that the health needs of women, children, and men must be given priority.

The Panel recognizes, however, that the embryo merits respect as a developing form of human life and should be used in research only for the most serious and compelling reasons. There is also a possibility that if researchers had broad permission to develop embryos for research, more embryos might be created than is truly justified. The Panel believes that the use of oocytes fertilized expressly for research should be allowed only under two conditions. The first condition is when the research by its very nature cannot otherwise be validly conducted. Examples of studies that might meet this condition include (1) oocyte maturation or oocyte freezing followed by fertilization and examination for subsequent developmental viability and chromosomal normalcy and (2) investigations into the process of fertilization itself (including the efficacy of new contraceptives). If oocyte maturation techniques were improved, eggs could be obtained without reliance on stimulatory drugs, lessening some of the potential risks for both patients and egg donors.

The second condition under which the fertilization of oocytes would be allowed expressly for research is when a compelling case can be made that this is necessary for the validity of a study that is potentially of outstanding scientific and therapeutic value. One member of the Panel dissented from the Panel conclusion that under this condition oocytes may be fertilized expressly for research purposes (see appendix A).

Panel members believe that special attention is warranted for such research because of their concern that attempts might be made to create embryos for reasons that relate solely to the scarcity of embryos remaining from infertility programs and because of their interest in preventing the creation of embryos for any but the most compelling reasons. An example of studies that might meet this second condition is research to ensure that specific drugs used in reproductive medicine, such as those for inducing ovulation, have no harmful effect on oocytes and their developmental potential and do not compromise the future reproductive health of women.

In another case, future discoveries might provide strong evidence that some forms of infertility, birth defects, or childhood cancer are due to chromosomal abnormalities, DNA modifications, or metabolic defects in embryos from gametes of men and women of a particular category—for example, those exposed to specific environmental agents or carrying specific genetic traits. In order to test or validate such hypotheses, a compelling case might be made for comparing embryos from at-risk couples with control embryos from "normal" couples. While embryos from many infertile couples in in vitro fertilization (IVF) programs might be suitable for this control group, in specific cases a compelling argument might be made that gametes donated by fertile individuals carefully matched for age and ethnic background to those in the at-risk group are necessary for the most accurate and informative comparative scientific data.

Sources of Gametes and Embryos for Research

Having concluded that Federal funding of certain areas of preimplantation embryo research is acceptable within stringent guidelines, the Panel went on to address another set of ethical dilemmas raised by the issue of acceptability of various sources of gametes and embryos. In considering these issues the Panel identified four concerns that require special vigilance: the need for informed consent, limits on commercialization, equitable selection of donors for research, and appropriate balancing of risks and benefits among subgroups of the population. These concerns parallel those addressed by well-established ethical guidelines for all human research. The selection of sources of gametes and embryos for research must be consistent with these established guidelines and in addition must show respect for the special qualities of the human gamete and embryo.

The Panel gave careful consideration to the two distinct means by which a preimplantation human embryo can become available for research. The first occurs when embryos already fertilized for infertility treatments are not used for that purpose but are donated by the progenitors for research (these embryos are sometimes referred to as "spare" embryos). The second occurs when an oocyte is fertilized expressly for the purpose of research. The Panel also considered the ethical acceptability of the various donor sources of oocytes for research involving transfer, research without transfer, and research involving parthenogenesis. These possible donor sources include women in IVF programs, healthy volunteers, women undergoing pelvic surgery, women and girls who have died, and aborted fetuses.

In analyzing the acceptability of donor sources of gametes and embryos for research, the Panel emphasized that the risks of the research, including the risks of gamete procurement, must be in proportion to the anticipated benefits. Risks that occur at various stages of research and in the context of diverse protocols restrict the acceptable sources of research gametes and embryos. For example, the need to consider the well-being of the future child when embryos are transferred to the uterus mandates particular attention to the acceptability of gamete and embryo sources, including a requirement that the gamete donors approve of the research as well as the transfer.

In general, the Panel concludes that, provided all conditions regarding consent and limits on commercialization are met, embryos donated by couples in IVF programs are acceptable sources for basic research that does not involve transfer, as well as for clinical studies that may involve transfer. Women undergoing IVF treatment may also donate oocytes not needed for their own treatment, provided other guidelines are met. In this regard, the Panel believes it is right for women and couples undergoing infertility treatment to assume a fair share of the burden of advancing research in this area given that they, as a class, stand to benefit most from the clinical applications that may result. However, the Panel also recognizes that infertility can cause great physical and psychological pain and that women and couples undergoing treatment may be more vulnerable as a result. For this reason one member of the Panel dissents from allowing women in IVF treatment the opportunity to donate oocytes for research that does not involve transfer (see appendix A). In order that women and couples in IVF programs are not made to feel compelled to donate, great care must be taken to ensure that there is no undue, or even subtle, pressure to donate. The voluntary nature of such donations is essential, and under no circumstances should individuals who do not wish to donate their gametes ever feel pressured to do so.

Donation of oocytes for research purposes without intent to transfer raises special concerns regarding risks to women. Some of the methods used to procure eggs, especially hyperstimulation, involve the use of powerful drugs and invasive procedures that could pose risks to the health of women. Women undergoing treatment for infertility consent to these risks in return for potential therapeutic benefit and are an acceptable source of oocytes for basic research that does not involve transfer, as well as for clinical studies that may involve transfer.

Women undergoing scheduled pelvic surgery are an additional permissible source of oocytes for research, provided that other guidelines are met and that no additional risks are imposed. Researchers must explain any changes from standard surgical procedures and, if hormonal stimulation is used, the risks of such drugs.

Women who are not scheduled to undergo a surgical procedure are *not* a permissible source of oocytes for embryos developed for research at this time, even if they wish to volunteer to donate their oocytes. The Panel, however, is willing to allow such volunteers to donate oocytes if the intent is to transfer the resulting embryo for the purpose of establishing a pregnancy. This is because the risks to the donor undergoing oocyte retrieval may be justified by the potential direct benefit to the infertile couple who hope to become parents as a result of the procedure. Absent the goal of establishing a pregnancy for an infertile couple, the lack of direct therapeutic benefit to the donor and the dangers of commercial exploitation do not justify exposing women to such risks.

Women who have died are a permissible source of oocytes for research without transfer, provided that the woman had not expressly objected to such use of her oocytes and that appropriate consent is obtained. If the woman had expressed no objection to such use of her oocytes, either she must have consented to donation before her death or, in the absence of explicit consent on her part, next of kin may give consent at the time of her death. One member of the Panel dissents from this recommendation based on the belief that consent must have been obtained from the woman before her death (see appendix A). Care must be taken to ensure that the consenting donors, or their next of kin who would be providing proxy consent, are clearly and specifically aware that the organ being donated is the ovary and that it might be used in research that could involve the fertilization of any oocytes derived from it. It should also be made clear to donors and next of kin that transfer of any embryo created from such material to the uterus is prohibited.

Because of strong concerns about the importance of parenthood and the orderly sequence of generations, as well as the need for detailed medical histories, the Panel concluded that research involving the transfer of embryos created from oocytes obtained from cadaveric sources, including aborted fetuses, should be unacceptable for Federal funding. The Panel also felt that it would be unwise public policy at this time to support, without additional review, research involving the fertilization of fetal oocytes, even if not intended for transfer to the uterus. Such research should not be supported until the ethical implications are more fully explored and addressed by a national advisory body.

Transfer of Embryos to a Uterus

In addition to these general guidelines, the Panel developed specific guidelines for research on preimplantation embryos intended for transfer and for those not intended for transfer, as well as guidelines for research involving parthenogenesis.

It is important to recognize that when transfer to a uterus is intended, research on the preimplantation embryo can result in harm to the child who could be born, a research subject whose treatment raises distinct ethical issues. In both law and ethics it is clear that fetuses who are brought to term are considered persons with full moral status and protectability. It would therefore be unacceptable to transfer an embryo if it is reasonable to believe that a child who might be born from these procedures will suffer harm as a result of the research. Even when research involves a diagnostic procedure, an embryo may not be transferred unless there is reasonable confidence that any child born as a result of these procedures has not been harmed by them. This distinction in treatment between embryos that will be transferred and those that will not is warranted by the need to avoid harm to the child who could be born.

Parthenogenesis

In keeping with its mandate, the Panel also considered the acceptability of Federal funding of research involving the parthenogenetic activation of eggs. Parthenogenesis is the activation of eggs to begin cleavage and development without fertilization. It has been shown in research involving parthenogenesis in mammals that when such parthenotes are transferred to the uterus, few reach the stage of implantation. The few that do reach implantation develop to various stages of early cell differentiation but then lose capacity for further development and die. Parthenotes fail to develop further because they lack expression of essential genes contributed by the sperm. All evidence therefore suggests that human parthenotes intrinsically are not developmentally viable human embryos. Thus, they do *not* represent a form of sexual reproduction.

Research on parthenotes, or activated eggs, might provide information on the specific role of the egg mechanisms in activating and sustaining early development, without generating a human embryo. Parthenotes may have research utility nearly identical to the normal embryo up to the blastocyst stage. In addition, a certain type of ovarian tumor originates from eggs that develop as parthenotes while still in the ovary. Research on parthenotes may shed light on problems arising during oocyte development that promote this type of tumor formation.

The Panel recommends that research proposals involving parthenogenesis be considered ethically acceptable on the conditions that they adhere to the general principles and that transfer of parthenogenetically activated oocytes not be permitted under any circumstances. The Panel wishes to allay fears expressed by members of the public who are concerned about the end point of research on parthenogenesis. To many, such research appears to represent a tampering with the natural order in unacceptable ways. Even though it is considered intrinsically impossible in humans, the Panel would preclude any attempts to develop a fetus or child without a paternal progenitor by prohibiting research involving the transfer of parthenotes.

Review and Oversight of Research

The Panel does not recommend that an Ethics Advisory Board (EAB) be reconstituted for the purpose of reviewing research protocols involving embryos and fertilized eggs. Although revisiting the EAB experience offers the potential for developing public consensus and a consistent application of the new guidelines, it nonetheless has significant disadvantages. These disadvantages include the creation of an additional standing government board, the likelihood of a significant delay before embryo research could be funded in order to meet legal requirements for new rulemaking prior to the official creation of the government body, and further possible delay if all proposals for embryo research were required to be considered individually by an EAB-type board, despite appearing to be consistent with a developed consensus at NIH about acceptability for funding.

The Panel wishes to retain the strengths of the old EAB—such as its assurance of consistent application of guidelines—without creating a new regulatory body. Therefore, the Panel recommends that all research proposals involving preimplantation human embryo research that are submitted to NIH for funding or that are proposed for conduct in the NIH intramural research program be subject to an additional review at the national level by an ad hoc body created with the discretionary authority of the Director of NIH. Two members of the Panel formally dissent from this recommendation, citing the adequacy of existing review through local IRBs and the possibility of such a review board being subject to undue pressures.

The purpose of the recommended review is to ensure that such research is conducted in accordance with guidelines established by NIH. This review is in addition to existing procedures and should occur after the standard reviews and approvals by the study section and council have been completed. The additional review process should continue for at least 3 years. If the NIH Director elects to dissolve this ad hoc review process after 3 years, a more decentralized review with certain additional oversight provisions, as specified further below, should begin.

When the ad hoc review body ceases to exist, the Panel recommends that all such research proposals continue to be specially monitored by the NIH councils and the NIH Office for Protection From Research Risks. This monitoring would include a commitment by the councils to pay particular attention to the protocols as they are presented for approval, in order to ensure that the local IRB and NIH study section have correctly applied the guidelines adopted by the NIH Director.

Categories of Research

Acceptable for Federal Funding

Consistent with its mandate, the Panel considered specific areas of research in terms of acceptability for Federal funding. While it is clearly impossible to anticipate every type of research project that might be proposed, the Panel was charged to divide types of embryo research into three categories: (1) acceptable for Federal funding, (2) warranting additional review, and (3) unacceptable for Federal funding.

A research proposal is presumed acceptable if it is in accordance with the guidelines described above and is not described below as warranting additional review or being unacceptable. A protocol not in the last two categories would be classified acceptable if it is scientifically valid and meritorious; relies on prior adequate animal studies and, where appropriate, studies on human embryos without transfer; uses a minimal number of embryos; documents that informed consent will be obtained from acceptable donor sources; involves no purchase or sale of gametes or embryos; does not continue beyond the time of the usual appearance of the primitive streak in vivo (14 days); and has passed the required review by a local IRB, appropriate NIH study section and council, and, for the immediate future, the additional ad hoc review body at the national level established at the discretion of the NIH Director.

Proposals in the acceptable category must also meet the specific guidelines set forth in this report concerning types of research (i.e., transfer, no transfer, parthenogenesis) (see chapter 5), and acceptable sources of gametes and embryos. Examples of such proposals include, but are not limited to the following:

- Studies aimed at improving the likelihood of a successful outcome for a pregnancy.
- Research on the process of fertilization.
- Studies on egg activation and the relative role of paternally derived and maternally derived genetic material in embryo development (parthenogenesis without transfer).
- Studies in oocyte maturation or freezing followed by fertilization to determine developmental and chromosomal normality.
- Research involving preimplantation genetic diagnosis with and without transfer.
- Research involving the development of embryonic stem cells, but only with embryos resulting from IVF for infertility treatment or clinical research that have been donated with the consent of the progenitors.
- Nuclear transplantation into an enucleated, fertilized or unfertilized (but activated) egg without transfer for research that aims to circumvent or correct an inherited cytoplasmic defect.

With regard to the last example, a narrow majority of the Panel believed such research should be acceptable for Federal funding. Nearly as many thought that the ethical implications of research involving the transplantation of a nucleus, whether transfer was contemplated or not, need further study before the research could be considered acceptable for Federal funding.

In addition to these examples, the Panel singled out two types of acceptable research for special consideration in the recommended ad hoc review process.

• Research involving the use of existing embryos where one of the progenitors was an anonymous gamete source who received monetary compensation. (This exception would apply only to embryos already in existence at the time at which this report is accepted by the Advisory Committee to the Director, NIH, should such acceptance occur.)
• A request to fertilize ova where this is necessary for the validity of a study that is potentially of outstanding scientific and therapeutic value.

In the first instance, for reasons explained in chapter 4 of this report, the Panel, with the exception of one member (see appendix C), would make an allowance for an interim period for research involving the use of existing embryos where one of the progenitors was anonymous and had received monetary compensation. However, the Panel believes that in order to determine whether the exception might apply, special attention must be given during the review process to ensure that payment has not been provided for the embryo itself and that all other proposed guidelines are met.

In the second instance, Panel members believe that special attention is warranted for such research because of concern that attempts might be made to create embryos for reasons that relate solely to the scarcity of embryos remaining from infertility programs and because of the Panel's interest in preventing the creation of embryos for any but the most compelling reasons.

Warrants Additional Review

The Panel places research of a particularly sensitive nature in this category. The Panel did not make a determination on the acceptability of these proposals and therefore recommends that there be a presumption against Federal funding of such research for the foreseeable future. This presumption could be overcome only by an extraordinary showing of scientific or therapeutic merit, together with explicit consideration of the ethical issues and social consequences. Such research proposals could be funded only after review by a broad-based ad hoc body created at the discretion of the Director, NIH, or by some other formal review process.

Research that the Panel determined should be placed in a category warranting additional review includes the following:

• Research between the appearance of the primitive streak and the beginning of neural tube closure.
• Cloning by blastomere separation or blastocyst splitting without transfer.
• Nuclear transplantation into an enucleated, fertilized or unfertilized (but activated) egg with transfer, with the aim of circumventing or correcting an inherited cytoplasmic defect.
• Research involving the development of embryonic stem cells from embryos fertilized expressly for this purpose. (One member of the Panel dissents from this categorization; see appendix B.)
• Research that uses fetal oocytes for fertilization without transfer.

The Panel wishes to note that it was extremely circumspect in its consideration of the appropriate classification of the last two research areas and that members were divided in their views about where to place the research. For research involving the development of embryonic stem cells from deliberately fertilized oocytes, a narrow majority of members agreed such research warranted further review. A number of other members, however, felt that the research was acceptable for Federal funding, while some believed that such research should be considered unacceptable for Federal funding. The Panel's deliberation about the use of fetal oocytes for research without transfer involved painstaking reflection about the ethical implications and public sensibilities. The decision to recommend that this research be placed in the further review category, rather than the unacceptable category, was made by a bare majority.

Unacceptable for Federal Funding

Four ethical considerations entered into the deliberations of the Panel as it determined what types of research were unacceptable for Federal funding: the potential adverse consequences of the research for children, women, and men; the respect due the preimplantation embryo; concern for public sensitivities about highly controversial research proposals; and concern for the meaning of humanness, parenthood, and the succession of generations.

Throughout its report, the Panel considered these concerns as well as the scientific promise and the clinical and therapeutic value of proposed research, particularly as it might contribute to the well-being of women, children, and men. Regarding the types of research considered unacceptable, the Panel determined that the scientific and therapeutic value was low or questionable, or that animal studies did not warrant progressing to human research.

Research proposals in the unacceptable category should not be funded for the foreseeable future. Even if claims were made for their scientific or therapeutic value, serious ethical concerns counsel against supporting such research. Such research includes the following:

- Cloning of human preimplantation embryos by separating blastomeres or dividing blastocysts (induced twinning), followed by transfer in utero.
- Studies designed to transplant embryonic or adult nuclei into an enucleated egg, including nuclear cloning, in order to duplicate a genome or to increase the number of embryos with the same genotype with transfer.
- Research beyond the onset of closure of the neural tube.
- Research involving the fertilization of fetal oocytes with transfer.
- Preimplantation genetic diagnosis for sex selection, except for sex-linked genetic diseases.
- Development of human-nonhuman and human-human chimeras with or without transfer.
- Cross-species fertilization, except for clinical tests of the ability of sperm to penetrate eggs.
- Attempted transfer of parthenogenetically activated human eggs.
- Attempted transfer of human embryos into nonhuman animals for gestation.
- Transfer of human embryos for extrauterine or abdominal pregnancy.

Need for Public Education

Finally, the Panel believes that any successful efforts in preimplantation embryo research depend on improving public understanding of the nature of preimplantation embryo research and therefore recommends that NIH undertake efforts toward public education as it simultaneously educates the scientific community about guidelines for acceptable research.

Appendix 3.10   National Center for Human Genome Research, Policy on Availability and Patenting of Human Genomic DNA Sequence Produced by NCHGR Pilot Projects (1996)

This document describes the policy of the National Center for Human Genome Research with respect to availability and patenting of human genomic DNA sequence produced under grants funded as a result of RFA HG-95-005. In conformity with the existing spirit and philosophy of the Human Genome Project and in response to the recommendations of advisors and the expressed wishes of the community, NCHGR seeks to make DNA sequence information available as rapidly and freely as possible.

Background

The Human Genome Project (HGP) is an international research effort, begun in 1990, which has the scientific goals of generating maps of the human genome and producing the complete sequence of the human DNA by the year 2005. The project was undertaken in the U.S. following the advice of several scientific committees that emphasized its importance in creating a resource that "will facilitate research in biochemistry, physiology and medicine", "have a major impact on health care and disease prevention" and provide "enormous scientific and technological advances . . . , having both basic and commercial applications". At NIH, the National Center for Human Genome Research (NCHGR) was founded to implement the HGP.

The HGP has progressed rapidly, even beyond optimistic expectations. The initial mapping goals are nearly completed and recent improvements in DNA sequencing technology and capacity have led many scientists, including NCHGR advisors, to conclude that complete sequencing of human genomic DNA should begin. Early in 1995, NCHGR issued RFA HG-95–005 to solicit grant applications for pilot projects to test strategies that can potentially scale up to sequence the human genome. The applications received in response to the RFA were peer reviewed in the fall of 1995 and approved by the National Advisory Council for Human Genome Research in January 1996. A set of grants will be funded by April 1996.

At the inception of the HGP, the planners emphasized that, in order to reap the maximum benefit from the HGP, human DNA sequence should be freely available in the public domain. The NIH Ad Hoc Program Advisory Committee on Complex Genomes stated that "Distribution of and free access to the databases (containing the sequence data) must be fully encouraged. Thus, the data must be in the public domain, and the redistribution of the data should remain free of royalties." Similarly, the National Research Council stated: ". . . access to all sequences and material generated by these publicly funded projects should and even must be made freely available . . .". Most recently, an international group of scientists, from both the public and private sectors, who are already involved in genomic DNA sequencing, passed a unanimous resolution that "all human genomic DNA sequence information, generated by centers funded for large-scale human sequencing, should be freely available and in the public domain in order to encourage research and development and to maximize its benefit to society."

There are very strong scientific arguments that human genomic DNA sequence should be freely available and in the public domain:

- The human genomic DNA sequence is unique. Although there are many other types of information that contribute to the understanding of human biology, e.g., DNA sequence of model organism genomes, in the end, the only source of definitive information about the human is the human sequence.
- The human genomic DNA sequence is a vast resource. It contains a very large number of genes and an enormous amount of additional biological information. It is anticipated that the sequence resource will be the basis for many useful inventions and patentable products. It will take many researchers years to find and characterize all of the genes and other functional elements within the sequence and to use that information to develop products and other approaches that will improve the health of the American people.
- The human genome is a bounded resource. Once the genome has been sequenced, few or no opportunities will exist for discovery of new information that will not make reference to, or be dependent on, that first sequence. Thus, it is important to ensure maximum access of a large number of parties to the initial genomic DNA sequence as it is generated, to provide a broad opportunity for development of new products.

Policy

It is therefore NCHGR's intent that human genomic DNA sequence data, generated by the projects funded under RFA HG-95-005, should be released as rapidly as possible and placed in the public domain where it will be freely available. In order to implement this policy, NCHGR will require that grantees under RFA HG-95-005 adopt a policy of rapid release of data to public databases. This policy will be made a condition of the award.

In NCHGR's opinion, raw human genomic DNA sequence, in the absence of additional demonstrated biological information, lacks demonstrated specific utility and therefore is an inappropriate material for patent filing. NIH is concerned that patent applications on large blocks of primary human genomic DNA sequence could have a chilling effect on the development of future inventions of useful products. Companies are not likely to pursue projects where they believe it is unlikely that effective patent protection will be available. Patents on large blocks of primary sequence will make it difficult to protect the fruit of subsequent inventions resulting from real creative effort. However, according to the Bayh-Dole Act, the grantees have the right to elect to retain title to subject inventions and are free to choose to apply for patents should additional biological experiments reveal convincing evidence for utility. The grantees are reminded that the grantee institution is required to disclose each subject invention to the Federal Agency providing research funds within two months after the inventor discloses it in writing to grantee institution personnel responsible for patent matters. NCHGR will monitor grantee activity in this area to learn whether or not attempts are being made to patent large blocks of primary human genomic DNA sequence.

During this pilot period, NCHGR will be soliciting opinions and collecting evidence from the broad scientific and commercial sectors to allow an evaluation of whether the approach described above is sufficient to ensure that sequence generated by these grants is maximally useful to the research and commercial sectors. If not, NIH will consider a determination of exceptional circumstance to restrict or eliminate the right of parties, under future grants, to elect to retain title.

Appendix 3.11   NIH Reauthorization Act (1993), Sections on Clinical Research Equity and on Research on Transplantation of Fetal Tissue

Sec. 131. Requirement of Inclusion in Research

Part G of title IV of the Public Health Service Act, as amended by section 101 of this Act, is amended by inserting after section 492A the following section:

Inclusion of Women and Minorities in Clinical Research

Sec. 492B.
    (a) Requirement of Inclusion.—
        (1) In general.—In conducting or supporting clinical research for purposes of this title, the Director of NIH shall, subject to subsection (b), ensure that—
            (A) women are included as subjects in each project of such research; and
            (B) members of minority groups are included as subjects in such research.
        (2) Outreach regarding participation as subjects.—The Director of NIH, in consultation with the Director of the Office of Research on Women's Health and the Director of the Office of Research on Minority Health, shall conduct or support outreach programs for the recruitment of women and members of minority groups as subjects in projects of clinical research.
    (b) Inapplicability of Requirement.—The requirement established in subsection (a) regarding women and members of minority groups shall not apply to a project of clinical research if the inclusion, as subjects in the project, of women and members of minority groups, respectively—
        (1) is inappropriate with respect to the health of the subjects;
        (2) is inappropriate with respect to the purpose of the research; or
        (3) is inappropriate under such other circumstances as the Director of NIH may designate.
    (c) Design of Clinical Trials.—In the case of any clinical trial in which women or members of minority groups will under subsection (a) be included as subjects, the Director of NIH shall ensure that the trial is designed and carried out in a manner sufficient to provide for a valid analysis of whether the variables being studied in the trial affect women or members of minority groups, as the case may be, differently than other subjects in the trial.

(d) Guidelines.—

(1) In general.—Subject to paragraph (2), the Director of NIH, in consultation with the Director of the Office of Research on Women's Health and the Director of the Office of Research on Minority Health, shall establish guidelines regarding the requirements of this section. The guidelines shall include guidelines regarding—

(A) the circumstances under which the inclusion of women and minorities as subjects in projects of clinical research is inappropriate for purposes of subsection (b);

(B) the manner in which clinical trials are required to be designed and carried out for purposes of subsection (c); and

(C) the operation of outreach programs under subsection (a).

(2) Certain provisions.—With respect to the circumstances under which the inclusion of women or members of minority groups (as the case may be) as subjects in a project of clinical research is inappropriate for purposes of subsection (b), the following applies to guidelines under paragraph (1):

(A) (i) In the case of a clinical trial, the guidelines shall provide that the costs of such inclusion in the trial is not a permissible consideration in determining whether such inclusion is inappropriate.

(ii) In the case of other projects of clinical research, the guidelines shall provide that the costs of such inclusion in the project is not a permissible consideration in determining whether such inclusion is inappropriate unless the data regarding women or members of minority groups, respectively, that would be obtained in such project (in the event that such inclusion were required) have been or are being obtained through other means that provide data of comparable quality.

(B) In the case of a clinical trial, the guidelines may provide that such inclusion in the trial is not required if there is substantial scientific data demonstrating that there is no significant difference between—

(i) the effects that the variables to be studied in the trial have on women or members of minority groups, respectively; and

(ii) the effects that the variables have on the individuals who would serve as subjects in the trial in the event that such inclusion were not required.

Sec. 111. Fetal Tissue Transplantation

Part G of title IV of the Public Health Service Act (42 U.S.C. 289 et seq.) is amended by inserting after section 498 the following section:

Research on Transplantation of Fetal Tissue

Sec. 498A.

(a) Establishment of Program.—

(1) In general.—The Secretary may conduct or support research on the transplantation of human fetal tissue for therapeutic purposes.

(2) Source of tissue.—Human fetal tissue may be used in research carried out under paragraph (1) regardless of whether the tissue is obtained pursuant to a spontaneous or induced abortion or pursuant to a stillbirth.

(b) Informed Consent of Donor.—

(1) In general.—In research carried out under subsection (a), human fetal tissue may be used only if the woman providing the tissue makes a statement, made in writing and signed by the woman, declaring that—

(A) the woman donates the fetal tissue for use in research described in subsection (a);

(B) the donation is made without any restriction regarding the identity of individuals who may be the recipients of transplantations of the tissue; and

(C) the woman has not been informed of the identity of any such individuals.

(2) Additional statement.—In research carried out under subsection (a), human fetal tissue may be used only if the attending physician with respect to obtaining the tissue from the woman involved makes a statement, made in writing and signed by the physician, declaring that—

(A) in the case of tissue obtained pursuant to an induced abortion—

(i) the consent of the woman for the abortion was obtained prior to requesting or obtaining consent for a donation of the tissue for use in such research;

(ii) no alteration of the timing, method, or procedures used to terminate the pregnancy was made solely for the purposes of obtaining the tissue; and

(iii) the abortion was performed in accordance with applicable State law;

(B) the tissue has been donated by the woman in accordance with paragraph (1); and

(C) full disclosure has been provided to the woman with regard to—

(i) such physician's interest, if any, in the research to be conducted with the tissue; and

(ii) any known medical risks to the woman or risks to her privacy that might be associated with the donation of the tissue and that are in addition to risks of such type that are associated with the woman's medical care.

(c) Informed Consent of Researcher and Donee.—In research carried out under subsection (a), human fetal tissue may be used only if the individual with the principal responsibility for conducting the research involved makes a statement, made in writing and signed by the individual, declaring that the individual—

(1) is aware that—

(A) the tissue is human fetal tissue;

(B) the tissue may have been obtained pursuant to a spontaneous or induced abortion or pursuant to a stillbirth; and

(C) the tissue was donated for research purposes;

(2) has provided such information to other individuals with responsibilities regarding the research;

(3) will require, prior to obtaining the consent of an individual to be a recipient of a transplantation of the tissue, written acknowledgment of receipt of such information by such recipient; and

(4) has had no part in any decisions as to the timing, method, or procedures used to terminate the pregnancy made solely for the purposes of the research.

Sec. 112. Purchase of Human Fetal Tissue

Prohibitions Regarding Human Fetal Tissue

Sec. 492B.

(a) Purchase of Tissue.—It shall be unlawful for any person to knowingly acquire, receive, or otherwise transfer any human fetal tissue for valuable consideration if the transfer affects interstate commerce.

(b) Solicitation or Acceptance of Tissue as Directed Donation for Use in Transplantation.—It shall be unlawful for any person to solicit or knowingly acquire, receive, or accept a donation of human fetal tissue for the purpose of transplantation of such tissue into another person if the donation affects interstate commerce, the tissue will be or is obtained pursuant to an induced abortion, and—

(1) the donation will be or is made pursuant to a promise to the donating individual that the donated tissue will be transplanted into a recipient specified by such individual;

(2) the donated tissue will be transplanted into a relative of the donating individual; or

(3) the person who solicits or knowingly acquires, receives, or accepts the donation has provided valuable consideration for the costs associated with such abortion.

Appendix 4
RESEARCH ETHICS POLICIES FROM OTHER COUNTRIES

Appendix 4.1 Royal College of Physicians, Research Involving Patients—Summary of Recommendations (1990)

Research involving patients is in the interests of patients and of society and should proceed without unnecessary impediment. Certain safeguards are, however, necessary to protect the patient from suffering physical or emotional harm or breach of confidentiality in the course of research.

Role of Research Ethics Committees

1. All research involving patients should be approved by a local Research Ethics Committee. This applies to research undertaken in hospitals and in other institutions, research conducted in general practice and elsewhere in the community and research carried out by doctors and non-medical health or other workers. Recommendations on the composition and function of Research Ethics Committees are set out in Chapter 4 (4.1–4.12).

Assessing the Aims, Quality, Risks and Benefits of Research

2. The Research Ethics Committee should be satisfied that the question addressed by the research activity is a worthwhile one and Research Ethics Committees should examine the overall design of proposed research that comes before them *(5.1–5.7)*.

3. Research Ethics Committees must assess whether, in proposed research, the risk or inconvenience caused to the patient is justifiable in relation to the value of the information sought *(5.8–5.26)*.

4. Research Ethics Committees and investigators have a duty to ensure that the risks inherent in proposed research have been reduced to the minimum necessary to achieve the research objective *(5.20)*.

5. Investigators must ensure that the study protocol effectively excludes special groups of patients in whom the risk of participation would be particularly great *(5.21, 6.16–6.17)*.

6. As a general rule, research involving patients should not incur risk greater than minimal (see *5.11*). An exception to the general rule may be justified where there is great potential benefit to the individual participating in therapeutic research (that is, research which offers the prospect of direct benefit to the patient taking part—see *5.14*). Non-therapeutic research involving greater than minimal risk might be approved by a Research Ethics committee but only under rare circumstances where i. the risk of the research procedure is still very small in comparison to the risks already incurred by the patient as a consequence of the disease itself; ii. the disease under study is a serious one; iii. there is great potential benefit in terms of the importance of the knowledge gained; iv. there is no other means of obtaining the knowledge, and v. the subject understands well what is involved and wishes to participate (see *5.26*.

Selection of Patients and Use of Medical Records

7. Any list of patients' names should be confidential to the person or institution responsible for its construction *(6.2)*.

8. Where records are used as a starting point in the recruitment of patients the person who approaches the patient should normally be the individual who was responsible for the clinical care at the time that the patient's relevant case records were generated *(6.3)*.

9. Research work based upon scrutiny of medical records should continue without unnecessary impediment but great care is required to avoid causing harm or distress to patients or their relatives, particularly through breach of confidentiality. Research which will involve access to personal medical records should receive approval by the local Research Ethics Committee *(6.12)*.

Recruitment of Patients

10. Arrangements should be made to exclude patients who may be at increased risk from proposed research procedures *(6.16–6.17)*.

11. Excessively frequent requests to patients to participate in research should be avoided *(6.18)*.

12. Patients should be invited to participate in research as volunteers in the same way as healthy individuals are invited to volunteer *(7.1, 7.2)*.

13. In the course of inviting a patient to participate in research, an investigator must make it clear that the patient is free to decline to participate without giving a reason, that a decision to decline will be accepted without question or displeasure and that the patient will then be treated as though the matter had not arisen and without any disadvantage to future care *(7.4)*.

14. The patient participating in research should understand that he will remain free to withdraw at any time, that no reason need be given for the withdrawal and that the withdrawal will be accepted without question, without incurring displeasure and without any disadvantage to future care *(7.5)*.

Consent

15. Patients should know that they are taking part in research *(7.6)*.

16. Research involving a patient should only be carried out with the patient's consent *(7.6)*. We have found it necessary to describe exceptions to this general rule in the case of some innocuous observations of behavior, research based on anonymous specimens or on medical records and some research into unheralded emergencies *(7.7)*.

17. The simple procedure of seeking oral consent after an oral explanation may need to be supported by additional measures.

> i *A Patient Information Sheet* may be used to back up the oral description of what is involved *(7.12–7.14)*.
>
> ii *Time to reflect* may be arranged to allow the patient to consider the question of enrolment *(7.16)*.
>
> iii *Written consent* may be sought *(7.17–7.21)*.
>
> iv *A third party* may act as adviser or friend to the patient *(7.22)*.
>
> v *Witnessed consent* may be a useful alternative in patients with impaired capacity to comprehend *(7.23)*.
>
> vi *Special arrangements* are necessary in the case of patients who may have impaired capacity to comprehend (eg children, the mentally handicapped and patients with mental illness) *(7.24)*.

18. Research involving minimal risk or greater than minimal risk should be described in a Patient Information Sheet which is given to patients when they are invited to participate and retained by them. The Information Sheet should be submitted to the Research Ethics Committee for approval *(7.12–7.14)*.

19. The use of written consent and a consent form is recommended in research projects associated with minimal or more than minimal risk or with significant discomfort. The Consent Form should be submitted to the Research Ethics Committee for approval *(7.19–7.12)*.

Research Involving Children

20. Research which could equally well be done on adults should never be done on children *(7.25)*.

21. Children should be consulted when the question of their participation in research arises *(7.32)*.

22. Even if an investigator believes that a child is capable of giving consent, the approval of a parent or guardian should be obtained before any research procedure is contemplated on a child under the age of 16 years. It may also be desirable to obtain parental consent in some older children *(7.32)*.

23. Where the research is for the benefit of children generally, and the child is incapable of giving consent, the investigator can properly rely on the consent of a parent or guardian. If, when the parental approval has been obtained, a child objects to the procedure itself, the investigator and the parent or guardian should reconsider whether it is appropriate to proceed *(7.34)*.

Research Involving Mentally Handicapped Patients

24. Research should never be carried out in mentally handicapped patients which could equally well be undertaken in adults who are not mentally handicapped *(7.36)*.

25. Research in mentally handicapped patients should be limited to that which is related to mental handicap *(7.36)*.

26. Research in mentally handicapped patients is subject to the usual constraints affecting all research in patients *(7.36)*.

27. Many mentally handicapped patients are capable of giving consent but consideration should be given to the use of simple tests of competence and to the use of 'two part' consent forms in which the first part comprises a test. Even if consent is forthcoming it is good practice to obtain the consent of the next-of-kin after proper explanation of the intended research *(7.37– 7.41)*. A strong ethical case can be made out for therapeutic and non-therapeutic research involving only minimal risk in mentally handicapped patients not competent to give consent. The best guidance might be that there should be agreement by close relatives and that the individual should seem to consent to the procedure, but the legal status of such research remains uncertain *(7.40–7.41)*.

Research Involving the Mentally Ill

28. Research should never be carried out in mentally ill patients which could equally well be undertaken in adults who are not mentally ill *(7.42)*.

29. Research in mentally ill patients should be limited to that which is related to the mental illness *(7.42)*.

30. Research in mentally ill patients is subject to the usual constraints affecting all research in patients. Most patients with mental illness are competent to make up their own minds as to whether they wish to take part in research and to comprehend the implications of the research *(7.42 and 7.44)*.

31. The Research Ethics Committee must be convinced that the inclusion of patients who are incompetent to give consent is acceptable and that it arises because the research is specifically directed to the condition of patients who might be incompetent *(7.47)*.

32. Where competence is in doubt or absent, due to psychosis, dementia or other causes, and in all patients detained under the Mental Health Act irrespective of competence, a procedure which seeks what is in effect a mixture of consent by the patient and consent by a relative or nominated individual may be the most satisfactory arrangement *(7.47)*. The same considerations that affect therapeutic and non-therapeutic research in mentally handicapped individuals who

are incompetent to give consent may also apply in mentally ill patients incompetent to give consent; the legal status of such research is at present uncertain *(7.40–7.41)*.

Research Involving Prisoners

33. Research should not be undertaken *solely* in prisoners who are patients unless the fact of being imprisoned is itself an essential component of the research topic *(7.48–7.50)*.

Research Involving Severely Ill Patients

34. Where the severity of a patient's illness renders him incompetent to give consent to participate in research the principles which should apply resemble those applicable to mentally handicapped and mentally ill patients. *(7.53–7.54)*.

35. In research involving severely ill patients the researcher should obtain as competent consent as possible. No patient who refused or, if incapable of refusing, resisted, should be included or continued in research. A near relative should be informed of the nature of the research and of the details of what is involved and should concur. In general, the patient should be told about the participation in research later when he recovers sufficiently to comprehend *(7.53–7.54)*. The same considerations apply here as those that affect therapeutic and non-therapeutic research in mentally handicapped and mentally ill individuals who are incompetent to give consent; the legal status of such research is at present uncertain *(7.40–7.41)*.

Research Involving Pregnant Patients

36. Research in pregnant patients should only be undertaken if pregnancy is an essential part of the research *(7.56)*.

37. Research into pregnancy and childbirth requires special consideration since two individuals, mother and child, are inevitably involved and the rights and concerns of the father may need to be taken into account *(7.56–7.57)*.

Research Involving Elderly Patients

38. The participation of elderly patients in research is desirable. Elderly patients present special problems because of their altered metabolism, the frequency of multiple ailments, and their reduced tolerance of invasive procedures. In general, elderly patients should be assumed to be competent to give consent unless there is evidence to the contrary. It should not be thought that, because of their age, they need to know any less about the intended research than a younger patient *(7.58–7.63)*.

Initiation of Research without Consent

39. There are some circumstances in which it is justifiable to initiate research without the consent of the patient. Such circumstances do not affect the duty of the investigator to obtain the prior approval of the Research Ethics Committee in the usual way *(7.64–7.74)*.

Inducements to Patients

40. Improved care should not be offered as an inducement to participate *(7.75–7.79)*.

41. Payments to patients are generally undesirable but are occasionally acceptable in studies which are lengthy and tedious *(7.81)*. Payments to patients should not be for undergoing risk and should not be such as to persuade patients to volunteer against their better judgement *(7.81)*.

42. Any payments to be made to patients should be reviewed by the Research Ethics Committee *(7.81)*.

Inducements to Researchers

43. Personal expenses incurred by a doctor in the course of undertaking research involving patients may be reimbursed by the sponsor of the research. It is proper for doctors engaged in research to be paid a fee for their services but doctors should not be paid a fee for carrying out research work in sessions for which they are already being paid from another source *(7.82–7.83)*.

44. The physician responsible for the project or trial is responsible for informing his employer of payments, for ensuring that proper accounting procedures are adopted with independent audit and for fulfilling all legal requirements. Financial arrangements should be made through the finance office of a Health Authority or a University and the accounts supervised by the financial officers *(7.84)*.

45. Payments made to doctors must be reasonable in terms of the time and effort given to the trial and openly declared *(7.84)*.

46. Payments made to doctors on a *per capita* basis (ie according to the number of patients that they recruit to a study) are unethical. Even fees paid to an institution on a *per capita* basis may lead to undue pressure to recruit patients *(7.86–7.87)*.

47. All financial arrangements and also *ad hoc* payments should be divulged to Research Ethics Committees *(7.87)*.

48. In the conduct of 'post-marketing surveillance' of medicines, the guidelines drawn up between the Association of the British Pharmaceutical Industry, the British Medical Association, the Committee on Safety of Medicines and the Royal College of General Practitioners should be followed *(7.89–7.92)*.

Randomised Controlled Therapeutic Trials

49. The randomised controlled therapeutic trial has proved extremely valuable as a tool for examining the effectiveness of treatments and we give special attention to it because of its importance and because of the special ethical issues it raises. We discuss amongst other things the use of placebo treatments, double-blind procedure and randomisation. Detailed recommendations are set out in paras *7.93–7.111*.

Conduct of Research

50. The ordinary requirements of patients—both medical and others—should not be neglected in the course of the involvement in research and the identity of the person in overall clinical charge of the patient's care must be clear *(8.1–8.3)*.

51. Where research activities will be delegated by the investigator, the investigator should delegate only to individuals who have the necessary skills and experience *(8.4–8.6)*.

52. The confidentiality of personal data must be preserved during the conduct of research *(8.8–8.9)*.

53. The rights of patients, other doctors and sponsors to have access to the results of research require special consideration *(9.1–9.4)*.

54. The results of research should be published free from any interference by financial sponsors of the research *(9.1)*.

Monitoring the Conduct of Research

55. Research Ethics Committees should require investigators in charge of approved research projects to submit a brief report of progress at least annually *(4.13 and 10.11)*.

56. Investigators should be requested to send copies of any published reports to the Research Ethics Committee *(10.11)*.

57. Ways in which patients and health workers may approach the Research Ethics Committee when there is concern about the conduct of research should be devised and made known. It will sometimes be appropriate for this information to be included on the Patient Information Sheet *(10.11)*.

Arrangements for Compensation

58. Although the chances of harm coming to patients in the course of carefully conducted research are very small, it is important that proper arrangements are made to compensate patients in the event of such harm occurring *(11.1–11.5)*.

59. Bodies that sponsor research, including both publicly funded bodies (such as the Research Councils, the Department of Health and the National Health Service), and the pharmaceutical industry, should now so arrange their affairs as to implement the principle that injury due to participation in research sponsored by them or conducted by their staff with the approval of a Research Ethics Committee shall be compensated by a simple, informal and expeditious procedure *(11.6–11.12)*.

60. In the event of any significant injury the patient must be entitled to receive compensation regardless of whether there may or may not have been negligence or legal liability on any other basis *(11.8)*.

Appendix 4.2   British Medical Research Council, The Ethical Conduct of Research in Children (1991)

6.1 General

6.1.1 There is thus a broad consensus, with which we concur, that a principled case can be made on ethical grounds for research on children. There are a number of situations in which knowledge that is badly needed for the sake of children suffering from various conditions can only be acquired by research on children.

6.1.2 At the same time, there is agreement on the need for strict safeguards for such research. In particular:

children should take part in research only if the relevant knowledge could not be gained by research in adults

all projects must be approved by the appropriate LREC(s)

either those included have given consent, or consent has been given on their behalf by a parent or guardian and those included do not object or appear to object in either words or action.

6.1.3 When a child has sufficient understanding to consent, his consent should of course be sought. The advisability from a legal standpoint of seeking parental consent in addition to that of a child who is able to consent is discussed in section 7 below. From an ethical standpoint, research workers and LRECs should consider carefully the maturity and independence of the children to be approached and the likely expectations of their parents. For example, an LREC may agree that it would be inappropriate to approach the parents of children who are living independently of them.

6.1.4 When a child lacks sufficient understanding to consent, his willing cooperation should be sought. The ethical grounds for including such children with parental consent in therapeutic and non-therapeutic research are discussed in sections 6.2 and 6.3 below. Section 7 discusses the legal considerations.

6.2 Therapeutic Research

6.2.1 We believe that subject to the safeguards listed at 6.1.2 above there is a strong ethical case for including children who cannot consent in therapeutic research; indeed we would argue that in circumstances where participation would be in their best interests their exclusion would be unethical.

6.2.2 When a child lacks sufficient understanding to consent, his inclusion in therapeutic re- search should be subject to his parents' or guardians' judgement that the benefits likely to accrue to him outweigh the possible risks of harm, and that participation is therefore in his best interests.

6.3 Non-therapeutic Research

6.3.1 Because it might infringe the rights of a group which society should take particular care to protect, the participation of children in non-therapeutic research raises more complex ethical issues. We do not seek to argue that a child's participation in non-therapeutic research is in his best interests. But we recognise that there are circumstances in which it is important to gain knowledge which may be of benefit to children in general and which can only be acquired as a result of research which involves children.

6.3.2 We therefore believe that there is a strong case for including children unable to consent in such research, but it is essential that the safeguards listed at 6.1.2 are observed, and that those included are placed at no more than negligible risk of harm.

6.3.3 The degree of risk involved in a particular project should be given particularly careful scrutiny by the LREC when children are to be included. There have been various attempts to describe and define degrees of risk. We use the term negligible risk to mean that the risks of harm anticipated in the proposed research are not greater, considering the probability and magnitude of physiological or psychological harm or discomfort, than those ordinarily en- countered in daily life or during the performance of routine physical or psychological exami- nation or tests. Examples of procedures involving negligible risk would include the observation of behaviour, non-invasive physiological monitoring, developmental assessments and physical examinations, changes in diet and obtaining blood and urine specimens. We discuss risk in non-therapeutic research in the context of the law in para 7.2.10 below.

6.3.4 We are clear that a child's participation in such research can only be ethical if his parents or guardians agree that it would place him at no more than negligible risk of harm and is therefore not against his interests.

* * *

Appendix 4.3   British Animals (Scientific Procedures) Act (1986)

Preliminary

1. (1) Subject to the provisions of this section, "a protected animal" for the purposes of this Act means any living vertebrate other than man.

(2) Any such vertebrate in its foetal, larval or embryonic form is a protected animal only from the stage of its development when—

(a) in the case of a mammal, bird or reptile, half the gestation or incubation period for the relevant species has elapsed; and

(b) in any other case, it becomes capable of independent feeding.

(3) The Secretary of State may by order—

(a) extend the definition of protected animal so as to include invertebrates of any description;

(b) alter the stage of development specified in subsection (2) above;

(c) make provision in lieu of subsection (2) above as respects any animal which becomes a protected animal by virtue of an order under paragraph (a) above.

(4) For the purposes of this section an animal shall be regarded as continuing to live until the permanent cessation of circulation or the destruction of its brain.

(5) In this section ''vertebrate'' means any animal of the Sub-phylum Vertebrata of the Phylum Chordata and ''invertebrate'' means any animal not of that Sub-phylum.

2.   (1) Subject to the provisions of this section, ''a regulated procedure'' for the purposes of this Act means any experimental or other scientific procedure applied to a protected animal which may have the effect of causing that animal pain, suffering, distress or lasting harm.

(2) An experimental or other scientific procedure applied to an animal is also a regulated procedure if—

(a) it is part of a series or combination of such procedures (whether the same or different) applied to the same animal; and

(b) the series or combination may have the effect mentioned in subsection (1) above; and

(c) the animal is a protected animal throughout the series or combination or in the course of it attains the stage of its development when it becomes such an animal.

(3) Anything done for the purpose of, or liable to result in, the birth or hatching of a protected animal is also a regulated procedure if it may as respects that animal have the effect mentioned in subsection (1) above.

(4) In determining whether any procedure may have the effect mentioned in subsection (1) above the use of an anaesthetic or analgesic, decerebration and any other procedure for rendering an animal insentient shall be disregarded; and the administration of an anaesthetic or analgesic to a protected animal, or decerebration or any other such procedure applied to such an animal, for the purposes of any experimental or other scientific procedure shall itself be a regulated procedure.

(5) The ringing, tagging or marking of an animal, or the application of any other humane procedure for the sole purpose of enabling an animal to be identified, is not a regulated procedure if it causes only momentary pain or distress and no lasting harm.

(6) The administration of any substance or article to an animal by way of a medicinal test on animals as defined in subsection (6) of section 32 of the Medicines Act 1968 is not a regulated procedure if the substance or article is administered in accordance with the provisions of subsection (4) of that section or of an order under section 35(8)(b) of that Act.

(7) Killing a protected animal is a regulated procedure only if it is killed for experimental or other scientific use, the place where it is killed is a designated establishment and the method employed is not one appropriate to the animal under Schedule 1 to this Act.

(8) In this section references to a scientific procedure do not include references to any recognised veterinary, agricultural or animal husbandry practice.

(9) Schedule 1 to this Act may be amended by orders made by the Secretary of State.

Personal and Project Licences

3. No person shall apply a regulated procedure to an animal unless—

(a) he holds a personal licence qualifying him to apply a regulated procedure of that description to an animal of that description;

(b) the procedure is applied as part of a programme of work specified in a project licence authorising the application, as part of that programme, of a regulated procedure of that description to an animal of that description; and

(c) the place where the procedure is carried out is a place specified in the personal licence and the project licence.

4. (1) A personal licence is a licence granted by the Secretary of State qualifying the holder to apply specified regulated procedures to animals of specified descriptions at a specified place or specified places.

(2) An application for a personal licence shall be made to the Secretary of State in such form and shall be supported by such information as he may reasonably require.

(3) Except where the Secretary of State dispenses with the requirements of this subsection any such application shall be endorsed by a person who—

(a) is himself the holder of a personal licence or a licence treated as such a licence by virtue of Schedule 4 to this Act; and

(b) has knowledge of the biological or other relevant qualifications and of the training, experience and character of the applicant;

and the person endorsing an application shall, if practicable, be a person occupying a position of authority at a place where the applicant is to be authorised by the licence to carry out the procedures specified in it.

(4) No personal licence shall be granted to a person under the age of eighteen.

(5) A personal licence shall continue in force until revoked but the Secretary of State shall review each personal licence granted by him at intervals not exceeding five years and may for that purpose require the holder to furnish him with such information as he may reasonably require.

5. (1) A project licence is a licence granted by the Secretary of State specifying a programme of work and authorising the application, as part of that programme, of specified regulated procedures to animals of specified descriptions at a specified place or specified places.

(2) A project licence shall not be granted except to a person who undertakes overall responsibility for the programme to be specified in the licence.

(3) A project licence shall not be granted for any programme unless the Secretary of State is satisfied that it is undertaken for one or more of the following purposes—

(a) the prevention (whether by the testing of any product or otherwise) or the diagnosis or treatment of disease, ill-health or abnormality, or their effects, in man, animals or plants;

(b) the assessment, detection, regulation or modification of physiological conditions in man, animals or plants;

(c) the protection of the natural environment in the interests of the health or welfare of man or animals;

(d) the advancement of knowledge in biological or behavioural sciences;

(e) education or training otherwise than in primary or secondary schools;

(f) forensic enquiries;

(g) the breeding of animals for experimental or other scientific use

(4) In determining whether and on what terms to grant a project licence the Secretary of State shall weigh the likely adverse effects on the animals concerned against the benefit likely to accrue as a result of the programme to be specified in the licence.

(5) The Secretary of State shall not grant a project licence unless he is satisfied that the applicant has given adequate consideration to the feasibility of achieving the purpose of the programme to be specified in the licence by means not involving the use of protected animals.

(6) The Secretary of State shall not grant a project licence authorising the use of cats, dogs, primates or equidae unless he is satisfied that animals of no other species are suitable for the purposes of the programme to be specified in the licence or that it is not practicable to obtain animals of any other species that are suitable for those purposes.

(7) Unless revoked and subject to subsection (8) below, a project licence shall continue in force for such period as is specified in the licence and may be renewed for further periods but (without prejudice to the grant of a new licence in respect of the programme in question) no such licence shall be in force for more than five years in all.

(8) A project licence shall terminate on the death of the holder but if—

(a) the holder of a certificate under section 6 below in respect of a place specified in the licence; or

(b) where by virtue of subsection (2) of that section the licence does not specify a place in respect of which there is such a certificate, the holder of a personal licence engaged on the programme in question,

notifies the Secretary of State of the holder's death within seven days of its coming to his knowledge the licence shall, unless the Secretary of State otherwise directs, continue in force until the end of the period of twenty-eight days beginning with the date of the notification.

• • •

Additional Controls

14. (1) Where a protected animal—

(a) has been subjected to a series of regulated procedures for a particular purpose; and

(b) has been given a general anaesthetic for any of those procedures and allowed to recover consciousness,

it shall not be used for any further regulated procedures.

(2) Subsection (1) above shall not preclude the use of an animal with the consent of the Secretary of State if—

(a) the procedure, or each procedure, for which the anaesthetic was given consisted only of surgical preparation essential for a subsequent procedure; or

(b) the anaesthetic was administered solely to immobilise the animal; or

(c) the animal is under general anaesthesia throughout the further procedures and not allowed to recover consciousness.

(3) Where a protected animal—

(a) has been subjected to a series of regulated procedures for a particular purpose; but

(b) has not been given a general anaesthetic for any of those procedures,

it shall not be used for any further regulated procedures except with the consent of the Secretary of State.

(4) Any consent for the purposes of this section may relate to a specified animal or to animals used in specified procedures or specified circumstances.

15. (1) Where a protected animal—

(a) has been subjected to a series of regulated procedures for a particular purpose; and

(b) at the conclusion of the series is suffering or likely to suffer adverse effects,

the person who applied those procedures, or the last of them, shall cause the animal to be immediately killed by a method appropriate to the animal under Schedule 1 to this Act or by such other method as may be authorised by the personal licence of the person by whom the animal is killed.

(2) Subsection (1) above is without prejudice to any condition of a project licence requiring an animal to be killed at the conclusion of a regulated procedure in circumstances other than those mentioned in that subsection.

16. (1) No person shall carry out any regulated procedure as an exhibition to the general public or carry out any such procedure which is shown live on television for general reception.

(2) No person shall publish a notice or advertisement announcing the carrying out of any regulated procedure in a manner that would contravene subsection (1) above.

17. No person shall in the course of a regulated procedure—

    (a) use any neuromuscular blocking agent unless expressly authorised to do so by the personal and project licences under which the procedure is carried out; or

    (b) use any such agent instead of an anaesthetic.

Appendix 4.4   British Human Fertilisation and Embryology Act (1990)

1.   (1) In this Act, except where otherwise stated—

    (a) embryo means a live human embryo where fertilisation is complete, and

    (b) references to an embryo include an egg in the process of fertilisation,

and, for this purpose, fertilisation is not complete until the appearance of a two cell zygote.

(2) This Act, so far as it governs bringing about the creation of an embryo, applies only to bringing about the creation of an embryo outside the human body; and in this Act—

    (a) references to embryos the creation of which was brought about *in vitro* (in their application to those where fertilisation is complete) are to those where fertilisation began outside the human body whether or not it was completed there, and

    (b) references to embryos taken from a woman do not include embryos whose creation was brought about *in vitro*.

(3) This Act, so far as it governs the keeping or use of an embryo, applies only to keeping or using an embryo outside the human body.

(4) References in this Act to gametes, eggs or sperm, except where otherwise stated, are to live human gametes, eggs or sperm but references below in this Act to gametes or eggs do not include eggs in the process of fertilisation.

2.   (1) In this Act—

    "the Authority" means the Human Fertilisation and Embryology Authority established under section 5 of this Act.

    "directions" means directions under section 23 of this Act,

    "licence" means a licence under Schedule 2 to this Act and, in relation to a licence, "the person responsible" has the meaning given by section 17 of this Act, and

    "treatment services" means medical, surgical or obstetric services provided to the public or a section of the public for the purpose of assisting women to carry children.

(2) References in this Act to keeping, in relation to embryos or gametes, include keeping while preserved, whether preserved by cryopreservation or in any other way; and embryos or gametes so kept are referred to in this Act as "stored" (and "store" and "storage" are to be interpreted accordingly).

(3) For the purposes of this Act, a woman is not to be treated as carrying a child until the embryo has become implanted.

3.   (1) No person shall—

    (a) bring about the creation of an embryo, or

    (b) keep or use an embryo,

except in pursuance of a licence.

(2) No person shall place in a woman—

    (a) a live embryo other than a human embryo, or

    (b) any live gametes other than human gametes.

(3) A licence cannot authorise—

    (a) keeping or using an embryo after the appearance of the primitive streak,

    (b) placing an embryo in any animal,

(c) keeping or using an embryo in any circumstances in which regulations prohibit its keeping or use, or

(d) replacing a nucleus or a cell or an embryo with a nucleus taken from a cell of any person, embryo or subsequent development of an embryo.

(4) For the purposes of subsection (3)(a) above, the primitive streak is to be taken to have appeared in an embryo not later than the end of the period of 14 days beginning with the day when the gametes are mixed, not counting any time during which the embryo is stored.

4. (1) No person shall—

(a) store any gametes, or

(b) in the course of providing treatment services for any woman, use the sperm of any man unless the services are being provided for the woman and the man together or use the eggs of any other woman, or

(c) mix gametes with the live gametes of any animal,

except in pursuance of a licence.

(2) A licence cannot authorise storing or using gametes in any circumstances in which regulations prohibit their storage or use.

(3) No person shall place sperm and eggs in a woman in any circumstances specified in regulations except in pursuance of a licence.

(4) Regulations made by virtue of subsection (3) above may provide that, in relation to licences only to place sperm and eggs in a woman in such circumstances, sections 12 to 22 of this Act shall have effect with such modifications as may be specified in the regulations.

(5) Activities regulated by this section or section 3 of this Act are referred to in this Act as "activities governed by this Act".

. . .

11. (1) The Authority may grant the following and no other licences—

(a) licences under paragraph 1 of Schedule 2 to this Act authorising activities in the course of providing treatment services,

(b) licences under that Schedule authorising the storage of gametes and embryos, and

(c) licences under paragraph 3 of that Schedule authorising activities for the purposes of a project of research.

(2) Paragraph 4 of that Schedule has effect in the case of all licences.

12. The following shall be conditions of every licence granted under this Act—

(a) that the activities authorised by the licence shall be carried on only on the premises to which the licence relates and under the supervision of the person responsible,

(b) that any member or employee of the Authority, on production, if so required, of a document identifying the person as such, shall at all reasonable times be permitted to enter those premises and inspect them (which includes inspecting any equipment or records and observing any activity),

(c) that the provisions of Schedule 3 to this act shall be complied with,

(d) that proper records shall be maintained in such form as the Authority may specify in directions,

(e) that no money or other benefit shall be given or received in respect of any supply of gametes or embryos unless authorised by directions,

(f) that, where gametes or embryos are supplied to a person to whom another licence applies, that person shall also be provided with such information as the Authority may specify in directions, and

(g) that the Authority shall be provided, in such form and at such intervals as it may specify in directions, with such copies of or extracts from the records, or such other information, as the directions may specify.

. . .

Schedule 2: Activities for Which Licences May Be Granted

1. (1) A licence under this paragraph may authorise any of the following in the course of providing treatment services—
    (a) bringing about the creation of embryos *in vitro,*
    (b) keeping embryos,
    (c) using gametes,
    (d) practices designed to secure that embryos are in a suitable condition to be placed in a woman or to determine whether embryos are suitable for that purpose,
    (e) placing any embryo in a woman,
    (f) mixing sperm with the egg of a hamster, or other animal specified in directions, for the purpose of testing the fertility or normality of the sperm, but only where anything which forms is destroyed when the test is complete and, in any event, not later than the two cell stage, and
    (g) such other practices as may be specified in, or determined in accordance with, regulations.
    (2) Subject to the provisions of this Act, a licence under this paragraph may be granted subject to such conditions as may be specified in the licence and may authorise the performance of any of the activities referred to in subparagraph (1) above in such manner as may be so specified.
    (3) A licence under this paragraph cannot authorise any activity unless it appears to the Authority to be necessary or desirable for the purpose of providing treatment services.
    (4) A licence under this paragraph cannot authorise altering the genetic structure of any cell while it forms part of an embryo.
    (5) A licence under this paragraph shall be granted for such period not exceeding five years as may be specified in the licence.

2. (1) A licence under this paragraph or paragraph 1 or 3 of this Schedule may authorise the storage of gametes or embryos or both.
    (2) Subject to the provisions of this Act, a licence authorising such storage may be granted subject to such conditions as may be specified in the licence and may authorise storage in such manner as may be so specified.
    (3) A licence under this paragraph shall be granted for such period not exceeding five years as may be specified in the licence.

3. (1) A licence under this paragraph may authorise any of the following—
    (a) bringing about the creation of embryos *in vitro,* and
    (b) keeping or using embryos,
    for the purposes of a project of research specified in the licence.
    (2) A licence under this paragraph cannot authorise any activity unless it appears to the Authority to be necessary or desirable for the purpose of—
    (a) promoting advances in the treatment of infertility,
    (b) increasing knowledge about the causes of congenital disease,
    (c) increasing knowledge about the causes of miscarriages,
    (d) developing more effective techniques of contraception, or
    (e) developing methods for detecting the presence of gene or chromosome abnormalities in embryos before implantation
    or for such other purposes as may be specified in regulations.
    (3) Purposes may only be so specified with a view to the authorisation of projects of research which increase knowledge about the creation and development of embryos, or about disease, or enable such knowledge to be applied.
    (4) A license under this paragraph cannot authorise altering the genetic structure of any cell while it forms part of an embryo, except in such circumstances (if any) as may be specified in or determined in pursuance of regulations.
    (5) A licence under this paragraph may authorise mixing sperm with the egg of a hamster,

or other animal specified in directions, for the purpose of developing more effective techniques for determining the fertility or normality of sperm, but only where anything which forms is destroyed when the research is complete and, in any event, not later than the two cell stage.

(6) No license under this paragraph shall be granted unless the Authority is satisfied that any proposed use of embryos is necessary for the purposes of the research.

(7) Subject to the provisions of this Act, a license under this paragraph may be granted subject to such conditions as may be specified in the licence.

(8) A licence under this paragraph may authorise the performance of any of the activities referred to in subparagraph (1) or (5) above in such manner as may be so specified.

(9) A licence under this paragraph shall be granted for such period not exceeding three years as may be specified in the licence.

4.   (1) A licence under this schedule can only authorise activities to be carried on on premises specified in the licence and under the supervision of an individual designated in the licence.

(2) A licence cannot—

(a) authorise activities falling within both paragraph 1 and paragraph 3 above,

(b) apply to more than one project of research,

(c) authorise activities to be carried on under the supervision of more than one individual, or

(d) apply to premises in different places.

Schedule 3: Consents to Use of Gametes or Embryos

1. A consent under this schedule must be given in writing and, in this Schedule, "effective consent" means a consent under this Schedule which has not been withdrawn.

2.   (1) A consent to the use of any embryo must specify one or more of the following purposes—

(a) use in providing treatment services to the person giving consent, or that person and another specified person together,

(b) use in providing treatment services to persons not including the person giving consent, or

(c) use for the purposes of any project of research,

and may specify conditions subject to which the embryo may be so used.

(2) A consent to the storage of any gametes or any embryo must—

(a) specify the maximum period of storage (if less than the statutory storage period), and

(b) state what is to be done with the gametes or embryo if the person who gave the consent dies or is unable because of incapacity to vary the terms of the consent or to revoke it,

and may specify conditions subject to which the gametes or embryo may remain in storage.

(3) A consent under this Schedule must provide for such other matters as the Authority may specify in directions.

(4) A consent under this Schedule may apply—

(a) to the use or storage of a particular embryo, or

(b) in the case of a person providing gametes, to the use or storage of any embryo whose creation may be brought about using those gametes,

and in the paragraph (b) case the terms of the consent may be varied, or the consent may be withdrawn, in accordance with this Schedule either generally or in relation to a particular embryo or particular embryos.

3.   (1) Before a person gives consent under this Schedule—

(a) he must be given a suitable opportunity to receive proper counselling about the implications of taking the proposed steps, and

(b) he must be provided with such relevant information as is proper.

(2) Before a person gives consent under this Schedule he must be informed of the effect of paragraph 4 below.

4. (1) The terms of any consent under this Schedule may from time to time be varied, and the consent may be withdrawn, by notice given by the person who gave the consent to the person keeping the gametes or embryo to which the consent is relevant.

(2) The terms of any consent to use of any embryo cannot be varied, and such consent cannot be withdrawn, once the embryo has been used—

(a) in providing treatment services, or

(b) for the purposes of any project of research.

5. (1) A person's gametes must not be used for the purposes of treatment services unless there is an effective consent by that person to their being so used and they are used in accordance with the terms of the consent.

(2) A person's gametes must not be received for use for those purposes unless there is an effective consent by that person to their being so used.

(3) This paragraph does not apply to the use of a person's gametes for the purpose of that person, or that person and another together, receiving treatment services.

6. (1) A person's gametes must not be used to bring about the creation of any embryo *in vitro* unless there is an effective consent by that person to any embryo the creation of which may be brought about with the use of those gametes being used for one or more of the purposes mentioned in paragraph 2(1) above.

(2) An embryo the creation of which was brought about *in vitro* must not be received by any person unless there is an effective consent by each person whose gametes were used to bring about the creation of the embryo to the use for one or more of the purposes mentioned in paragraph 2(1) above of the embryo.

(3) An embryo the creation of which was brought about *in vitro* must not be used for any purpose unless there is an effective consent by each person whose gametes were used to bring about the creation of the embryo to the use for that purpose for the embryo and the embryo is used in accordance with those consents.

(4) Any consent required by this paragraph is in addition to any consent that may be required by paragraph 5 above.

7. (1) An embryo taken from a woman must not be used for any purpose unless there is an effective consent by her to the use of the embryo for that purpose and it is used in accordance with the consent.

(2) An embryo taken from a woman must not be received by any person for use for any purpose unless there is an effective consent by her to the use of the embryo for that purpose.

(3) This paragraph does not apply to the use, for the purpose of providing a woman with treatment services, of an embryo taken from her.

8. (1) A person's gametes must not be kept in storage unless there is an effective consent by that person to their storage and they are stored in accordance with the consent.

(2) Any embryo the creation of which was brought about *in vitro* must not be kept in storage unless there is an effective consent, by each person whose gametes were used to bring about the creation of the embryo, to the storage of the embryo and the embryo is stored in accordance with those consents.

(3) An embryo taken from a woman must not be kept in storage unless there is an effective consent by her to its storage and it is stored in accordance with the consent.

Appendix 4.5   British Guidance on the Research Use of Fetuses and Fetal Material (1989) Conclusion: Summary of Principles

We are conscious that we cannot predict what the future will hold in terms of changes in society and in the growth of scientific knowledge. It has not been our purpose to attempt any consideration of particular contemporary developments. Instead, we have sought to express our Report in terms of ethical principles which provide general guidelines against which specific proposals can be evaluated.

In summary, these may be expressed as:

1. On the basis of its potential to develop into a human being, a fetus is entitled to respect, according it a status broadly comparable to that of a living person. Thus, the relevant categories of ethical significance are "alive" and "dead", and the category of "pre-viable", used in the Peel Report, is not of ethical relevance.

2. The stated intention to abort a fetus does not of itself abrogate that status. It follows that in general, with the exception of abortion permitted under the 1967 Abortion Act, intervention on a living fetus in *utero* should carry only minimal risk of harm or, if a greater risk than that is involved, the action is intended, on balance, for the benefit of the fetus. In the case of the fetus in *utero* this consideration has, of course, to be weighed against consideration of the well-being of the mother. The delicate ethical issues relating to the trial of procedures carrying greater than minimal risk (eg trials of diagnostic procedures for conditions which may cause serious handicap) but which may be of great potential benefit to the group to which the subject of the trial belongs, must be considered in a manner broadly similar to the way such issues are considered for children and adults. All clinical research into techniques for the termination of pregnancy must take place only in the context of the act of abortion itself.

3. Tissue from therapeutic abortions may be used, provided any decision concerning this use is separated from the decision to induce abortion. The mother's decision to terminate her pregnancy, and the method and timing of that abortion, must not be influenced by consideration of possible use which might be made of the tissue. There should be barriers between the process of procuring the tissue and its subsequent use in order to ensure ethically acceptable procedures. We describe this as "separation". Although separation is, in our view, a necessity to make the use of tissue from therapeutic abortions ethically acceptable, it is equally our recommendation that the clinical management of a mother whose fetus dies in *utero* or whose fetus is aborted spontaneously, should not be influenced by any considerations other than the mother's welfare.

Necessarily, our detailed recommendations are framed in terms of the legislative, administrative and medical practice of today. In time, we can expect our report to need reconsideration, just as we have had to undertake a reassessment of matters considered in 1972 by the Peel Committee. It is desirable that subsequent revision should be undertaken as it becomes necessary and not have to await the arousal of considerable public concern before being taken in hand. Accordingly, we recommend that the Health Departments should take steps to keep these issues under regular review, perhaps in consultation with the MRC and the professions.

Appendix 4.6   British Committee on the Ethics of Gene Therapy, Summary of Main Conclusions and Recommendations on the Ethics of Gene Therapy (1989)

8.1 The Committee on the Ethics of Gene Therapy, a non-statutory body, was set up by the Government on 28 November 1989 with the following terms of reference:

"To draw up ethical guidance for the medical profession on treatment of genetic disorders in adults and children by genetic modification of human body cells; to invite and consider proposals from doctors wishing to use such treatment on individual patients; and to provide advice to United Kingdom Health Ministers on scientific and medical developments which bear on the safety and efficacy of human gene modification.''

8.2 Although there are effective treatments for some genetic disorders, conventional treatments for most of them are inadequate and, for many, are limited to the relief of symptoms. Gene therapy offers for the first time the prospect of effective treatment and cure in many genetic disorders.

Ethical Basis

8.3 Before gene therapy is introduced into medical practice it must be ethically acceptable. To find an ethical position which would command acceptance for the foreseeable future we have consulted widely. We have also taken careful notice of the treatment of these matters in other countries of similar cultural heritage. Unsurprisingly, the same questions have been discussed elsewhere, with a consistency in approach and underlying ethical conviction which have made our task easier. Our discussions and enquiries confirmed our tentative view that gene therapy should initially be regarded as research involving human subjects. It should therefore conform with accepted ethical codes whose purposes, together with the means of giving them force, are to:

(a) facilitate justifiable advancement of biomedical knowledge;
(b) maintain ethical standards of practice;
(c) protect the subjects of research from harm;
(d) preserve subjects' rights and liberties; and
(e) provide reassurance to the public, to the professions and to Parliament that these are being done.

We consider what in gene therapy research is justifiable, and the conditions that should be met for such research to be ethical and seen to be so.

Somatic Cell Gene Therapy

8.4 The purpose of somatic cell gene therapy in an individual patient is to alleviate disease in that individual, and that individual alone. We conclude that the development and introduction of safe and effective means of gene modification for this purpose is a proper goal for medical science. We therefore recommend that the necessary research should continue.

8.5 Somatic cell gene therapy may hold great potential benefit for some patients; but it may also carry risks. To ensure that the benefits are assessed and the risks are identified as expeditiously as possible, we recommend that somatic cell gene therapy should, for the present, be conducted according to the discipline of research and governed by the exacting requirements which already apply in the United Kingdom to research involving human subjects.

8.6 The first candidates for somatic cell gene therapy should be patients who are suffering from a disorder which is life threatening, or causes serious handicap, and for which treatment is unavailable or unsatisfactory, but which has not already progressed so far as to reduce significantly the potential for benefit. Some genetic disorders lead to irreversible and cumulative effects from early childhood, and even before birth. In such instances therapy must be given correspondingly early in life.

8.7 We are firmly of the view that gene therapy should be directed to alleviating disease in individual patients, although wider application may soon call for attention. In the current state of knowledge any attempt to change human traits not associated with disease would not be acceptable.

8.8 Somatic cell gene therapy will be a new kind of treatment, but it does not represent a major departure from established medical practice, nor does it, in our view, pose new ethical challenges. However, because of the special qualities of an individual's genetic make-up and the complex nature of genetic disorders, familiar issues assume greater prominence. They are:

(a) questions of safety, which are heightened by the possibility of inadvertent and unpredictable consequences of gene therapy to the patient, and the possible long term consequences;

(b) the need for long term surveillance and follow-up;

(c) the matter of consent, especially in view of (a) above;

(d) the probability that children will be among the first candidates for therapy;

(e) confidentiality, and any necessary disclosure in respect of genetic information which may be important to kindred.

Germ Line Gene Therapy

8.9 The purpose of gene modification of sperm or ova or cells that produce them would be to prevent the transmission of defective genes to subsequent generations. Gene modification at an early stage of embryonic development might be a way of correcting gene defects in both the germ line and somatic cells. However, we have concluded that there is insufficient knowledge to evaluate the risks to future generations. We recommend, therefore, that gene modification of the germ line should not yet be attempted.

Supervision of Gene Therapy

8.10 A decision on whether gene therapy research on human subjects should proceed must depend on the careful assessment of the scientific merits of the proposal, the competence of those wishing to carry it out and the potential benefits and risks. This assessment should include a critical examination of arrangements for the conduct of therapy and subsequent monitoring. It will necessarily call upon a uncommon degree and range of scientific and medical expertise. Similar expertise is required to provide advice to Ministers. No existing body is constituted for this task. Accordingly, we recommend that a supervisory body with the necessary collective expertise, experience and authority be set up, having the responsibility for making such assessments in conjunction with local research ethics committees (LRECs).

We recommend that this supervisory body should have a responsibility for:

(1) advising on the content of proposals, including the details of protocols, for therapeutic research in somatic cell gene modification;

(2) advising on the design and conduct of the research;

(3) advising on the facilities and service arrangements necessary for the proper conduct of the research;

(4) advising on the arrangements necessary for the long term surveillance and follow-up of treated patients;

(5) receiving proposals from doctors who wish to conduct gene therapy in individual patients and making an assessment of:

(a) the clinical status of the patient;

(b) the scientific quality of the proposal, with particular regard to the technical competence and scientific requirements for achieving therapy effectively and safely;

(c) whether the clinical course of the particular disorder is known sufficiently well

— for sound information, counselling and advice to be given to the patient or those acting on behalf of the patient;

— for the outcomes of therapy to be assessable;

(d) the potential benefits and risks for the patient;

(e) the ethical acceptability of the proposal.

In the light of this assessment the expert supervisory body should make a recommendation on whether the proposal should be approved, and if so on what, if any, conditions. The supervisory body should also have a responsibility for:

(6) acting in co-ordination with LRECs;

(7) acting as a repository of up-to-date information on research in gene therapy internationally;

(8) setting up and maintaining a confidential register of patients who have been the subjects of gene therapy;

(9) oversight and monitoring of the research;

(10) providing advice to Health Ministers in the United Kingdom, on scientific and medical developments which bear on the safety and efficacy of human gene modification.

8.11 We recommend that any proposal for gene therapy should be approved by the new body as well as by a properly constituted LREC, and that anyone wishing to conduct such research should submit proposals simultaneously to both.

8.12 We recommend that the attention of the Advisory Committee on Genetic Modification (ACGM) be drawn to our report.

Control and discipline

8.13 We also recommend that there should be an effective means of control and discipline. If it comes to the attention of a LREC that research is being carried out which it has not been asked to consider, or which it has considered but its recommendations have been ignored, then that ethics committee should bring the matter to the attention of its appointing authority, the relevant NHS body, and to the appropriate professional body; and the supervisory body should bring it to the attention of Ministers.

8.14 The arrangements that we recommend are, we submit, adequate to provide the safeguards necessary to ensure ethical practice when gene therapy is proposed. They should also be flexible enough to adapt to foreseeable changes in research and clinical practice in the field of gene therapy. Therefore, we recommend that the proposed supervisory body should be nonstatutory and, lest it be thought that the body would not be sufficiently independent of medical research interests, we recommend that it should be funded by, and be under the aegis of, the Department of Health.

8.15 As with other very specialised medical interventions we recommend that gene therapy be confined to a small number of centres whilst experience is gained.

Appendix 4.7   German Embryo Protection Law (1990)

Improper Use of Reproductive Technologies

1. (1) A penalty of up to three years' imprisonment or a fine shall be imposed on any person who:

    1. transfers, into a woman, an unfertilized egg cell produced by another woman;

    2. attempts to fertilize artificially an egg cell for any purpose other than bringing about a pregnancy of the woman from whom the egg cell originated;

    3. attempts, within one treatment cycle, to transfer more than three embryos into a woman;

    4. attempts, by means of gamete intrafallopian transfer, to fertilize more than three egg cells within one treatment cycle;

    5. attempts to fertilize more egg cells from a woman than may be transferred to her within one treatment cycle;

    6. removes an embryo from a woman before completion of implantation in the uterus, with a view to transferring it to another woman or to using it for another purpose that is not conductive to its preservation; or

    7. attempts to carry out artificial fertilization of a woman who is prepared to give up her child permanently after birth (surrogate mother) or to transfer a human embryo into her.

(2) The same penalty shall be imposed on any person who:

1. Brings about artificially the penetration of a human egg cell by a human sperm cell; or

2. transfers a human sperm cell into a human egg cell artificially, without intending to bring about a pregnancy in the woman from whom the egg cell originated.

(3) No penalties shall be imposed on:

1. in the case of items 1, 2, and 6 of subsection 1, the woman from whom the egg cell or embryo originated, as well as the woman into whom the egg or embryo [is] to be transferred; and

2. in the case of item 7 of subsection 1, the surrogate mother as well as the person wishing to assume responsibility for the long-term care of the child.

(4) In the case of item 6 of subsection 1 and Section 2, attempts shall be punishable.

Improper Use of Human Embryos

2. (1) Any person who transfers a human embryo that is derived from extracorporeal procreation or that has been removed from a woman before its nidation in the uterus, or who disposes of, acquires, or uses it for a purpose other than its preservation, shall be punished by up to three years' imprisonment or by a fine.

(2) The same penalty shall be imposed upon any person who is responsible for the extracorporeal development of a human embryo, for purposes other than pregnancy.

(3) Attempts shall be punishable.

Prohibited Sex Selection

3. Any person who attempts to artificially fertilize a human egg cell with a sperm cell, that is selected for the sex chromosome contained in it, shall be punished by up to one year's imprisonment or by a fine. This shall not apply if the selection of a sperm cell is made by a physician in order to prevent the child from developing Duchenne-type muscular dystrophy or a sex-linked hereditary disease of similar severity, and if the disease threatening the child is recognized as being of appropriate severity by the authority that is competent for this matter under *Land* law.

Unauthorized Fertilization, Unauthorized Embryo Transfer, and Artificial Fertilization After Death

4. (1) A penalty of up to three years' imprisonment or a fine shall be imposed on any person who:

1. attempts to artificially fertilize an egg cell without the woman whose egg cell is to be fertilized, and the man whose sperm cell is to be used for fertilization, having given consent;

2. attempts to transfer an embryo into a woman without her consent; or

3. knowingly fertilizes artificially an egg cell with the sperm of a man after his death.

(2) In the case of item 3 of subsection 1, no penalties shall be imposed on the woman upon whom the artificial fertilization was performed.

Artificial Alteration of Human Germline Cells

5. (1) Any person who artificially alters the genetic information of a human germline cell shall be punished by up to five years' imprisonment or by a fine.

(2) The same penalty shall be imposed on any person who uses a human germ cell with artificially modified genetic information for fertilization.

(3) Attempts shall be punishable.

(4) Subsection 1 shall not apply to:

    1. the artificial modification of the genetic information of a germline cell situated outside the body, if there is no possibility of its being used for fertilization;

    2. the artificial modification of the genetic information of germline cells from a different body, that have been removed from a dead conceptus, from a living person, or from a deceased person, if there is no possibility that:

        (a) they will be transferred to an embryo, fetus, or human being, or

        (b) a germ cell will develop from them; and

    3. vaccination, radiation, chemotherapeutic, or other treatments, by which a modification of the genetic information of germline cells is not intended.

Clones

6.   (1) Any person who artificially causes a human embryo to develop with the same genetic information as another embryo, fetus, living person, or deceased person shall be punished by up to five years' imprisonment or by a fine.

    (2) The same penalty shall be imposed on a person who transfers an embryo as specified in subsection 1 into a woman.

    (3) Attempts shall be punishable.

Creation of Chimeras and Hybrids

7.   (1) A penalty of up to five years' imprisonment or a fine shall be imposed on any person who attempts:

    1. to unite in one syncytium embryos with different genetic information, involving the use of at least one human embryo;

    2. to combine a human embryo with a cell that contains different genetic information from the embryo cells, and which is capable of subsequent differentiation; or

    3. by fertilization of a human egg cell with the sperm of an animal or by fertilization of an animal's egg cell with the sperm of a man, to produce an embryo capable of differentiation.

    (2) The same penalty shall be imposed on any person who attempts:

    1. to transfer an embryo produced by a procedure as specified in subsection 1 into:

        (a) a woman; or

        (b) an animal; or

    2. to transfer a human embryo into an animal.

Definitions

8.   (1) For the purpose of this Law, the term "embryo" means the human egg cell, fertilized and capable of development, from the time of fusion of the nuclei, as well as each totipotent cell removed from an embryo that is capable, in the presence of other necessary conditions, of dividing and developing into an individual.

    (2) In the first 24 hours after fusion of the nuclei, the fertilized human egg cell shall be considered to be capable of development, unless it is established before the end of this period that it is not capable of developing beyond the single-cell stage.

    (3) "Germline cells", for the purposes of this Law, means all cells that lead in a cell line from the fertilized egg cell to the egg cells and sperm cells of the human being produced, as well as the egg cell from the moment of introduction or penetration of the sperm cell to the completion of fertilization through the fusion of nuclei.

• • •

Appendix 4.8   French Law on the Protection of Persons to Whom Medical Experiments are Performed (1989–91)

Title I, General Provisions

Article L. 209-2.—No biomedical research may be made on human beings:

— If it is not founded on the latest scientific knowledge or on sufficient preclinical experimentation;
— If the foreseeable risk incurred by participants in the research is out of proportion with the benefits anticipated for these persons or the interests of the research;
— If it does not have as a goal the broadening of scientific knowledge of human beings and of means capable of improving the condition of human beings.

Article L. 209-3.—Biomedical research may only be made:

— Under the direction and supervision of a doctor with the proper experience;
— In material and technical conditions adapted to the experiment which are compatible with the imperatives of scientific rigor and of the security of the persons participating in the research.

Article L. 209-4.—Research without direct individual benefit on women who are pregnant or nursing is only allowed if it presents no foreseeable risk to the health of the woman or child and if it adds to the knowledge of phenomena linked to pregnancy and/or to nursing.

Article L. 209-5.—Persons deprived of liberty by judicial or administrative order may not be solicited to participate in biomedical research unless a direct and major benefit on the health of said persons is expected from the research.

Article L. 209-6.—Minors, majors under guardianship, persons staying at public or social health institutions, and the critically ill may not be solicited to participate in biomedical research unless one might expect a direct benefit on the health of said persons from the research.

However, research without direct, individual benefit is permitted if the following three conditions are satisfied:

— the research presents no serious risk to the health of the individual;
— the research is useful to other persons having the same characteristics of age, sickness, or handicap;
— the research is in no other way possible.

Article L. 209-7—For biomedical research without direct, individual benefit, the sponsor assumes, even without fault, responsibility for compensation for injurious consequences of the research to the person who volunteers. The assumption of said responsibility may not be opposed by a third party and is not nullified by the voluntary withdrawal of the person who had initially volunteered for the research.

For biomedical research with direct, individual benefit, the sponsor assumes responsibility for compensation for injurious consequences of the research to the person who volunteers, except for where the sponsor proves that the injury is not his/her fault, or that of all others taking part in the research. The assumption of said responsibility may not be opposed by a third party and is not nullified by the voluntary withdrawal of the person who had initially volunteered for the research.

For all biomedical research, the sponsor secures insurance guaranteeing his/her legal responsibility such as it is defined by the present article and that of all others taking part in the research, independently of the nature of the relationship between all others taking part in the research and the sponsor. The points of the present article are of public domain.

Article L. 209-8—Biomedical research gives rise to no direct or indirect financial compensation for persons participating in research outside of reimbursement for reported expenses and under provision of the particular points outlined by article L 209-15 of the current code relating to research without direct, therapeutic ends.

Title II, Of Consent

Article L. 209-9—Before undertaking biomedical research on a person, the free, clear, and express consent of the person must be obtained after a researcher, or a doctor representing him/her, has made the person aware of:

— the objective of the research, its methodology, and the duration of the research;
— the benefits expected, the constraints and possible risks, including the possibility of the premature end of the research;
— the opinion of the committee mentioned in article L. 209-12 of the present code.

The researcher or doctor representing him/her informs the person whose consent is sought of his/ her right to refuse to participate in the research or to withdraw from the research at any moment without incurring any penalty.

As an exception, when in the interest of an ill person to whom one was not able to reveal his/ her diagnosis, the researcher may, in respecting his confidence, withhold certain information linked to the diagnosis. In this case, the research protocol must mention this possibility.

The information given to the patient is summarized in a written document which is given to the person whose consent is solicited.

Consent is given in writing, or, if this is impossible, by a third party who must be completely independent from the researcher and the sponsor.

However, in the case of biomedical research conducted in emergency situations which do not allow one to solicit the prerequisite consent of the person who will take part in the research, the protocol presented for approval by the committee installed by article L. 209–11 of the current code may anticipate that the consent of the person will not be sought and that the only consent sought will be that of those close to the person who are present, in the conditions outlined above. The person will be informed as soon as possible and his/her consent will be asked for the continuation of the research.

Article L. 209-10—When biomedical research is practiced on minors or majors under guardianship:

— consent must be given, following the rules outlined in article L. 209-9 of the current code, by those exercising parental authority over non-independent minors. For minors or majors under guardianship, consent is given by the guardian for research with direct, individual benefit which does not present any foreseeable serious risk, and, in other cases, consent is given by the guardian authorized by the family council or the guardianship judge.
— The consent of the minor or major under guardianship must also be sought when he/she is apt to express his/her will. The refusal or revocation of consent of said person may not be overridden.

· · ·

Title IV, Provisions Particular to Research Without Direct Therapeutic Ends

Article L. 209-14—Biomedical research without direct, individual benefit must not entail any serious, foreseeable risk to the health of the persons who volunteer for the research.

Research must be preceded by a medical exam of the volunteers. The results of this exam are given to the volunteers by a doctor of their choice.

Article L. 209-15—In the case of research without direct, individual benefit to those who volunteer for the research, the sponsor reimburses these persons an indemnity for losses suffered. The total of these indemnities that a person might receive over the course of a year is limited by the Minister of Health.

Research on minors, majors under guardianship, or people staying at public or social health institutions may not give rise to such an indemnity.

Article L. 209-16 All biomedical research without direct, individual benefit on a person who is not affiliated with a Social Security plan or who is not a beneficiary of such a plan is forbidden.

The Social Security system holds an action against the sponsor for the payment of benefits deposited or furnished to the volunteer.

Article L. 209-17—No one may simultaneously volunteer for several biomedical research projects without direct, individual benefit.

For each research project without direct, individual benefit, the protocol submitted to the consulting committee for the protection of persons in biomedical research for its opinion establishes a period of exclusion during which a person who volunteers for research may not participate in other research without direct, therapeutic ends. The length of this period varies in relation to the nature of the research.

In order to apply the above provisions, the Minister of Health establishes and maintains a national file.

Article L. 209-18.—Biomedical research without direct, individual benefit may only take place in a location equipped with the material and technical means adapted for the research and which are compatible with the requirements for the safety of the persons who volunteer for the research, as authorized by the Minister of Health.

Appendix 4.9   Canadian Council on Animal Care, Ethics of Animal Investigation (1989)

The use of animals in research, teaching, and testing is acceptable only if it promises to contribute to understanding of fundamental biological principles, or to the development of knowledge that can reasonably be expected to benefit humans or animals.

Animals should be used only if the researcher's best efforts to find an alternative have failed. A continuing sharing of knowledge, review of the literature, and adherence to the Russell-Burch "3R" tenet of "Replacement, Reduction and Refinement" are also requisites. Those using animals should employ the most humane methods on the smallest number of appropriate animals required to obtain valid information.

The following principles incorporate suggestions from members of both the scientific and animal welfare communities, as well as the organizations represented on Council. They should be applied in conjunction with CCAC's "Guide to the Care and Use of Experimental Animals."

1. If animals must be used, they should be maintained in a manner that provides for their physical comfort and psychological well-being, according to CCAC's "Policy Statement on Social and Behavioural Requirements of Experimental Animals."

2. Animals must not be subjected to unnecessary pain or distress. The experimental design must offer them every practicable safeguard, whether in research, in teaching or in testing procedures; cost and convenience must not take precedence over the animal's physical and mental well-being.

3. Expert opinion must attest to the potential value of studies with animals. The following procedures, which are restricted, require independent, external evaluation to justify their use:

   i) burns, freezing injuries, fractures, and other types of trauma investigation in anesthetized animals, concomitant to which must be acceptable veterinary practices for the relief of pain, including adequate analgesia during the recovery period;

   ii) staged encounters between predator and prey or between conspecifics where prolonged fighting and injury are probable.

4. If pain or distress is a necessary concomitant to the study, it must be minimized both in intensity and duration. Investigators, animal care committees, grant review committees and referees must be especially cautious in evaluating the proposed use of the following procedures:

   a) experiments involving withholding pre and post-operative pain-relieving medication;

   b) paralyzing and immobilizing experiments where there is no reduction in the sensation of pain;

   c) electric shock as negative reinforcement;

d) extreme environmental conditions such as low or high temperatures, high humidity, modified atmospheres, etc., or sudden changes therein;

e) experiments studying stress and pain;

f) experiments requiring withholding of food and water for periods incompatible with the species specific physiological needs; such experiments should have no detrimental effect on the health of the animal;

g) injection of Freund's Complete Adjuvant (FCA). This must be carried out in accordance with "CCAC Guidelines on Acceptable Immunological Procedures."

5. An animal observed to be experiencing severe, unrelievable pain or discomfort should immediately be humanely killed, using a method providing initial rapid unconsciousness.

6. While non-recovery procedures involving anesthetized animals, and studies involving no pain or distress are considered acceptable, the following experimental procedures inflict excessive pain and are thus unacceptable:

a) utilization of muscle relaxants or paralytics (curare and curare-like) alone, without anesthetics, during surgical procedures;

b) traumatizing procedures involving crushing, burning, striking or beating in unanesthetized animals.

7. Studies such as toxicological and biological testing, cancer research and infectious disease investigation may, in the past, have required continuation until the death of the animal. However, in the face of distinct signs that such processes are causing irreversible pain or distress, alternative endpoints should be sought to satisfy both the requirements of the study and the needs of the animal.

8. Physical restraint should only be used after alternative procedures have been fully considered and found inadequate. Animals so restrained must receive exceptional care and attention, in compliance with species specific and general requirements as set forth in the "Guide."

9. Painful experiments or multiple invasive procedures on an individual animal, conducted solely for the instruction of students in the classroom, or for the demonstration of established scientific knowledge, cannot be justified. Audiovisual or other alternative techniques should be employed to convey such information.

Appendix 4.10 Canadian Council on Animal Care, Categories of Invasiveness in Animal Experiments (1991)

Investigators and teachers who consider it essential to use vertebrates or invertebrates in their research, teaching or testing in the laboratory or in the field, must adhere to humane principles, and take cognizance of the Canadian Council on Animal Care's (CCAC) Ethics of Animal Investigation and other CCAC documentation in assigning a category. Protocols must be submitted to an appropriate review committee for all studies and courses which involve the use of vertebrates and some invertebrates in Categories B through E. Cephalopods and some other higher invertebrates have nervous systems as well developed as in some vertebrates, and may therefore warrant inclusion in Category B, C, D, or E.

The following list of categories provides possible examples of experimental procedures which are considered to be representative of each category.

A. Experiments on Most Invertebrates or on Live Isolates.

Possible examples: the use of tissue culture and tissues obtained at necropsy or from the slaughterhouse; the use of eggs, protozoa or other single-celled organisms; experiments involving containment, incision or other invasive procedures on metazoa.

B. Experiments Which Cause Little or No Discomfort or Stress.

Possible examples: domestic flocks or herds being maintained in simulated or actual commercial production management systems; the short-term and skilful restraint of animals for purposes of observation or physical examination; blood sampling; injection of material in amounts that will not cause adverse reactions by the following routes: intravenous, subcutaneous, intramuscular, intra-peritoneal, or oral, but not intrathoracic or intracardiac (Category C); acute non-survival studies in which the animals are completely anesthetized and do not regain consciousness; approved methods of euthanasia following rapid unconsciousness, such as anesthetic overdose, or decapitation preceded by sedation or light anesthesia; short periods of food and/or water deprivation equivalent to periods of abstinence in nature.

C. Experiments Which Cause Minor Stress or Pain of Short Duration.

Possible examples: cannulation or catheterization of blood vessels or body cavities under anesthesia; minor surgical procedures under anesthesia, such as biopsies, laparoscopy; short periods of restraint beyond that for simple observation or examination, but consistent with minimal distress; short periods of food and/or water deprivation which exceed periods of abstinence in nature; behavioural experiments on conscious animals that involve short-term, stressful restraint; exposure to non-lethal levels of drugs or chemicals. Such procedures should not cause significant changes in the animal's appearance, in physiological parameters such as respiratory or cardiac rate, or fecal or urinary output, or in social responses.

Note: During or after Category C studies, animals must not show self-mutilation, anorexia, de-hydration, hyperactivity, increased recumbency or dormancy, increased vocalization, aggressive-defensive behaviour or demonstrate social withdrawal and self-isolation.

D. Experiments Which Cause Moderate to Severe Distress or Discomfort.

Possible examples: major surgical procedures conducted under general anesthesia, with subsequent recovery; prolonged (several hours or more) periods of physical restraint; induction of behavioural stresses such as maternal deprivation, aggression, predator-prey interactions; procedures which cause severe, persistent or irreversible disruption of sensorimotor organization; the use of Freund's com-plete adjuvant (see *CCAC Guidelines on Acceptable Immunological Procedures*).

Other examples include induction of anatomical and physiological abnormalities that will result in pain or distress; the exposure of an animal to noxious stimuli from which escape is impossible; the production of radiation sickness; exposure to drugs or chemicals at levels that impair physio-logical systems.

Note: Procedures used in Category D studies should not cause prolonged or severe clinical distress as may be exhibited by a wide range of clinical signs, such as marked abnormalities in behavioural patterns or attitudes, the absence of grooming, dehydration, abnormal vocalization, prolonged an-orexia, circulatory collapse, extreme lethargy or disinclination to move, and clinical signs of severe or advanced local or systemic infection, etc.

E. Procedures Which Cause Severe Pain Near, At, or Above the Pain Tolerance Threshold of Unanesthetized Conscious Animals.

This Category of Invasiveness is not necessarily confined to surgical procedures, but may include exposure to noxious stimuli or agents whose effects are unknown; exposure to drugs or chemicals at levels that (may) markedly impair physiological systems and which cause death, severe pain, or extreme distress; completely new biomedical experiments which have a high degree of invasiveness; behavioural studies about which the effects of the degree of distress are not known; use of muscle relaxants or paralytic drugs without anesthetics; burn or trauma infliction on unanesthetized animals;

a euthanasia method not approved by the CCAC; any procedures (e.g. the injection of noxious agents or the induction of severe stress or shock) that will result in pain which approaches the pain tolerance threshold and cannot be relieved by analgesia (e.g. when toxicity testing and experimentally-induced infectious disease studies have death as the endpoint).

Appendix 4.11   Canadian Federal Center for AIDS, Guidelines on Ethical and Legal Considerations in Anonymous Unlinked HIV Seroprevalence Research (1990)

This document provides guidelines on the ethical and legal considerations in anonymous unlinked human immunodeficiency virus (HIV) seroprevalence research. The guidelines are intended as a resource for researchers, grant reviewers, government agencies and institutional ethics committees. The Department of National Health and Welfare does not accept responsibility for their use in studies funded by other agencies.

Anonymous unlinked HIV seroprevalence research ("blinded surveys") is the least biased method of estimating the extent of HIV infection in a population. Serum left over from that routinely collected for other purposes and permanently unlinked from any information that could identify individuals is tested for HIV antibodies. The accuracy of the estimated rate of HIV infection in the population depends on the random selection of the blood samples tested.

The National Health Research and Development Program (NHRDP) and the Federal Centre for AIDS (FCA) released a joint Request for Research Proposals for National HIV Seroprevalence Studies in October 1988. Recognizing the importance of ethical and legal considerations in such research the FCA convened a multidisciplinary Working Group on Anonymous Unlinked HIV Seroprevalence Studies, which met Dec. 13 and 14, 1988. Participants included experts in ethics, law, medicine, theology, nursing, philosophy and public health. These guidelines reflect the deliberations of this expert group.

The Canadian Situation

In 1988 the Royal Society of Canada recommended that "to replace assumptions with data . . . epidemiological surveys be carried out to estimate the number of HIV-infected persons in Canada" and that "anonymous sample surveys, approved by institutional ethics or human experimentation committees, [be] the preferred avenue for achieving the goal of HIV epidemiologic surveillance".

At its meeting on Oct. 19, 1987, the National Advisory Committee on AIDS recommended that the Department of National Health and Welfare be encouraged to obtain or support the collection of HIV seroprevalence data adhering to the following criteria: testing should be conducted anonymously on specimens obtained for other routine tests; only the demographic information attached to these specimens should be collected; and voluntary HIV antibody testing should be available to all subjects under conditions of informed consent, pretest and posttest counseling, and confidentiality.

The Medical Research Council of Canada has stated that "consent is generally unnecessary for research undertaken, for example, upon surplus blood, urine, tissue, and similar samples obtained for diagnostic or treatment purposes if the patient is not identifiable, and the requirements of the research do not influence the procedures used for obtaining the samples".

The International Situation

Unlinked HIV seroprevalence research began in the United States in 1986 with the use of serum left over from sentinel hospitals and neonatal metabolic screening programs. The US Centers for Disease Control (CDC) now oversee a variety of such studies involving sentinel physicians, women's health centres, sexually transmitted disease clinics, addiction treatment facilities, prisons and emergency rooms, as well as a national nutrition survey.

The CDC and the Office for Protection from Research Risks, National Institutes of Health, have determined that anonymous unlinked surveys "that cause no collection of information or specimens that would not otherwise be obtained for routine medical purposes and obtain no data which can be linked to identifiable individuals can be considered blinded, or unlinked surveys, not involving 'human subjects'. Since patient identifying information will not be linked to HIV test results, informed consent will not be required."

In Britain the government funded the Medical Research Council in 1988 to conduct a variety of anonymous unlinked HIV seroprevalence studies.

Purpose of HIV Seroprevalence Research

Although monitoring the number of identified AIDS cases on a national basis provides one important measure of the AIDS epidemic, such surveillance misses cases of asymptomatic HIV infection. Consequently, this information cannot be used to assess current seroprevalence rates. Identifying and monitoring changes in the prevalence of HIV infection among Canadians are necessary steps in assessing the need for prevention programs, designing and targeting such programs, evaluating their effectiveness, identifying priority groups for screening should a vaccine or early treatment be developed, and planning and allocating resources for future health and social service needs with respect to HIV infection and AIDS.

Consensus of the Working Group

The working group agreed that the related ethical and legal concerns do not constitute an insurmountable barrier to anonymous unlinked HIV seroprevalence research, provided that specific requirements are met.

Rationale

The working group agreed that the anonymous unlinked methodology would be the most scientifically acceptable and feasible research design and would offer several advantages.

- It would provide accurate estimates of the prevalence of HIV infection because it would avoid the self-selection bias inherent in all voluntary studies.
- It would be noninvasive.
- It would ensure personal privacy because individuals could not be linked to HIV antibody test results.
- It would be cost-effective.

Adoption of the anonymous unlinked methodology raises three important issues. First, individual informed consent would not be obtained. However, seroprevalence studies on populations of unidentified people can be distinguished from testing on an individual basis. The working group agreed that it would be reasonable not to require individual informed consent when testing leftover, permanently unlinked serum for HIV antibodies.

Second, HIV-seropositive individuals would not be identified. The objective of the anonymous unlinked research design is to produce accurate seroprevalence estimates, a goal independent of voluntary individual testing and subsequent contact tracing. The HIV antibody test is available to Canadians through the health care system and should be given under conditions of informed consent, pretest and posttest counselling, and confidentiality.

Third, there is a potential for indirect harm to groups or individuals—for example, through stigmatization. This could be minimized by appropriate research requirements and would be outweighed by the benefits to the public of accurate HIV seroprevalence data. Such data would constitute an early warning system to detect changes in the pattern of spread of HIV infection in specific populations. Planning preventive or screening measures on the basis of inaccurate, particularly low, estimates would bring greater harm to groups and individuals.

Requirements for Anonymous Unlinked HIV Seroprevalence Research

The working group agreed that the following basic requirements must be met.

- Universal access to individual voluntary testing under prescribed conditions of informed consent, pretest and posttest counselling, and confidentiality would be a prerequisite.
- Only leftover serum routinely collected for other purposes would be used.
- Records would be permanently unlinked before testing, so that it would be impossible at any time to identify individual test results.
- No sample size small enough to identify individuals would be reported.
- No information that might lead to the identification of individuals would be used.
- The research would have to meet the approval of the relevant institutional ethics review committees.
- The public would be made aware of the research.

The working group also agreed on the following requirements related to communication issues.

- Communication with the public should be clear and balanced.
- Methods of informing the public about plans for anonymous unlinked research will vary from study to study. Researchers should be prepared to determine the most appropriate medium to use. Mass mailings, video recordings, toll-free telephone numbers, special seminars and ethnic language newspapers are all potential tools for informing the public.
- Researchers would be responsible for anticipating to a reasonable extent the special communication needs of the population being tested.
- Physicians should be informed through their provincial associations and colleges about unlinked HIV antibody testing and its nontherapeutic purpose. Voluntary individual testing remains an option within the patient-physician relationship and would not be affected by this research.
- The researcher's contact number should be readily available so that a physician or a patient, or both, can discuss the research in more detail. After learning more about the research some patients may request that their leftover serum not be included in the random selection of samples. Physicians must be informed of how this issue is addressed in the research protocol.
- Researchers would be responsible for anticipating to a reasonable extent the potential for indirect harm to groups or individuals. Special interest groups should be involved in developing the communication plan for potentially sensitive research results.

Appendix 4.12   Australian National Health and Medical Research Council, Statement on Human Experimentation and Supplementary Notes (1992)

The collection of data from planned experimentation on human beings is necessary for the improvement of human health. Experiments range from those undertaken as a part of patient care to those undertaken either on patients or on healthy subjects for the purpose of contributing to knowledge, and include investigations on human behaviour. Investigators have ethical and legal responsibilities toward their subjects and should therefore observe the following principles:

1. The research must conform to generally accepted moral and scientific principles. To this end institutions in which human experimentation is undertaken should have a committee con-

cerned with ethical aspects and all projects involving human experimentation should be submitted for approval by such a committee (see supplementary note 1 on institutional ethics committees).

2. Protocols of proposed projects should contain a statement by the investigator of the ethical considerations involved.

3. The investigator after careful consideration and appropriate consultation must be satisfied that the possible advantage to be gained from the work justifies any discomfort or risks involved.

4. The research protocol should demonstrate knowledge of the relevant literature and wherever possible be based on prior laboratory and animal experiments.

5. In the conduct of research, the investigator must at all times respect the personality, rights, wishes, beliefs, consent and freedom of the individual subject.

6. Research should be conducted only by suitably qualified persons with appropriate competence, having facilities for the proper conduct of the work; clinical research requires not only clinical competence but also facilities for dealing with any contingencies that may arise.

7. New therapeutic or experimental procedures which are at the stage of early evaluation and which may have long-term effects should not be undertaken unless appropriate provision has been made for long-term care, observation and maintenance of records.

8. Before research is undertaken the free consent of the subject should be obtained. To this end the investigator is responsible for providing the subject at his or her level of comprehension with sufficient information about the purpose, methods, demands, risks, inconveniences and discomforts of the study. Consent should be obtained in writing unless there are good reasons to the contrary. If consent is not obtained in writing, the circumstances under which it is obtained should be recorded.

9. The subject must be free at any time to withdraw consent to further participation.

10. Special care must be taken in relation to consent, and to safeguarding individual rights and welfare where the research involves children, the mentally ill and those in dependant relationships or comparable situations (see supplementary note 2 on research on children, the mentally ill and those in dependant relationships or comparable situations, including unconscious patients).

11. The investigator must stop or modify the research program or experiment if it becomes apparent during the course of it that continuation may be harmful.

12. Subject to maintenance of confidentiality in respect of individual patients, all members of research groups should be fully informed about projects on which they are working.

13. Volunteers may be paid for inconvenience and time spent, but such payment should not be so large as to be an inducement to participate.

Supplementary Note 1—Institutional Ethics Committees

1. All research projects involving human subjects and relating to health must be considered and approved by a committee constituted in accordance with this supplementary note.

2. Institutions in which such research is undertaken should establish and maintain an institutional ethics committee (IEC) composed and functioning in accordance with this supplementary note.

Where an institution can not maintain a properly constituted IEC, approval of research proposals should be sought from an IEC established and maintained by another institution.

3. An IEC must ensure that ethical standards are maintained in research projects to protect the interests of the research subjects, the investigator and the institution.

4. Composition

(i) An IEC shall be composed of men and women of different age groups, and include at least one member from each of the following categories:

• laywoman not associated with the institution

• layman not associated with the institution

• minister of religion
• lawyer
• medical graduate with research experience

(ii) Persons may be appointed to stand-in for members when necessary.

(iii) An institution may appoint more persons than those specified in 4 (i) as members of an IEC.

(iv) Members and stand-in members shall be appointed by an institution on such terms and conditions as the institution determines and in such manner as to ensure that the committee will fulfil its responsibilities.

(v) Members shall be appointed as individuals for their expertise and not in a representative capacity.

(vi) A layperson is one who is not closely involved in medical, scientific or legal work.

(vii) A minister of religion may be of any faith.

5. Functions

(i) A research project may be approved and may continue only if an IEC is satisfied that:
• the project as set out in the protocol is acceptable on ethical grounds; and
• the project continues to conform to the approved protocol.

(ii) An IEC shall maintain a record of all proposed research projects including:
• name of responsible institution;
• project identification number;
• principal investigator(s);
• short title of project;
• ethical approval or non-approval with date;
• the relevance of the Privacy Guidelines, which address the use of data from Commonwealth agencies;
• approval or non-approval of any changes to the protocol; and
• action taken by the IEC to monitor the conduct of the research.

The protocols of research projects shall be preserved in the form in which they are approved.

(iii) The NHMRC accepts the responsibility to communicate with and audit the activities of IECs to ensure compliance with this supplementary note.

An IEC shall accept an obligation to provide information from its records to the NHMRC on request.

6. Application of Functions

In carrying out these functions, an IEC shall:

(i) conform with the *NHMRC Statement on Human Experimentation and Supplementary Notes* as published from time to time;

(ii) while promoting the advance of knowledge by research, ensure that the rights of the subjects of research take precedence over the expected benefits to human knowledge;

(iii) ensure that, in all projects involving human subjects and relating to health, the free and informed consent of the subjects will be obtained;

(iv) ensure that no member of the committee adjudicates on projects in which they may be personally involved;

(v) ensure that research projects take into consideration local cultural and social attitudes;

(vi) give its own consideration to projects that involve research in more than one institution;

(vii) require the principal investigator to disclose any previous decisions regarding the project made by another IEC and whether the protocol is presently before another IEC; and

(viii) determine the method of monitoring appropriate to each project.

7. Meeting Procedures

(i) Wherever possible, a decision by an IEC shall be made after a person from each of the categories listed in section 4 (i) of this supplementary note has had an opportunity to contribute their views during the decision making process;

(ii) An IEC should seek to reach decisions by general agreement which need not involve unanimity;

(iii) In the absence of general agreement that a project is ethically acceptable, an IEC shall either establish a procedure to arrive at a decision, for example a simple majority, or inform the principal investigator of necessary amendments to the protocol;

(iv) An IEC may invite the investigator(s) to be present for discussions of the project; and

(v) An IEC may seek advice and assistance from experts to assist with consideration of a proposal.

8. Monitoring

An IEC shall ensure that there is appropriate monitoring of research projects until their completion. To achieve this a committee shall:

(i) at regular periods, and not less frequently than annually, require principal investigators to provide reports on matters including:

- security of records
- compliance with approved consent procedures and documentation
- compliance with other special conditions;

(ii) as a condition of approval of the protocol; require that investigators report immediately anything which might affect ethical acceptance of the protocol, including:

- adverse effects on subjects
- proposed changes in the protocol
- unforeseen events that might affect continued ethical acceptability of the project; and

(iii) establish confidential mechanisms for receiving complaints or reports on the conduct of the project:

Supplementary note 2—Research on children, the mentally ill, those in dependent relationships or comparable situations (including unconscious patients)

Ethics of Research on Children

In these notes the principles and guidelines that are set out largely reflect the 'Report on the Ethics of Research in Children' prepared by the Council of the Australian College of Paediatrics and published in the *Australian Paediatric Journal* 17:162, 1981.

1. Scientific research is essential to advance knowledge of all aspects of childhood disease. Such research, however, may be performed only when the information sought cannot in practice be obtained by other means.

2. All research must be based on sound scientific concepts and must be planned and conducted in such a fashion as will reasonably ensure that definite conclusions will be reached. Some programs may offer direct benefit to the individual child, while others may have a broader community purpose. In appropriate circumstances both may be ethical.

3. In all centres undertaking research in children, the following special responsibilities of the institutional ethics committee are emphasized:

(i) protecting the rights and welfare of children involved in research procedures;

(ii) determining the acceptability of the risk/benefit relationship of any research study conducted;

(iii) ensuring that informed consent from parents/guardian and where appropriate the child, is obtained in a manner appropriate to the study;

(iv) encouraging the performance of necessary and appropriate research; and

(v) preventing unscientific or unethical research.

4. Consent to research should be obtained from:

(i) the parents/guardian in all but exceptional circumstances (e.g. emergencies); and

(ii) the child where he or she is of sufficient maturity and intelligence to make this practicable.

In this context 'consent' means consent following a full and clear explanation of the research planned, its objectives and any risks involved.

5. Risk of research may be considered in terms of:
    (i) therapeutic research (where the procedure may be of some benefit to the child).
        In determining whether there is an acceptable relationship between potential benefit and the risk involved, it is essential to weigh the risk of the proposed research against customary therapeutic measures and the natural hazards of the disease or condition.
    (ii) non-therapeutic research (where the procedure is of no direct benefit to the child).
        The risk to the child should be so minimal as to be little more than the risks run in everyday life.

Risks of research in this context include the risk of causing physical disturbance, discomfort, anxiety, pain or psychological disturbance to the child or the parents rather than the risk of serious harm, which would be unacceptable.

The Mentally Ill

It is always desirable to obtain informed consent from a person who has the intelligence or capacity to make this practicable. In the case of those who lack legal capacity due to mental illness, consent should also be obtained from the person who stands legally in the position of guardian, next friend, or the like.

Those in Dependant Relationships or Comparable Situation

Some people merit special attention before inclusion in a project in order to ensure that consent is both informed and free. It is not possible to define them exhaustively, but in addition to children and the mentally ill they may include the following:

• elderly persons who may have legal capacity but may nonetheless be in a position where they are unable to give a free or comprehending consent;
• wards of state;
• those in doctor and patient, and teacher and student relationships;
• prisoners;
• members of the Services; and
• hospital and laboratory staff.

Unconscious and Critically Ill Patients

Unconscious, semi-conscious or critically ill patients from whom or on behalf of whom consent cannot be obtained for treatment or other intervention, because of the urgency of their condition, also merit special attention.

A person might be in such a situation, for example, following a drug overdose or a cardiac arrest. Two kinds of experimental intervention may be envisaged. The first is intended or expected to benefit the person. The second is intended or expected to yield important scientific information but is not intended or expected to benefit the person. (The taking of a sample of blood for studies not directly relevant to the diagnosis or treatment of the patient would be an example of the latter.)

1. Experimental intervention intended or expected to benefit the patient.
Before approving a research protocol an institutional ethics committee should satisfy itself:
    (i) that the guidelines, other than those bearing on consent, in the statement on human experimentation are followed; and
    (ii) that in the light of available knowledge it is reasonable to adopt the experimental intervention as being in the interests of the patient.
2. Experimental intervention is neither intended nor expected to benefit a patient.
Before approving a research protocol, an institutional ethics committee should satisfy itself:
    (i) that the guidelines, other than those bearing on consent, in the statement on human experimentation are followed;

(ii) that there are good reasons why the experimental intervention cannot be limited to persons from whom, or on behalf of whom, consent can be obtained;

(iii) that the experimental intervention will be one which will involve no material risks beyond those associated with procedures that are clinically indicated for the patient;

(iv) that the requirements of the research do not influence the procedures that are clinically indicated; and

(v) that the confidentiality of information identifying the patient will be preserved.

Supplementary Note 3—Clinical Trials

A clinical trial is a study done in humans to find out if a treatment or diagnostic procedure, which it is believed may benefit a patient, actually does so. A clinical trial can involve testing a drug, a surgical or other procedure, or a therapeutic or diagnostic device.

The drug procedure or device may be a new or an old one. It may be under trial in new clinical circumstances, or its conventional use may be under review. It is not always possible to make a clear distinction between ordinary diffusion of clinical knowledge and the medical and surgical circumstances that warrant a formal clinical trial. Clinicians should be aware of the benefits that come from (a) designing and conducting clinical trials, and (b) sharing ethical responsibility for innovation in medical practice.

The *NHMRC Statement on Human Experimentation and Supplementary Notes* are applicable to all clinical trials.

Following are some particular matters concerning the design and conduct of clinical trials that need to be taken into account when ethical aspects are being considered. Clinical trials involving DNA (gene) therapy are subject to additional requirements (see supplementary note 7).

1. Trials should be conducted according to written protocols, which should be approved by institutional ethics committees.

2. When an institutional ethics committee is reviewing a proposal for a clinical trial involving a drug it should be assured:

(i) that a pharmacologist or clinical pharmacologist has been involved in preparing the protocol;

(ii) that for trials involving new drugs the protocol includes a full investigational profile of the drug or drugs to be used;

(iii) that the protocol contains precise information on dosage, formulation, frequency of administration and methods of assessing safety; and

(iv) that all suspected adverse drug effects observed in the course of a trial will be reported to the Commonwealth Department of Health, Housing and Community Services.

3. When an institutional ethics committee is reviewing a proposal for a clinical trial involving a therapeutic or diagnostic device it should be assured:

(i) that persons suitably qualified to assess the technical and clinical aspects of the device have been involved in preparing the protocol;

(ii) that the protocol contains adequate information on methods of use, risks and benefits expected; and

(iii) that the guidelines for investigational use of therapeutic devices prepared by the Commonwealth Department of Health, Housing and Community Services are taken into account

4. The aims of every trial should be precisely stated and important enough to be worth achieving, having in mind the time, effort, cost and possible discomfort that may be involved.

5. The experimental design should be such as to ensure that it will be possible to answer the question asked. In particular institutional ethics committees should be assured of the statistical validity of the design of a proposed trial.

6. Some trials involve the use of control groups for purposes of comparison. Patients in control

groups should receive what is considered to be the best treatment currently available; in some cases this may be simply observation or administration of placebo.

7. When informed consent is being sought, costs which may be incurred by subjects as a result of participation in the trial should be discussed with them.

8. There should be a reasonable expectation that the objectives of a clinical trial will be achieved within a defined period of time. In some circumstances it may be unethical to continue a trial for the full period that was planned. For example, it would be wrong to continue if there were substantial deviations from the trial protocol, or if side effects of unexpected type or frequency were encountered. It would also be wrong to continue if one of several treatments or procedures being compared proved, as the trial progressed, to be so much better, or worse, than other(s) that continued adherence to the trial would disadvantage some of the subjects enrolled.

The progress of a trial should generally, therefore, be monitored. Monitoring should be done by an independent person or small committee. Independence is necessary because it is often important, in order to minimise observer and patient bias, for those conducting a trial to remain unaware of the trends in the results during the study; it may also be hard for them to take a detached view of the merits of continuing a trial already under way. Those conducting the trial should give the monitoring body such information as it may request to enable it to be satisfied that the trial protocol is being followed and that the outcome of treatment, including side effects, is not such as to warrant premature termination of the study.

Supplementary Note 4—In Vitro Fertilization and Embryo Transfer

In vitro fertilisation (IVF) of human ova with human sperm and transfer of the early embryo to the human uterus (embryo transfer, ET) can be a justifiable means of treating infertility. While IVF and ET is an established procedure, much research remains to be done and the *NHMRC Statement on Human Experimentation and Supplementary Nores* should continue to apply to all work in this field.

Particular matters that need to be taken into account when ethical aspects are being considered follow.

1. Every centre or institution offering an IVF and ET program should have all aspects of the program approved by an institutional ethics committee. The IEC should ensure that a register is kept of all attempts made at securing pregnancies by these techniques. The register should include details of parentage, the medical aspects of treatment cycles, and a record of success or failure with:
- ovum recovery
- fertilization
- cleavage
- embryo transfer
- pregnancy outcome

These institutional registers, as medical records, should be confidential. Summaries for statistical purposes, including details of any congenital abnormalities among offspring, should be available for collation by a national body.

2. Although IVF and ET as techniques have an experimental component, the clinical indications for their use, treatment of infertility within an accepted family relationship, are well established. IVF and ET will normally involve the ova and sperm of the partners.

3. An ovum from a female partner may either be unavailable or unsuitable (e.g. severe genetic disease) for fertilization. In such a situation the following restrictions should apply to ovum donation for embryo transfer to that woman:
(i) the transfer should be part of treatment within an accepted family relationship;
(ii) the recipient couple should intend to accept the duties and obligations of parenthood;
(iii) consent should be obtained from the donor to the recipient couple;
(iv) there should be no element of commerce between the donor and recipient couple.

4. A woman could produce a child for an infertile couple from ova and sperm derived from that couple. Because of current inability to determine or define motherhood in this context, this situation is not yet capable of ethical resolution.

5. Research with sperm, ova or fertilized ova has been and remains inseparable from the development of safe and effective IVF and ET; as part of this research other important scientific information concerning human reproductive biology may emerge. However continuation of embryonic development in vitro beyond the stage at which implantation would normally occur is not acceptable.

6. Sperm and ova produced for IVF should be considered to belong to the respective donors. The wishes of the donors regarding the use, storage and ultimate disposal of the sperm, ova and resultant embryos should be ascertained and as far as is possible respected by the institution. In the case of the embryos, the donors' joint directions (or the directions of a single surviving donor) should be observed; in the event of disagreement between the donors the institution should be in a position to make decisions.

7. Storage of human embryos may carry biological and social risks. Storage for transfer should be restricted to early, undifferentiated embryos. Although it may be possible technically to store such embryos indefinitely, time limits for storage should be set in every case. In defining these time limits, account should be taken both of the wishes of the donors and of a set upper limit, which would be of the order of ten years, but which should not be beyond the time of conventional reproductive need or competence of the female donor.

8. Cloning experiments designed to produce from human tissues viable or potentially viable offspring that are multiple and genetically identical are ethically unacceptable.

9. In this, as in other experimental fields, those who conscientiously object to research projects or therapeutic programs conducted by institutions that employ them should not be obliged to participate in those projects or programs to which they object, nor should they be put at a disadvantage because of their objection.

Supplementary Note 5—the Human Fetus and the Use of Human Fetal Tissue

Introduction

1. This supplementary note, which should be read in conjunction with the *NHMRC Statement on Human Experimentation and Supplementary Notes*, is intended as a guide on ethical matters for research involving the human fetus or human fetal tissue. Included in this research is the possible usefulness of transplantation of fetal tissue for the treatment of disease.

2. For the purpose of these guidelines the terms fetus and fetal tissue include respectively the whole or part of what is called the embryo, fetus or neonate, from the time of implantation to the time of complete gestation, whether born alive or dead. The fetal membranes, placenta, umbilical cord and amniotic fluid are regarded as part of the fetus prior to separation; after separation they are also subject to certain guidelines.

The Fetus in Utero

3. There are two circumstances in which it may be ethical to carry out experiments on the fetus in utero:
   (i) where experiments are consistent with the promotion of life or health of the fetus;
   (ii) where research on antenatal fetal diagnosis provides the mother with information about the health or normality of the fetus and so gives her choices between continuation of the pregnancy, treatment for the fetus, and lawful termination of the pregnancy.

4. There may be risks to both mother and fetus in research on the fetus in utero, and insti-

tutional ethics committees (IECs) should carefully consider the risks and benefits to both in every case.

5. It is unethical to administer drugs to, or to carry out any procedure on, the mother with the intention of ascertaining harmful effects that these may have on the fetus, whether in anticipation of induced abortion or otherwise. Some research procedures may be allowable once the physical process of abortion is irrevocably in train.

The Separated Previable Fetus and Fetal Tissues

6. For the purposes of medical research, a separated previable fetus is at present regarded as one that has not attained a gestational age of 20 weeks and does not exceed 400g in weight. Adoption of this description will prevent inadvertent withholding of life-sustaining treatment from a separated fetus that may in fact be viable.

7. The following conditions should be observed:

(i) the fetus should be available for research only as a result of separation by natural processes or by lawful means;

(ii) dissection of the fetus should not be carried out while a heart beat is still apparent or there are other obvious signs of life;

(iii) research procedures should not be performed in the immediate area in which clinical procedures are carried out; and

(iv) those concerned with research involving the use of tissue from a fetus should have no part in the management of either the mother or the fetus, or in deciding if the fetus is previable.

General Conditions for Research on the Fetus and Fetal Tissue

8. The research must be conducted only in institutions that have a properly constituted ethics committee, and only according to written protocols approved by the ethics committees of all institutions involved.

9. The consent of the mother and, whenever practicable that of the father, should be obtained before research is undertaken. If fetal cells including cells from fetal membranes, placenta, umbilical cord and amniotic fluid are to be stored or propagated in tissue culture, or tissues or cells are to be transplanted into a recipient human, consent for this should be obtained specifically.

10. The decisions (a) whether it is appropriate in a particular instance to approach the mother about the possible use of fetal tissue for research and (b) whether a fetus or its tissue is in a category that may be used for research, must rest with the attending clinician and not with the intending research worker.

The obtaining of consent for research should also be through the attending clinician.

11. When an IEC is reviewing a proposal for research it should also take particular account of the following:

(i) the required information should not be obtainable by other means or by using other species;

(ii) the investigators should have the necessary special facilities and skills;

(iii) there should be no element of commerce involved in the transfer of human fetal tissue;

(iv) that the separation of clinical and research responsibilities that is crucial to the ethical basis for research in this area clearly exists; and

(v) a record of all attempts to transplant human fetal tissue, including a description of the outcome, should be maintained by the institution.

12. In this, as in other experimental fields, those who conscientiously object to research projects or therapeutic programs conducted by institutions that employ them should not be obliged

to participate in those projects or programs to which they object, nor should they be put at a disadvantage because of their objection.

Supplementary Note 6—Epidemiological Research

1. This supplementary note should be read in conjunction with the *NHMRC Statement on Human Experimentation and Supplementary Notes*. It is intended as a guide on ethical matters arising in medical research using the methods of epidemiology.

2. Epidemiological research is necessary for measuring the frequency and severity of disease in populations, identifying harmful effects from the environment, and establishing the effectiveness and safety of drugs, and other forms of medical and surgical treatment. It is concerned with the improvement of human health; it can provide new knowledge which is unobtainable in any other way.

3. In epidemiological research, medically relevant information about individuals is accumulated so that features of groups of persons may be investigated. These guidelines refer to the use in research of such information whether or not it was originally obtained for research purposes.

4. All epidemiological research should be conducted according to written protocols that state the aims of the study, the data needed and the way in which the data will be collected, used and protected.

5. Protocols for epidemiological research must be approved by properly constituted ethics committees of all the institutions involved in that research. If no institutions with ethics committees are involved, the investigators should secure ethical approval from a properly constituted ethics committee of an institution that is appropriate to the subjects or community concerned.

6. Access to medical records for research should normally be restricted to medically qualified investigators and research associates responsible to them.

7. Consent of subjects should generally be obtained for the use of their records for medical research, but in certain circumstances an ethics committee may approve the granting of access to records without consent. This course should only be adopted if the procedures required to obtain consent are likely either to cause unnecessary anxiety or to prejudice the scientific value of the research and if, in the opinion of the ethics committee, it will not be to the disadvantage of the subjects.

8. The use in an epidemiological study of confidential or personal information should not be allowed to cause material, emotional or other disadvantage to any individual.

9. Information that is confidential or personal, obtained for research, must not be used for purposes other than those specified in the approved protocol (see para. 5). If the information is to be used for new research, a new protocol must first be approved by an institutional ethics committee (IEC).

10. Investigators and their associates must preserve the confidentiality of information about research subjects. The confidentiality of records used in epidemiological research, both in the short and long term, must be at least as secure as it was in the sources from which the records were obtained.

11. Results of research must not be published in a form that permits identification of individual subjects.

12. In epidemiological research consent must be obtained specifically for clinical procedures and these must only be carried out by properly qualified persons and in accordance with the *NHMRC Statement on Human Experimentation and Supplementary Notes*.

13. If in the course of epidemiological research new information of clinical relevance is obtained, or existing treatment is thought to need alteration, the patient and his or her usual medical attendant must be informed.

14. The relationships between subjects and their usual medical attendants must not be adversely

affected by the research and confidential relationships between doctors and patients must be preserved.

15. When an IEC is reviewing a proposal for epidemiological research it should also be satisfied that:

(i) the research is likely to contribute to the acquisition of knowledge that may improve the health of the community; and

(ii) the investigators have the necessary skills in epidemiology and facilities for the research.

Supplementary Note 7—Somatic Cell Gene Therapy and Other Forms of Experimental Introduction of DNA and RNA into Human Subjects

1. Somatic cell gene therapy involves the introduction of pieces of DNA or RNA into human somatic (non-reproductive) cells. The aim is to improve the health of people with certain grave inherited diseases or with certain forms of cancer or some virus infections. Pieces of DNA or RNA may also be introduced into somatic cells to mark their distribution and fate in certain forms of research on serious diseases. There may also be other well justified non-therapeutic reasons for introducing pieces of DNA or RNA. While the development of methods of introducing DNA or RNA into somatic cells is acceptable, the introduction of pieces of DNA or RNA into germ (reproductive) cells or fertilised ova is not, because there is insufficient knowledge about the possible consequences, hazards, and effects on future generations.

2. All attempts to introduce pieces of DNA or RNA into human cells should be considered to be experimental and subject to the NHMRC Statement on Human Experimentation and Supplementary Notes.

3. The following particular matters need to be taken into account when protocols for somatic cell gene therapy or research are being considered by an institutional ethics committee:

(a) the therapy should be attempted only in genetic diseases in which the cause is a defect in a single pair of genes or in cancers in which there is a good reason to believe that it may improve clinical outcomes. Gene therapy to correct defects in multiple genes should not be attempted.

(b) introduction of pieces of DNA or RNA for research reasons should have a sound basis in current knowledge of the biological system involved.

(c) the choice of diseases for clinical trials or research is critical. For the present, evidence of hazards associated with the treatment can only be estimated and evaluated from experiments on animals. Initial trials in patients should therefore be limited:

(i) to diseases for which there is no effective treatment, and which cause a severe burden of suffering. Diseases causing a lesser burden, when account is taken of currently available treatment, should become candidates for somatic cell gene therapy or research only after the risks associated with this therapy have been determined by experience in humans over some years.

(ii) to diseases in which the effects of treatment or research can be measured, and

(iii) to patients for whom long-term follow-up is assured.

4. When considering a proposal for somatic cell gene therapy, or introduction of pieces of DNA or RNA for research reasons, an institutional ethics committee should also be satisfied:

(a) that the research team has the necessary depth and breadth of knowledge of, and experience in, molecular genetics;

(b) that the purity of the DNA or RNA to be inserted and the methods of handling it during its preparation are in accord with current regulations and official guidelines; and

(c) that the technique of insertion has been shown by experiments in animals:

(i) to confine the inserted DNA or RNA to the intended somatic cells, without entry into germ cells;

(ii) to achieve the intended function in a high proportion of attempts, and

(iii) rarely to cause undesirable side effects.

In seeking to satisfy itself on (a), (b) and (c) above, and on all technical aspects of any proposal for research on gene therapy, or introduction of pieces of DNA or RNA for research reasons, the institutional ethics committee shall consult with the biosafety committee of the institution, which as necessary shall consult the official national body concerned with monitoring the safety of innovative genetic manipulation techniques.

Appendix 4.13   Health Sciences Council of Japan, Guidelines for Gene Therapy Clinical Research (1993)

Chapter 1. General Rules

Article 1. The purpose of these guidelines is to specify the matters to be followed, to ensure scientific validity and ethics, and promote proper conduct of gene therapy clinical research. (Definition)

Article 2. The definitions of the terms used in these guidelines are the following:

1. *Gene therapy.* Introducing genes or gene transferred-cells into the human body for the purpose of treating diseases and gene marking.

2. *Gene marking.* Introducing genes or gene-transferred cells as a marker into the human body for the purpose of developing treatment methods of diseases.

3. *Researchers.* Persons who conduct gene therapy clinical research.

4. *Director.* The researcher who is in a position to have general control over gene therapy clinical research.

5. *Institutions.* Institutions where gene therapy clinical research is carried out.

Chapter 2. Requirements for Gene Therapy Clinical Research

Article 3. Gene therapy clinical research should be limited to those types of research whose effectiveness and safety can be predicted based on sufficient scientific knowledge.

Article 4.

1. Diseases targeted by gene therapy clinical research (excluding gene-marking clinical research: also excluded in the text following) should be limited to those which meet all of the following requirements:

(1) they are fatal hereditary diseases or life-threatening diseases such as cancer and AIDS.

(2) the effectiveness of treatment is sufficiently predicted to be better than currently available alternative methods.

(3) the benefits which subjects of gene therapy clinical research receive from it are sufficiently predicted to be greater than adverse effects on them.

2. Diseases targeted by gene marking clinical research should be limited to those which meet all of the following requirements:

(1) they are fatal hereditary diseases or life-threatening diseases such as cancer and AIDS;

(2) knowledge acquired from gene marking clinical therapy is sufficiently predicted to be better than that from currently available methods;

(3) gene marking can be carried out in combination with currently existing treatment methods.

Article 5. Substances used *in vivo* such as genes in gene therapy clinical research should be limited exclusively to those whose effectiveness and safety is assured.

Article 6. Gene therapy clinical research for the purpose of genetically altering human germ cells and gene therapy clinical research in which there is a possibility of genetic alteration of human germ cells is prohibited.

Article 7. The protection of public health should be adequately considered in conducting gene therapy clinical research.

Article 8. Informed consent should be ensured in conducting gene therapy clinical research.

Chapter 3. Protecting the Human Rights of Research Subjects

Article 9. Subjects of gene therapy clinical research should be selected carefully with consideration of the health condition, age, ability to consent and so on in order to protect human rights.

Article 10.

1. The director or a researcher so ordered by the director ('director and others' in following text) should, in conducting gene therapy clinical research, inform the subjects of the matters specified in the next article and obtain voluntary consent in written form or orally. When consent is oral, a record about the consent should be made.

2. When it is difficult to obtain the consent of the subject because of lack of ability to consent or other reasons, but it is reasonably expected that subjects will benefit from gene therapy clinical research, consent can be obtained in written form from the person, such as a legal representative, qualified to give consent on behalf of the subject. In such cases, a record of the consent and the records which indicate the relationship between the person who consented and the subject should be kept.

Article 11. To obtain informed consent as discussed in the article above, the director and others should inform subjects (or the person who gives consent, in cases where Article 10.2 applies) of the following matters in a plain manner, as much as possible using terms which are not technical:

1) the purpose and method of gene therapy clinical research;
2) expected benefit and harm;
3) the existence, nature, and expected benefit and harm of alternative treatment methods;
4) that subjects will not be disadvantaged if they do not give consent to gene therapy clinical research;
5) that subjects can terminate consent to gene therapy clinical research at any time after giving it;
6) other matters necessary to protect the human rights of subjects.

Chapter 4. System of Research and Review

Article 12. The director carries out tasks specified as follows:

1) Considers the scientific validity and ethics of gene therapy clinical research based on the data and information available when conducting gene therapy clinical research.
2) Based on the results in 1), prepares the document constituting the project proposal of gene therapy clinical research ('project proposal' in the following text) and seeks the permission of the institution head.
3) Confirms that gene therapy clinical research is carried out properly as planned in the project proposal.
4) Has general control over gene therapy clinical research and gives the necessary directions to researchers.
5) Does things other than those specified above which are necessary to direct gene therapy clinical research generally.
   2. The director should be qualified to have general control over gene therapy clinical research and to give the necessary directions to researchers.
   3. Each gene therapy clinical research project shall have one director.

Article 13.

1. Researchers (excluding the director) plan and conduct the gene therapy clinical research project under the direction of the director and inform the director of necessary matters.

2. Researchers should have professional knowledge or clinical experience sufficient to properly conduct gene therapy clinical research.

Article 14. Institutions should fulfill the following requirements:

1) Possession of human resources and equipment sufficient to do adequate clinical observation, examination, as well as analysis and evaluation of the data resulting from them.

2) Possession of human resources and equipment to take necessary actions in case of emergency.

3) Possession of a committee as provided in Article 16.

Article 15. The institution head has tasks specified as follows:

1) When a director requests permission to conduct gene therapy clinical research, the institution head seeks the opinions of the review committee and the Minister of Health and Welfare concerning the conduct of gene therapy clinical research, and based on the opinions, gives the necessary instructions or permission for the research to be conducted.

2) Is informed and is provided with opinions from the director or the committee about the progress and the results of gene therapy clinical research and, when necessary, gives instructions to the director about points to consider or to improve, or to inform the Ministry of Health and Welfare.

Article 16.

1. The review committee, at the request of the institution head, has the following tasks:

   1) Examines the planned gene therapy clinical research based on the project proposal, etc., following these guidelines, and submits opinions about the appropriateness of the research, the points to consider and the points to be improved.

   2) Examines the important changes in the planned gene therapy clinical research in accordance with these guidelines and submits opinions about the appropriateness of the research, the points to consider and the points to be improved.

2. The committee should meet the following requirements:

   1) The committee should consist of medical professionals in basic fields such as molecular biology, cell biology, genetics, clinical pharmacology, pathology, and professionals in areas of clinical medicine which are related to the diseases targeted by the planned gene therapy clinical research, and legal specialists who are qualified to examine comprehensively scientific and ethical issues related to the conduct of gene therapy clinical research.

   2) In order to carry out fair reviews, the freedom and independence of the committee must be ensured, and a researcher who submitted a proposal should not be allowed to participate in the review of that same gene therapy clinical research project.

   3) The rules governing the required procedures for examining gene therapy clinical research, such as the constitution, organization and activities of the committee, should be open to the public.

   4) The review process of the committee should be recorded, preserved and open to the public.

Chapter 5. Procedures for Conducting and Concluding Research

Article 17.

1. The director should obtain the permission of the institution head before conducting gene therapy clinical research.

2. The director should prepare a project proposal and submit it to the institution head to obtain the permission mentioned above.

Article 18.

1. The matters specified in the attached table should appear in the project proposal.

2. A summary of the project written as much as possible in plain words other than technical terms should be added to the project proposal.

Article 19.

1. Immediately after confirming that the gene therapy clinical research has been completed, the director should compile and submit to the institution head a final report which should contain the items specified below:

   1) the purposes and the period during which the gene therapy clinical research was conducted;

   2) the name and address of the institution at which the research was conducted;

   3) the name of the director and researchers of the gene therapy clinical research project;

   4) the results and a discussion of gene therapy clinical research.

2. The final report should be signed and stamped by the director.

Chapter 6. Opinions of the Minister of Health and Welfare

Article 20.

1. Upon request by the institution head, the Minister of Health and Welfare shall provide opinions on the conduct of gene therapy clinical research in the institution.

2. In giving the above-mentioned opinions, the Minister of Health and Welfare shall listen to the views of professionals.

3. The institution head shall submit the following documents:

   1) the project proposal;

   2) a document showing the review committee's process of examining the research plan and its findings, written by the committee;

   3) a document showing the organization, structure and methods of work of the review committee.

Article 21.

1. When deemed necessary, the Minister of Health and Welfare should ask the institution head to submit information such as that specified in paragraph three of the previous article along with other data, and should investigate the institution with the consent of the institution head in order to provide the opinions mentioned above.

Article 22.

1. When the institution head receives the final report from the director, s/he should immediately submit a copy of the report to the Minister of Health and Welfare.

2. If the director reports occurrences of a serious nature, such as the death of subjects in the course of gene therapy clinical research, the institution head must immediately inform the Minister of Health and Welfare.

Chapter 7. Miscellaneous

Article 23. Records of the gene therapy clinical research should be kept under appropriate conditions by the person designated as responsible for record-keeping.

Article 24. Researchers, members of the review committee and the institution head should not disclose personal secrets they come to know in the conduct of gene therapy clinical research without justifiable reason.

Article 25. The director and the institution head should make efforts to promote the disclosure of appropriate and accurate information to the public about planned or presently conducted gene therapy clinical research.

Article 26. Researchers should make efforts to educate and popularize by using any occasion to provide information and education on gene therapy.

NOTES

Many of the citations refer to official policy statements not included in the appendices to the book. These documents will be referred to by the following abbreviations. Included in this list is the abbreviation, the name of the policy document, and the relevant bibliographical information:

AUS, ANIMALS   *Australian Code of Practice for the Care and Use of Animals for Scientific Purposes* (Australia Government Publishing Service: Canberra, 1990)

CANADA, 1996   Tri-Council Working Group, *Code of Conduct for Research Involving Humans* (Medical Research Council: Ottawa, 1996)

CANADA, 1997   Tri-Council Working Group, *Code of Ethical Conduct for Research Involving Humans* (Medical Research Council: Ottawa, 1997)

EURCOUNCIL, GENENG   Parliamentary Assembly of the Council of Europe, Recommendation 934 (1982) on genetic engineering, reprinted in A. Rogers and D. de Bousingen, *Bioethics in Europe* (Council of Europe Press: Strasbourg, 1995)

EURUNION, EPI COMAC   Working Group on Ethical Issues in Epidemiology, "Ethical Issues in Epidemiological Research" in M. Hallen and K. Vuylsteek (eds.), *Workshop on Issues on the Harmonization of Protocols for Epidemiological Research in Europe* (Office for Official Publications of the European Communities: Luxembourg, 1992)

EURUNION, GENENG   Council Directives 90/219/EEC and 90/220/EEC of 23 April 1990 and 90/679/EEC of 26 November 1990 reprinted in T. Cook, C. Doyle, and D. Jabbari, *Pharmaceuticals, Biotechnology, and the Law* (Stockton Press: New York, 1991) pp. 429–87 supplemented by Commission Directive 94/51/EC of November 7 1994 and Commission Directive 94/730/EC of November 4, 1994, *Official Journal of the European Communities* (No. L 292/31, 12.11.94)

EURUNION, PRIVACY   Directive 95/46/EC of the European Parliament and of the Council of 24 October 1995 on the Protection of Individuals with Regard to the Processing of Personal Data and on the Free Movement of such Data, *Official Journal of the European Communities* (Nov. 23, 1995) No L. 281, p. 31

FRANCE, ANIMALS   "Summary of 1987 French Decree on Experimentation," Animal Welfare Institute, *Animals and their Legal Rights* (Animal Welfare Institute: Washington, 1990), pp. 328–35

FRANCE, REPRODUCTION   Law No. 94–654 of 29 July 1994 on the donation and use of elements and products of the human body, medically assisted procreation, and prenatal diagnosis, translated in *International Digest of Health Legislation* vol. 45 (1994), pp. 473–82

GERMANY, ANIMALS   Federal Republic of Germany, "Law on Animal Protection" Animal Welfare Institute, *Animals and their Legal Rights* (Animal Welfare Institute: Washington, 1990), pp. 336–52

UK, GEN   Gene Therapy Advisory Committee, "Guidance on Making Proposals to Conduct Gene Therapy Research on Human Subjects" *Human Gene Therapy* vol. 6 (March 1995), pp. 335–46

UK, MRC   Medical Research Council, *Responsibility in Investigations on Human Participants and Materials and on Personal Information* (Medical Research Council: London, 1992)

UK, RCP   Royal College of Physicians, *Guidelines on the Practice of Ethics Committees in Medical Research Involving Human Subjects*, 3rd. edition (Royal College of Physicians: London, 1996)

UK, REPRODUCTION   Human Fertilisation and Embryology Authority, "Code of Practice—Part 9/Research," reprinted in C. Foster (ed.), *Manual for Research Ethics Committees*, 3rd. edition (King's College: London, 1995)

USA, GENRES   Department of Health and Human Services, "Guidelines for Research Involving Recombinant DNA Molecules," *Federal Register* vol. 59 #127 (July 5, 1994) 34496-Appendix M contains the regulations on gene therapy protocols; this appendix will be referred to as USA, Points to Consider.

Introduction

1. D. Butler and M. Wadman, "Calls for Cloning Ban Sell Science Short," *Nature* vol. 386 (March 6, 1997), pp. 8–9
2. M. de Wachter, "The European Convention on Bioethics," *Hastings Center Report* vol. 27 (January–February, 1997), pp. 13–23
3. USA, GENRES
4. E. Clayton, K. Steinberg, M. Khoury, *et.al.*, "Informed Consent for Genetic Research on Stored Tissue Samples," *JAMA* vol. 274 (Dec. 13, 1995), pp. 1786–92
5. "Proposed Recommendations of the Task Force on Genetic Testing," *Federal Register* vol. 62 (Jan. 30, 1997), pp. 4539–47.
6. CANADA, 1996
7. CANADA, 1997. It is this draft, in an edited fashion, that is likely to become the final version.
8. The bill, House of Commons bill C-47, was introduced on June 14, 1996.
9. AUS, ANIMALS
10. The earlier bill was the Victoria Infertility (Medical Procedures) Act of 1984. The later bill was the Victoria Infertility Treatment Act of 1995. The differences are described in a note "New Victorian IVF Law Changes Pioneering Legislation," *Monash Bioethics Review* vol. 14 (July, 1995) p. 6
11. EURCOUNCIL, GENENG
12. EURUNION, GENENG

13. EURUNION, PRIVACY
14. FRANCE, ANIMALS
15. FRANCE, REPRODUCTION
16. GERMANY, ANIMALS
17. This initiative is described in H. P. Graf and D. Cole, "Ethics Committee Authorization in Germany," *Journal of Medical Ethics* vol. 21 (1995), pp. 229–33
18. UK, MRC
19. UK, GEN
20. UK, REPRODUCTION
21. M. Warnock, *A Question of Life* (Basil Blackwell: Oxford, 1985)
22. UK, RCP
23. Two particularly important reports are *Genetic Screening: Ethical Issues* (Nuffield Council on Bioethics: London, 1993) and *Animal-to-Human Transplants* (Nuffield Council on Bioethics: London, 1996). These can be ordered from the Council at 28 Bedford Square, London.

Chapter One

1. A good summary history is found in Chapter One of F. B. Orlans, *In the Name of Science* (Oxford University Press: New York, 1993)
2. C. Bernard, *Introduction to the Study of Experimental Medicine* (translated by H. C. Greene in 1957 and currently available in an undated paper edition from Dover Press, New York)
3. R. Leader and D. Stark, "The Importance of Animals in Biomedical Research," *Perspectives in Biology and Medicine* vol. 30 (Summer, 1987), pp. 470–85
4. The source of these data is a 1994 summary from the Canadian Council on Animal Care entitled "Scientific Use of Animals in Canada" and printed as a supplement to the journal *Resource* in its Spring 1994 issue.
5. The British data come from "1990 Animal Research Figures" *Bulletin of Medical Ethics* (September 1991, pp. 6–7) and "Home Office Reports a Further Decline in Experiments on Animals" *The Veterinary Record* (February 25, 1995), pp. 182–83.
6. These data are presented, with considerable discussion of the controversy surrounding them and their interpretation, in F. B. Orlans, "Data on Animal Experimentation in the United States" *Perspectives in Biology and Medicine* vol. 37 (Winter, 1994), pp. 217–31
7. D. Blum, *The Monkey Wars* (New York: Oxford University Press, 1994), is a useful history of those primate debates.
8. A. Lawler, "Panel Backs Joint Bion Mission" *Science* vol. 273 (July 12, 1996), p. 175
9. J. Bentham, *Introduction to the Principles of Morals and Legislation* reprinted in *The Works of Jeremy Bentham* vol. I (Russell and Russell: New York, 1962), pp. 142–3
10. This act is the ancestor of the 1986 British Act reprinted as Appendix 4.3 in this book
11. An outstanding account of the early philosophical discussions from antiquity through the nineteenth century is to be found in R. Sorabji, *Animal Minds and Human Morals*

(Cornell University Press: Ithaca, 1993). An excellent but brief summary of the recent discussions is presented in Chapter One of D. deGrazia, *Taking Animals Seriously* (Cambridge University Press: New York, 1996).

12. J. Passmore, *Man's Responsibility for Nature* (Duckworth: London, 1974)

13. An available edition is Henry Salt's *Animals' Rights* (ISAR, 1980)

14. T. Regan, *The Case for Animal Rights* (University of California Press: Berkeley and Los Angeles, 1983)

15. W. Russell and R. Burch, *The Principles of Humane Experimental Technique* (Methuen: London, 1959)

16. P. Singer, *Animal Liberation* (New York: Avon, 1975)

17. The report was published as J. Smith and K. Boyd, *Lives in the Balance* (Oxford University Press: Oxford, 1991)

18. A. Abbott, "Delays in Alternative Tests Defer Animal Ban" *Nature* vol. 383 (October 31, 1996) p. 748

19. GERMANY, ANIMALS Article 7(3)

20. OPRR, *Public Health Service Policy on Humane Care and Use of Laboratory Animals* (Department of Health and Human Services: Washington, 1986)

21. National Research Council, *Guide for the Care and Use of Laboratory Animals* (National Academy Press: Washington, 1996)

22. Section 205 of the Act (PL103–43)

23. PL 99–198

24. S. Burd, "U.S. Told it Needn't Monitor Care of Lab Mice, Rats, and Birds" *The Chronicle of Higher Education* (June 1, 1994)

25. OPRR, *Institutional Animal Care and Use Committee Guidebook* (NIH 92–3415; Washington, 1992)

26. AUS, ANIMALS

27. *Ibid.*, p. 1

28. *Ibid.*, p. 6, section 1.5

29. Office of Terchnology Assessment, *Patenting Life* (U.S. Government Printing Office, Washington, 1989)

30. *Ibid.*, pp. 31–33

31. H. R. Jaenichen, *The European Patent Office's Case Law on the Patentability of Biotechnology Inventions* (Carl Heymanns Verlag: Koln, 1993) pp. 20–27

32. Two major sources for this event are Richard Stone, "Religious Leaders Oppose Patenting Genes and Animals," *Science* vol. 268 (May 26, 1995) p. 1126 and E. Andrews, "Religious Leaders Prepare to Fight Patents on Genes" *The New York Times* (May 13, 1995), p. 1.

33. A. Abbott, "European Proposal Reopens Debate Over Patenting of Human Genes," *Nature* vol. 378 (December 21/28, 1995), p. 756

34. *Supra* note 32

35. *Supra* note 31

36. Institute of Medicine, *Xenotransplantation: Science, Ethics, and Public Policy* (National Academy Press: Washington, 1996)

37. The Nuffield Council report was cited *supra*, Chapter One, note 23. A summary of the more official Kennedy Report is to be found on pp. 8–11 of the February 1997 *Bulletin of Medical Ethics*.

Chapter Two

1. H. K. Beecher, "Ethics and Clinical Research," *The New England Journal of Medicine* vol. 274 (June 16, 1966), pp. 1354–60
2. This case is fully discussed on pp. 9–43 of J. Katz, *Experimentation with Human Beings* (Russell Sage Foundation: New York, 1972)
3. Background information is provided on pp. 77–81 of D. Rothman, *Strangers at the Bedside* (Basic Books: New York, 1991)
4. J. Jones, *Bad Blood* (The Free Press: New York, 1981)
5. M. H. Pappworth, *Human Guinea Pigs* (Beacon: Boston, 1967)
6. The case is discussed on p. 5 of Medical Research Council of Canada, *Guidelines on Research Involving Human Subjects* (MRC: Ottawa, 1987), a predecessor to CANADA, 1996 and 1997
7. This case is discussed on pp. 76–81 of P. McNeill, *The Ethics and Politics of Human Experimentation* (Cambridge University Press: Cambridge, 1993)
8. M. Grodin, "Historical Origins of the Nuremburg Code" in G. Annas and M. Grodin, *The Nazi Doctors and the Nuremberg Code* (New York: Oxford University Press, 1992), pp. 121–44
9. 21 *Code of Federal Regulations* 50, 60
10. "Good Clinical Practice for Trials on Medicinal Products in the European Community," *The Rules Governing Medicinal Products in the European Community*, vol. III Addendum of July 1990 (Office for Official Publications of the European Communities: Luxembourg, 1990) pp. 57–98
11. UK, RCP
12. UK, MRC
13. This document is reprinted in section V of C. Foster, *Manual for Research Ethics Committees*, 3rd. edition (King's College: London). This manual contains a great deal of additional U.K. and European material.
14. *Supra*, Chapter One, note 17
15. Nordic Council on Medicines, *Good Clinical Trial Practice* (Nordic Council: Uppsala, 1989)
16. *Supra*, note 6
17. CANADA, 1996, 1997
18. Notification 1–27 of the Pharmaceutical Affairs Bureau (October 2, 1989) translated and reprinted in *Clin. Eval.* vol. 18 (1990). This approach is being developed by a Committee on How Informed Consent Should be Practiced in the Future. I want to thank NASA for making available to me a translation of its preliminary 1995 report.
19. These issues are discussed extensively on pp. 21–23 of UK, RCP.
20. *Supra*, note 7
21. *The Blue Sheet* (January 15, 1997) p. 2
22. rt-PA Stroke Study Group, "Tissue Plasminogen Activator for Acute Ischemic Stroke" *The New England Journal of Medicine* vol. 333 (December 14, 1995), pp. 1581–7
23. N. Abramson, A. Meisel, and P. Safar, "Deferred Consent," *JAMA* vol. 255 (May 9, 1986), pp. 2466–71
24. *OPRR Reports* 93–3 (August 12, 1993)
25. M. Biros, R. Lewis, C. Olson, *et.al.* "Informed Consent in Emergency Research," *JAMA* vol. 273 (April 26, 1995), pp. 1283–7

26. CANADA, 1997, Article 1.7
27. UK, RCP sections 4.6–4.9
28. CANADA, 1997, Article 2.3
29. *Supra*, note 7, especially Part Four
30. This is found in the commentary on Guideline 14 (the guideline is found in Appendix 1.8 of this book). The commentary is found in the 1992 draft document circulated by CIOMS (the numbering of some of the guidelines has been changed).
31. UK, RCP, sections 2.2–2.3
32. CANADA, 1996, pp. 2–4 and 2–5
33. CANADA, 1997, pp. 17–19
34. President's Advisory Committee, *The Human Radiation Experiments* (Oxford University Press: New York, 1996), especially Part III "Contemporary Projects"
35. GAO, *Scientific Research: Continued Vigilance Critical to Protecting Human Subjects* (GAO/HEHS-96-72: Washington, 1996)
36. OPRR, *Protecting Human Research Subjects: Institutional Review Board Guidebook* (NIH: Washington, 1993), pp. 3–45
37. CANADA, 1997, Article 1.9
38. *Supra*, note 18, Chapter 10.6
39. UK, RCP, section 7.44
40. Commentary on Guideline 8 (the guideline is found in Appendix 1.8 of this book). The commentary is found in the 1992 draft document circulated by CIOMS (the numbering of some of the guidelines has been changed).
41. CANADA, 1996, Article 13.6. I cannot find such an explicit affirmation in CANADA, 1997.
42. H. Edgar and D. J. Rothman, "New Rules for New Drugs" *Milbank Quarterly*, vol. 68 (1990), pp. 111–41
43. *Supra*, note 40
44. Commentary on Guideline 13 (the guideline is found in Appendix 1.8 in this book). The commentary is found in a document distributed by CIOMS in 1992 (the numbering of the guidelines has been changed).

Chapter Three

1. This paragraph is based upon the useful historical summary presented in Chapter Three of T. Timmreck, *An Introduction to Epidemiology* (Jones and Bartlett: Boston, 1994)
2. *Ibid.*, pp. 70–73
3. *Ibid.*, pp. 85–6
4. 5 *USC* Section 552a
5. The European situation prior to the adoption of EURUNION, PRIVACY is analyzed in C. G. Wesrin, "Ethical, Legal, and Political Problems Affecting Epidemiology in European Countries" *IRB* vol. 15 (May–June, 1993) pp. 6–8
6. L. Gordis, E. Gold, and R. Seltser, "Privacy Protection in Epidemiologic and Medical Research" *American Journal of Epidemiology* vol. 105 (1977), pp. 163–8
7. EURUNION, EPI
8. M. Susser, Z. Stein, and J. Kline, "Ethics in Epidemiology," *Annals of the American Academy of Political and Social Science* vol. 437 (1978), pp. 128–41

9. The fullest rationale for this proposal was presented some years later in C. L. Soskolne, "Epidemiology: Questions of Science, Ethics, Morality, and Law," *American Journal of Epidemiology* vol. 129 (1989), pp. 1–18

10. J. M. Last, "Guidelines on Ethics for Epidemiologists" *International Journal of Epidemiology* vol. 19 (1990), pp. 226–29. An interesting account of why this project was never completed, together with many other related developments, is found in Chapter Three of S. Coughlin and T. Beauchamp (eds.) *Ethics and Epidemiology* (New York: Oxford University Press, 1996). S. Coughlin has also edited an important collection, *Ethics in Epidemiology and Clinical Research* (Epidemiology Resources: Newton, 1995), which contains many of the primary documents.

11. T. Beauchamp, R. Cook, W. Fayerweather, et.al., "Ethical Guidelines for Epidemiologists," *Journal of Clinical Epidemiology* vol. 44 (1991), pp. 151S–169S

12. "Guidelines for Good Epidemiology Practices for Occupational and Environmental Epidemiologic Research," *Journal of Occupational Medicine* vol. 33 (December 1991), pp. 1221–29

13. EURUNION, PRIVACY

14. *Supra*, Chapter Two, note 36, pp. 4–8 to 4–10

15. *Supra*, note 11, section 1.6

16. Probably the most important is K. Rothman, "The Rise and Fall of Epidemiology: 1950–2000 A. D." *New England Journal of Medicine* vol. 304 (March 5, 1981) pp. 600–602. It contains the example of the food additive cancer study.

17. UK, RCP Appendix B

18. CANADA, 1997, Section III. There is a subtle difference between the two; the Canadian emphasis is on whether the records consulted contain the identifying information whereas the U.S. emphasis is on whether the researchers record in their data the identifying information.

19. This act, which did not pass, was introduced as H. R. 1271

20. CANADA, 1997, Article 3.5

21. EURUNION, PRIVACY, especially Articles 8 and 11.

22. The French statute is translated and reprinted in *International Digest of Health Legislation* vol. 45 (1994), pp. 495–6, while the German statute is summarized in the same issue of the same journal on p. 500.

23. See the brief summary in P. Mitchell, "Drug Industry Lobbies Against European Research-Data Directive," *The Lancet* vol. 349 (May 10, 1997), p. 1378

24. This bill was introduced as S 1360. The relevant section is Section 209.

25. *Supra*, note 6

26. *Supra*, note 11, section 1.5

27. *Supra*, note 10, section 5.3

28. E. Clayton, K. Steinberg, M. Khoury, et.al., "Informed Consent for Genetic Research on Stored Tissue Samples," *JAMA* vol. 274 (December 13, 1995), pp. 1786–92

29. "Stored Tissue Sample Research Policy Proposals Fail to Include Scientific Input" *The Blue Sheet* (January 15, 1997) pp. 5–6

30. UK, RCP, Appendix B

31. CANADA, 1997, Article 10.3; the commentary on this section is particularly valuable.

32. *Supra*, note 28, p. 1791

33. UK, RCP, Appendix B

34. *Supra*, note 28, p. 1791

35. "Pathologists to Argue Second Informed Consent Not Needed for Genetic Research on Stored Tissues" *The Blue Sheet* (July 17, 1996) pp. 12–14

36. That seems to be the import of CANADA, 1997, article 10.3 (a)

37. *Supra*, note 28

38. CANADA, 1997, section 10.2

39. R. Bayer, L. H. Lumey, and L. Wan, "The American, British, and Dutch Responses to Unlinked Anonymous HIV Seroprevalence Studies," *Law, Medicine, and Health Care* vol. 19 (Fall-Winter, 1991), pp. 222–30

40. *Ibid.*, p. 226

41. Council of Europe, "Recommendation No. R (89) 14 of the Council of Ministers to Member States on the Ethical Issues of HIV Infection in the Health Care and Social Settings" *International Digest of Health Legislation* vol. 41 (1990), pp. 39–48, section IV

42. "Symposium on Community Intervention Trials," *American Journal of Epidemiology* vol. 142 (September 15, 1995), pp. 567–599

43. The study was described in COMMIT Research Group, "Community Intervention Trial for Smoking Cessation (COMMIT): Summary of Design and Intervention," *Journal of the National Cancer Institute* vol. 83 (1996), pp. 1620–28. Its results were presented in two papers in *American Journal of Public Health*, vol. 85 (February, 1995), pp. 183–92 and 193–200.

Chapter Four

1. An excellent history of the major developments in the early years of genetic engineering is S. Wright, *Molecular Politics* (University of Chicago Press: Chicago, 1994). Pages 129–59 contain a detailed account of the Gordon Conference and its aftermath.

2. Paul Berg, et.al., "Potential Biohazards of Recombinant DNA Molecules" *Science* vol. 185 (July 26, 1974), p. 303. The same letter was published in *Nature* for July 19, 1974, and in the July 1974 issue of the *Proceedings of the National Academy of Sciences*.

3. The latest version of those guidelines is USA, GENRES

4. The latest major revision of these occurred in 1992 in response to general European developments. The Health and Safety Executive issued in that year *A Guide to the Genetically Modified Organisms (Contained Use) Regulations*; its latest version is obtainable directly from the Executive.

5. EURCOUNCIL, GENENG

6. Wright, *supra* note 1, pp. 157–9

7. EURUNION, GENENG

8. This requirement was imposed by section 8 of the Genetically Modified Organisms (Deliberate Release) Regulations of 1992, enforced by the Department of the Environment.

9. Office of Science and Technology Policy, "Coordinated Framework for Regulation of Biotechnology" *Federal Register* vol. 51 (June 26, 1986), pp. 23302–23350

10. USA, GENRES

11. 7 *CFR (Code of Federal Regulations)* 340

12. Wright, *supra* note 1, chapter 12, especially pp. 455–6

13. L. Walters and J. Palmer, *The Ethics of Human Gene Therapy* (Oxford University Press: New York, 1997), pp. 145–6

14. *Ibid.*, pp. 17–24

15. An excellent summary of the early years of gene therapy and of the resulting feeling that more basic research is needed is found in E. Marshall, "Gene Therapy's Growing Pains," *Science* vol. 269 (August 25, 1995), pp. 1050–5

16. The latest version of which is USA, POINTS TO CONSIDER

17. UK, GEN

18. "RAC Retained Without Individual Protocol Approval Authority Under New Proposal Presented by NIH," *The Blue Sheet*, November 27, 1996, pp. 9–10

19. USA, POINTS TO CONSIDER

20. "Points to Consider in Human Somatic Cell Therapy and Gene Therapy" *Human Gene Therapy* vol. 2 (1991) pp. 251–6. The background of the FDA's involvement in this issue is presented in D. Kessler, J. Siegel, P. Noguchi, et.al., "Regulation of Somatic-Cell Therapy and Gene Therapy by the Food and Drug Administration," *New England Journal of Medicine* vol. 329 (October 14, 1993), pp. 1169–1173.

21. UK, GEN

22. *ibid.*, section 7.2.2

23. D. Kevles, *In the Name of Eugenics* (Alfred A. Knopf: New York, 1985)

24. For a full discussion of these issues, see Chapter Four of Walters and Palmer, *supra* note 13

25. "RAC Approves First Protocol in Normal Subjects; Policy Conference on Enhancement Recommended," *The Blue Sheet* (March 12, 1997) pp. 4–5

26. A full discussion of these arguments is found in Walters and Palmer, *supra* note 13, Chapter Three

27. An excellent history and analysis is to be found in R. Cook-Deegan, *The Gene Wars* (W. W. Norton: New York, 1994)

28. Z. Bankowski and A. M. Capron (eds.), *Proceedings of the 24th. CIOMS Round Table Conference* (CIOMS: Geneva, 1991) pp. 1–3

29. N. Lenoir, "UNESCO, Genetics, and Human Rights" *Kennedy Institute of Ethics Journal*, vol. 7 (1997) pp. 31–42

30. "Guidelines for the Molecular Genetics Predictive Test in Huntington's Disease," *Neurology* vol. 44 (1994) pp. 1533–6, Recommendations 2 and 2.1

31. Three recent statements about the current data and about the ethical issues are: National Institute on Aging, "Apolipoprotein E Genotyping in Alzheimer's Disease," *The Lancet* vol. 347 (April 20, 1996), pp. 1091–5; ACMG/ASHG, "Statement on Use of Apolipoprotein E Testing for Alzheimer Disease," *JAMA* vol. 274 (November 22/29, 1995), pp. 1627–9; and S. Post, P. Whitehouse, R. Binstock, et.al., "The Clinical Introduction of Genetic Testing for Alzheimer Disease," *JAMA* vol. 277 (March 12, 1997), pp. 832–6.

32. For a good discussion of the issues, see "Statement of the American Society of Clinical Oncology: Genetic Testing for Cancer Susceptibility," *Journal of Clinical Oncology* vol. 14 (May, 1996), pp. 1730–6 and the accompanying editorials.

33. G. Kolata, "Breaking Ranks, Lab Offers Test to Assess Risk of Breast Cancer," *New York Times* (April 1, 1996), p. 1

34. A useful historical and analytical account is B. Wilfond and K. Nolan, "National Policy Development for the Clinical Application of Genetic Diagnostic Technologies: Lessons from Cystic Fibrosis," *JAMA* vol. 270 (December 22/29, 1993), pp. 2948–54

35. E. M., "ELSI's Cystic Fibrosis Experiment," *Science* vol. 274 (October 25, 1996), p. 489
36. "NIH Panel Favors Prenatal Testing," *The Blue Sheet* (April 23, 1997), pp. 2–4
37. T. Lieu, S. Watson, and A. E. Washington, "The Cost-Effectiveness of Prenatal Carrier Screening for Cystic Fibrosis," *Obstetrics and Gynecology* vol. 84 (December, 1994), pp. 903–12.
38. *Supra*, Introduction, note 23
39. Council of Europe, "Recommendation No. R (94) 11 of the Committee of Ministers to Member States on Screening as a Tool of Preventive Medicine," *International Digest of Health Legislation* vol. 46 (1995), pp. 13–18.
40. "Proposed Recommendations of the Task Force on Genetic Testing," *Federal Register* vol. 62 (January 30, 1997), pp. 4539–47
41. OTA, *The Role of Genetic Testing in the Prevention of Occupational Disease* (Government Printing Office: Washington, 1983)
42. Task Force on Genetic Information and Insurance, *Genetic Information and Health Insurance* (NIH: Washington, 1993), Publication No. 93–3686
43. *Supra*, Introduction, note 23
44. K. Hudson, K. Rothenberg, L. Andrews, et al., "Genetic Discrimination and Health Insurance" *Science* vol. 270 (October 20, 1995), pp. 391–3, especially footnote 9
45. The Health Insurance Portability and Accountability Act of 1996 (P. L. 104–191)
46. *Supra*, note 42, p. v
47. These decisions, and the background to them, are analyzed in OTA, *Patenting Life* (Government Printing Office: Washington, 1989)
48. H. R. Jaenichen, *The European Patent Office's Case Law on the Patentability of Biotechnology Inventions* (Carl Heymanns Verlag: Koln, 1993)
49. B. Healy, "On Gene Patenting" *New England Journal of Medicine* vol. 327 (August 27, 1992), pp. 664–8
50. "EST Patents Will Proceed Despite "Obviousness" Dispute within Patent and Trademark Office" *The Blue Sheet* (February 19, 1997), pp. 3–5
51. "Council Directive on the Legal Protection of Biotechnological Inventions" (Brussels, December 16, 1992)
52. C. O'Brien, "European Parliament Axes Patent Policy" *Science* vol. 267 (March 10, 1995), pp. 1417–8 and A. Abbott, "European Proposal Reopens Debate over Patenting of Human Genes," *Nature* vol. 378 (December 21/8, 1995), p. 756. See also Opinion #8 in *Opinions of the Group of Advisers on the Ethical Implications of Biotechnology of the European Commission* (European Commission: Brusselles, 1996)
53. R. Stone, "Religious Leaders Oppose Patenting Genes and Animals," *Science* vol. 268 (May 26, 1995), p. 1126

Chapter Five

1. E. Connor, R. Sperling, R. Gelber, et al., "Reduction of Maternal-Infant Transmission of Human Immunodeficiency Virus Type 1 with Zidovudine Treatment" *New England Journal of Medicine* vol. 331 (November 3, 1994), pp. 1173–80
2. Appendix to Recommendation 1046 of the Parliamentary Assembly of the Council of Europe on The Use of Human Embryos and Fetuses, point B.i., reprinted on pp.

310–11 of A. Rogers and D. de Bousingen, *Bioethics in Europe* (Council of Europe Press: Strassbourg, 1995)

3. C. Byk, "A Proposed Draft Protocol for the European Convention on Biomedicine Relating to Research on the Human Embryo and Fetus," *Journal of Medical Ethics* vol. 23 (1997), pp. 32–7

4. Royal College of Physicians, *Research Involving Patients* (Royal College: London, 1990), section 7.56.

5. CANADA, 1997, p. IX–4

6. Commentary on Guideline 11 (the guideline is found in Appendix 1.8 of this book). The commentary is found in the 1992 draft document circulated by CIOMS (the numbering of some of the guidelines has been changed).

7. Royal Commission on New Reproductive Technologies, *Proceed with Care* (Minister of Government Services: Ottawa, 1993)

8. *Supra*, note 2

9. G. Boer on behalf of NECTAR, "Ethical Guidelines for the Use of Human Embryonic or Fetal Tissue for Experimentation and Clinical Neurotransplantation and Research" *Journal of Neurology* vol. 242 (1994), pp. 1–13

10. *Supra*, note 7

11. CANADA, 1997

12. M. C. Coutts, "Fetal Tissue Research," *Kennedy Institute of Ethics Journal* vol. 3 (1993), pp. 81–100

13. D. Branch, L. Ducat, A. Fantel, et al., "Suitability of Fetal Tissues from Spontaneous Abortions and from Ectopic Pregnancies for Transplantation," *JAMA* vol. 273 (January 4, 1995) pp. 66–8

14. GAO, *Therapeutic Human Fetal Tissue Transplantation Projects Meet Federal Requirements* (General Accounting Office: Washington, 1997–GAO/HEHS-97-61)

15. *The Use of Fetuses and Fetal Material for Research* (HMSO: London, 1972), especially Clause 1 of the appended Code of Practice.

16. *Review of the Guidance on the Research Use of Fetuses and Fetal Material* (HMSO: London, 1989) pp. 6–7

17. *Supra*, note 9, p. 4

18. *Supra*, note 16, section 6

19. C. Cohen and A. Jonsen, "The Future of the Fetal Tissue Bank" *Science* vol. 262 (December 10, 1993) pp. 1663–5

20. *Supra*, note 7. CANADA, 1997 is silent on this important recommendation.

21. B. Gustavii, "Fetal Brain Transplantation for Parkinson's Disease: Technique for Obtaining Donor Tissue," *The Lancet* (March 11, 1989), p. 565

22. See the three reports, and the accompanying editorials, in the November 26, 1992, issue of the *New England Journal of Medicine*.

23. *Supra*, note 9, p. 6

24. A good preliminary attempt, with reference to the fetal tissue debate, is to be found in J. Childress, "Ethics, Public Policy, and Human Fetal Tissue Transplantation Research," *Kennedy Institute of Ethics Journal* vol. 1 (1991), pp. 93–121

25. A. Caplan (ed.), *When Medicine Went Mad* (Humana Press: Totowa, 1992)

26. CANADA, 1996 article 16.11. This attitude about dealing with an area in which there is no consensus is missing from the corresponding section in CANADA, 1997, section 9.4

27. *Supra*, Introduction, note 21

28. *Ibid.*, section 11.22.

29. C. Byk, "France: Law Reform and Human Reproduction" in S. McLean (ed.), *Law Reform and Human Reproduction* (Dartmouth: Aldershot, 1992)
30. FRANCE, REPRODUCTION
31. D. Butler, "France is Urged to Loosen Ban on Embryo Research," *Nature*, vol. 387 (May 15, 1997) p. 218
32. "Extracts from the Infertility (Medical Procedures) Act 1984 (Victoria) in P. Singer, H. Kuhse, S. Buckle, et al. (eds.) *Embryo Experimentation* (Cambridge University Press: Cambridge, 1990) pp. 237–45
33. L. Waller, "Australia: The Law and Infertility—The Victorian Experience" in S. McLean (ed.), *Law Reform and Human Reproduction* (Dartmouth: Aldershot, 1992), pp. 17–45
34. *Supra*, note 32, clause 29 (7)
35. *Supra*, Introduction, note 10
36. *Supra*, note 7
37. CANADA, 1996, and CANADA, 1997
38. *Supra*, Introduction, note 8
39. *Supra*, note 7, pp. 635–6
40. *Ibid.*, pp. 639–40
41. CANADA, 1996, Articles 16.8 and 16.9
42. CANADA, 1997, Articles 9.4 and 9.5
43. *Supra*, Introduction, note 8
44. E. Marshall, "Embryologists Dismayed by Sanctions Against Geneticist," *Science* vol. 275 (January 24, 1997), p. 472
45. NABER, "Report on Human Cloning Through Embryo Splitting" *Kennedy Institute of Ethics Journal* vol. 4 (1994), pp. 251–82
46. Opinion No. 9 (May 28, 1997), distributed by the European Commission
47. Resolution of March 12, 1997, *Bulletin of Medical Ethics* (May, 1997), pp. 10–11
48. National Bioethics Advisory Commission, *Cloning Human Beings*, (NBAC: Rockville, 1997)
49. G. Annas, A. Caplan, and S. Elias, "The Politics of Human-Embryo Research—Avoiding Ethical Gridlock," *New England Journal of Medicine* vol. 334 (May 16, 1996), pp. 1329–32

Chapter Six

1. S. Lederer and M. Grodin, "Historical Overview: Pediatric Experimentation" in M. Grodin and L. Glantz (eds.), *Children as Research Subjects* (Oxford University Press: New York, 1994), pp. 3–25
2. *Supra*, Chapter Two, note 1
3. J. Vollmann and R. Winau, "The Prussian Regulation of 1900" *IRB* vol. 18 (July–August, 1996), pp. 9–11
4. "Guidelines for the Ethical Conduct of Studies to Evaluate Drugs in Pediatric Populations," *Pediatrics* vol. 95 (1995), pp. 286–294
5. National Council on Bioethics in Human Research, *Reflections on Research Involving Children* (National Council: Ottawa, 1993)
6. CANADA, 1996, and CANADA, 1997
7. British Paediatric Association, "Guidelines for the Ethical Conduct of Medical Re-

search Involving Children'' reprinted in C. Foster (ed.), *Manual for Research Ethics Committees* 3rd. ed. (King's College: London, 1994)

8. UK, RCP
9. *Supra*, note 7, p. 3
10. *Supra*, note 4, p. 287
11. "NIH Will Require Researchers to Address Inclusion of Children in New Grant Applications to Agency" *The Blue Sheet* (January 29, 1997), pp. 8–9
12. J. Morrissey, A. Hofmann, J. Thrope, *Consent and Confidentiality in the Health Care of Children and Adolescents* (Free Press: New York, 1986)
13. *Supra*, note 7, p. 12
14. UK, RCP, p. 36
15. *Supra*, note 5, p. 3
16. See, for example, Articles 1.3–1.4 of CANADA, 1997
17. *Supra*, note 4, p. 290
18. *Supra*, note 5, p. 3
19. *Supra*, note 7, p. 13
20. *Supra*, Chapter Two, note 36, pp. 6–22
21. *Supra*, note 5, p. 3
22. CANADA, 1997, Article 1.4
23. The history of this debate, and of its implications for the official regulations, is summarized in W. Bartholome, "Ethical Issues in Pediatric Research," in H. Vanderpool (ed.), *The Ethics of Research Involving Human Subjects* (University Publishing Group: Frederick, 1996), pp. 339–70
24. *Supra*, note 7, p. 9. It is important to take note, however, of the accompanying letter, dated December 10, 1992, from the Association's president clarifying that this is not an absolute classification, but one depending upon the reaction of the child.
25. *Supra*, note 5, p. ii
26. B. McNutt, "The Under-Enrollment of HIV-Infected Foster Children in Clinical Trials and Protocols and the Need for Corrective State Action," *American Journal of Law and Medicine* vol. 20 (1994), pp. 231–49
27. OPRR, *Evaluation of Human Subjects Protections in Schizophrenia Research Conducted by the University of California Los Angeles* (May 11, 1994)—this document contains the Institution's response in Attachment L
28. A. Shamoo and T. Keay, "Ethical Concerns about Relapse Studies," *Cambridge Quarterly of Healthcare Ethics* vol. 5 (1996), pp. 373–86
29. R. Levine, *Ethics and Regulation of Clinical Research* (Urban & Schwarzenberg: Baltimore, 1981) Chapter 10.
30. American College of Physicians, "Cognitively Impaired Subjects," *Annals of Internal Medicine* vol. 111 (1989) pp. 843–48.
31. "The Ethical Conduct of Research on the Mentally Incapacitated," reprinted in C. Foster (ed.), *Manual for Research Ethics Committeees*, 3rd. ed. (King's College: London, 1994)
32. B. A. Brody, *Life and Death Decision Making* (Oxford University Press: New York, 1988), section 5.1
33. *Supra*, note 31, section 6.1.1
34. A. Capron, "Incapacitated Research" *Hastings Center Report* vol. 27 (March–April, 1997), pp. 25–7
35. *Supra*, note 31, section 6.1.3
36. *Supra*, note 30, p. 844

37. *Ibid.*, p. 845
38. *Supra*, note 31, sections 6.1.3 and 6.1.4
39. *Supra*, note 30, p. 844
40. CANADA, 1997, Article 1.4
41. *Supra*, note 30, p. 845
42. *Supra*, note 31, section 6.3.2
43. *Supra*, note 30, p. 845
44. *Ibid.*, p. 846
45. *Supra*, note 29

Chapter Seven

1. J. Bull, "The Historical Development of Clinical Therapeutic Trials," *Journal of Chronic Diseases* vol. 10 (1959), pp. 218–48, and A. Lilienfeld, "Ceteris Parabus: The Evolution of the Clinical Trial," *Bulletin of the History of Medicine* vol. 56 (1982), pp. 1–18
2. Medical Research Council, "Streptomycin Treatment of Pulmonary Tuberculosis," *British Medical Journal* (1948), pp. 769–82
3. UK, RCP, p. 23
4. CANADA, 1997, Article 2.9
5. J. Lantos and J. Frader, "Extracorporeal Membrane Oxygenation and the Ethics of Clinical Research in Pediatrics," *New England Journal of Medicine* vol. 323 (August 9, 1990), pp. 409–13, and S. Elliott, "Neonatal Extracorporeal Membrane Oxygenation: How Not to Assess Novel Technologies," *The Lancet* vol. 337 (Feb. 23, 1991), pp. 476–8
6. UK Collaborative ECMO Trial Group, "UK Collaborative Randomised Trial of Neonatal Extracorporeal Membrane Oxygenation," *The Lancet* vol. 348 (July 13, 1996), pp. 75–82
7. R. Soll, "Neonatal Extracorporeal Membrane Oxygenation—A Bridging Technique" *The Lancet* vol. 348 (July 13, 1996), p. 70
8. Their efforts are described in a letter by D. Field, the chair of the study, on p. 1370 of *The Lancet* for May 27, 1995. My own concerns about their efforts are related to the fact that ECMO had been made unavailable in the United Kingdom outside the trial, raising questions about voluntariness, and the fact that the information sheets provided to the parents provide no information about the registry data, raising questions about whether the parents were fully informed.
9. C. Fried, *Medical Experimentation* (North Holland: Amsterdam, 1974)
10. B. Freedman, "Equipoise and the Ethics of Clinical Research," *New England Journal of Medicine* vol. 317 (July 16, 1987), pp. 141–5
11. *Supra*, Chapter Two note 36, p. 4–16
12. P. Meier, "Terminating a Trial-The Ethical Problem" *Clinical Pharmacology and Therapeutics* vol. 25 (1979), pp. 633–40. See my discussion on pp. 123–4 of B. Brody, *Ethical Issues in Drug Testing, Approval, and Pricing* (Oxford University Press: New York, 1995)
13. K. Zahka, M. Spector, and D. Hanisch, "Hypoplastic Left-Heart Syndrome: Norwood Operation, Transplantation, or Compassionate Care" *Clinics in Perinatology* vol. 20 (1993), pp. 145–54

14. CANADA, 1997, Article 5.4
15. *NCBHR Communique* vol. 7(2) (1996), pp. 20–21
16. *CEJA REPORT* 2-A-96
17. J. Cohen, "Ethics of AZT Studies in Poorer Countries Attacked," *Science* vol. 276 (May 16, 1997) p. 1022
18. M. Angell, "Patients' Preferences in Randomized Clinical Trials" *New England Journal of Medicine* vol. 310 (May 24, 1984), pp. 1385–7
19. B. Fisher, M. Bauer, R. Margolese et.al., "Five Year Results of a Randomized Clinical Trial Comparing Total Mastectomy and Segmental Mastectomy With or Without Radiation in the Treatment of Breast Cancer" *New England Journal of Medicine* vol. 312 (March 14, 1985), pp. 665–73. See p. 667 for the details of the consent process.
20. *Supra*, note 18
21. Royal College of Physicians, *Research Involving Patients* (Royal College: London, 1990). This is the document whose summary is reprinted as Appendix 4.1 to this book. The discussion of these issues is to be found on p. 32.
22. R. Chang, J. Falconer, S. Stulberg et.al., "Prerandomization: An Alternative to Classical Randomization," *Journal of Bone and Joint Surgery* vol. 72-A (1990), pp. 1451–55
23. These trials, and the related issues, are discussed on pp. 325–6 of B. Spilker, *Guide to Clinical Trials* (Raven Press: New York, 1991)
24. These issues are discussed on pp. 129–31 of the grant application for that research project, kindly supplied to me by the Principal Investigator
25. *Supra*, Chapter Two, note 36, pp. 3–39 to 3–40
26. *Supra*, note 21, pp. 32–3
27. See Volume 12 Number 5/6 of *Statistics in Medicine* (March, 1993), which is devoted entirely to the use of such monitoring committees
28. One good review of them is D. DeMets, "Practical Aspects in Data Monitoring," *Statistics in Medicine* vol. 6 (1987), pp. 753–60
29. *Supra*, Chapter Five, note 1
30. M. Simberkoff, P. Hartigan, J. Hamilton, et.al., "Ethical Dilemmas in Continuing a Zidovudine Trial after Early Termination of Similar Trials," *Controlled Clinical Trials* vol. 14 (1993), pp. 6–18

Chapter Eight

1. B. Brody, *Ethical Issues in Drug Testing, Approval, and Pricing* (Oxford University Press: New York, 1995). Chapter III provides a full history of the three periods.
2. 21 *CFR* 312.34
3. *Federal Register* vol. 57 (April 15, 1992) pp. 13250–59
4. "Reinventing the Regulation of Cancer Drugs," a document released by the FDA in March of 1996 as part of the National Performance Review
5. R. A. Merrill, "Regulation of Drugs and Devices," *Health Affairs* (Summer, 1994), pp. 47–69
6. This report is summarized in an FDA Talk Paper (T93-12) issued on March 5, 1993. The actual report, obtainable from the FDA, is entitled "Final Report of the Committee for Clinical Review."

7. A brief history and description of the U.K. system is provided in A. Watt, "Medicines Regulation in the United Kingdom" *Health Bulletin* vol. 48 (September, 1990), pp. 219–24. A fuller account is provided in Part II of T. Cook, C. Doyle, and D. Jabbari, *Pharmaceuticals Biotechnology and the Law* (Stockton: New York, 1991)

8. This literature is summarized in Brody, *supra* note 1

9. D. Kessler, A. Hass, K. Feiden, et al., "Approval of New Drugs in the United States" *JAMA* vol. 276 (Dec. 11, 1996), pp. 1826–31

10. K. Kaitin, "FDA Reform," *Drug Information Journal* vol. 31 (1997), pp. 27–33

11. I first called attention to this problem in Brody, *supra* note 1

12. The best history of that controversy is M. Angell, *Science on Trial* (Norton: New York, 1996)

13. The most recent version of this proposal is N. Campbell, *Making Drugs Safe and Available Without the FDA* (National Center for Policy Analysis: Dallas, 1997)

14. T. Smith, J. Lee, H. Kantarjian et al., "Design and Results of Phase I Cancer Clinical Trials," *Journal of Clinical Oncology* vol. 14 (1996) pp. 287–95

15. These surveys are summarized in C. Daugherty, M. Ratain, E. Grochowski, et al., "Perceptions of Cancer Patients and their Physicians Involved in Phase I Trials," *Journal of Clinical Oncology* vol. 13 (1995), pp. 1062–72.

16. *Ibid.*

17. Advisory Committee on Human Radiation Experiments, "Research Ethics and the Medical Profession," *JAMA* vol. 276 (1996), pp. 403–9

18. Useful discussions are found in E. Emanuel, "A Phase I Trial on the Ethics of Phase I Trials," *Journal of Clinical Oncology* vol. 13 (1995), pp. 1049–51, B. Freedman, "Cohort-Specific Consent," *IRB* (Jan./Feb., 1990) pp. 5–7, and Y. Willems and C. Sessa, "Informing Patients about Phase I Trials," *Acta Oncologica* vol. 28 (1989), pp. 106–7

19. J. O'Quigley, M. Pepe, and L. Fisher, "Continual Reassessment Method: A Practical Design for Phase I Clinical Trials in Cancer," *Biometrics* vol. 46 (1990), pp. 33–48

20. E. Korn, D. Midthune, T. Chen et al., "A Comparison of Two Phase I Trial Designs," *Statistics in Medicine* vol. 13 (1994), pp. 1799–1806

21. B. Brody, "Ethical and Legal Issues in Pediatric Oncology" in D. Fernbach and T. Vietti (eds.), *Clinical Pediatric Oncology* 4th. ed. (St. Louis: Mosby, 1991)

22. S. Coney, "Gene Trial Causes Ethical Storm in New Zealand," *The Lancet* vol. 347 (June 22, 1996), p. 1759. The researcher's response is M. During, "Gene Trial in New Zealand," *The Lancet* vol. 348 (August 31, 1996), p. 618

23. T. Ackerman, "The Ethics of Phase I Pediatric Oncology Trials," *IRB* vol. 17 (Jan.–Feb., 1995), pp. 1–5

24. The classical eloquent presentation of this perspective is Myra Bluebond-Langner, *The Private Worlds of Dying Children* (Princeton: Princeton University Press, 1978)

25. "Adverse Experience Reporting Requirements for Human Drug and Licensed Biological Products" *Federal Register* vol. 59 (October 27, 1994) pp. 54046–64

26. P. Hilts, "Panel Finds Researchers Free of Blame in 5 Deaths" *New York Times* (March 17, 1995), p. A10

27. WHO, "Guidelines for Good Clinical Practices" *International Digest of Health Legislation* vol. 46 (3) (1995), pp. 404–422

28. *Supra*, note 25

29. "Flexible Clinical Trial Monitoring, Improved Design Should Replace FDA Proposal," *The Blue Sheet* (March 1, 1995) pp. 14–5

30. *Supra*, Chapter Six, note 4

31. *Federal Register*, vol. 59 (Dec. 13, 1994), p. 64240
32. *Supra*, Chapter Six, note 5
33. Commentary to Guideline 5 (the guideline is found in Appendix 1.8 of this book). The commentary is found in the 1992 draft document circulated by CIOMS (the numbering of some of the guidelines has been changed).
34. CANADA, 1997, Article 6.6
35. C. Cote, R. Kauffman, G. Troendle, and G. Lambert, "Is the 'Therapeutic Orphan' About to be Adopted?" *Pediatrics* vol. 98 (1996), pp. 118–123 The proposed regulation is to be found in the *Federal Register* for August 15, 1997 pp. 43899–43916.
36. S. Stapleton, "Paving the Way for Pediatric Drug Trials" *American Medical News* (June 2, 1997), p. 3
37. *Guidelines for the Study of Drugs Likely to be Used in the Elderly* (FDA: Washington, 1989)
38. ICH Harmonized Tripartite Guidelines, *Studies in Support of Special Populations: Geriatrics* (ICH: Geneva, 1993)
39. Concorde Coordinating Committee, "CONCORDE: MRC/ANRS Randomized Double-Blind Controlled Trial of Immediate and Deferred Zidovudine in Symptom-Free HIV Infection," *The Lancet* vol. 343 (April 9, 1994), pp. 871–81
40. The details of all of these trials are to be found in Brody, *supra* note 1, Chapter One.
41. T. Fleming and D. DeMets, "Surrogate End Points in Clinical Trials" *Annals of Internal Medicine* vol. 125 (1996), pp. 605–13

Chapter Nine

1. D. DeBruin, "Justice and the Inclusion of Women in Clinical Studies," *Kennedy Institute of Ethics Journal* vol. 4 (1994), pp. 117–46.
2. *Federal Register* vol. 59 (March 9, 1994), pp. 11146–51
3. "Women in NIH Clinical Protocols Top 50% in FY 1994," *The Blue Sheet* (April 9, 1997), pp. 5–6
4. *Supra*, note 2
5. J. C. Bennett, "Inclusion of Women in Clinical Trials" *New England Journal of Medicine* vol. 329 (July 22, 1993), pp. 288–92
6. *Guidelines for the Format and Content of the Clinical and Statistical Sections of New Drug Applications* (FDA: Washington, 1988)
7. The data from both sides is presented in *Federal Register* vol. 58 (July 22, 1993), pp. 39411–416
8. *Supra*, note 3
9. "Women's Health Initiative Backgrounder" downloaded from the WHI Home Page (odp.od.nih.gov/whi/)
10. CANADA, 1997, Articles 6.3–6.4
11. *General Considerations for the Clinical Evaluation of Drugs* (FDA: Washington, 1977)
12. J. Jacobson, J. Greenspan, J. Spritzler, et al., "Thalidomide for the Treatment of Oral Aphthous Ulcers in Patients with Human Immunodeficiency Virus Infection" *New England Journal of Medicine*, vol. 336 (1997), pp. 1487–93. The discussion of the inclusion of the women of child-bearing potential is on p. 1492.

13. P. Walker, "Government May Ease Limits on Research on Pregnant Women," *The Chronicle of Higher Education* (June 21, 1996) p. A23
14. *Ibid.*
15. At one conference at which I discussed the issue with many who were critical of the regulations, it became clear that their misunderstanding was due to their mistaking the "or" before clause (2) for "and"
16. CANADA, 1997, p. VI–4. CANADA, 1996 was clearer on this balancing in that it explicitly stated (Article 12.8) the conditions (minimal benefits to women and substantial harms to fetuses) under which the research would not be allowed.
17. CANADA, 1996, Article 12.10
18. W. El-Sadr and L. Capps, "The Challenge of Minority Recruitment in Clinical Trials for AIDS," *JAMA* vol. 267 (February 19, 1992), pp. 954–7
19. *Supra*, note 6
20. *Supra*, note 3
21. CANADA, 1997, Article 6.2
22. *Ibid.*, section vii
23. This protocol was downloaded from their home page (www.leland.stanford.edu/group/morrinst/Protocol.html)

Chapter Ten

1. E. Westermarck, *Ethical Relativity* (Greenwood Press, 1970)
2. A. Jonsen and S. Toulmin, *The Abuse of Casuistry* (U.S. of California Press: Berkeley, 1988)
3. See B. Brody, "Intuitions and Objective Moral Knowledge," *The Monist* vol. 62 (1979) 446–56, and B. Brody, *Life and Death Decision Making* (Oxford University Press: New York, 1988)
4. *Ibid.*
5. Further useful evidence in support of this point is provided in R. Levine, "International Codes and Guidelines for Research Ethics" in H. Vanderpool (ed.), *The Ethics of Research Involving Human Subjects* (University Publishing: Frederick, 1996), especially p. 243

ACKNOWLEDGMENT OF SOURCES

Appendices 1.2–1.4 are reproduced with the permission of the Secretariat of the World Medical Association.

Appendices 1.6–1.8 are reproduced with the permission of the Office of the Secretary General of CIOMS.

Appendix 2.1 is reproduced with the permission of the Office for Official Publications of the European Communities.

Appendices 2.2–2.5 are reproduced with the permission of the Secretariat General of the Council of Europe. Full English versions are available from Council of Europe Publishing.

Appendix 2.6 is reproduced with the permission of the Lancet. It appeared as European Medical Research Councils, "Gene Therapy in Man" vol. 84 (June 4, 1988) pp. 1271–72.

Appendix 4.1 is reproduced with the permission of the Royal College of Physicians. It appeared as Chapter 12 of *Research Involving Patients* (London: Royal College of Physicians, 1990).

Appendix 4.2 is reproduced with the permission of the Medical Research Council. © Medical Research Council 1991.

Appendices 4.3–4.6 are crown copyright reproduced with the permission of the Controller of Her Majesty's Stationery Office.

Appendix 4.7 is reproduced with the permission of the editor in chief of *The Annual Review of Population Law*.

Appendices 4.9–4.10 are reproduced with the permission of the Canadian Council on Animal Care.

Appendix 4.11 is reproduced with the permission of the Canadian Federal Centre for AIDS.

Appendix 4.12 is reproduced with the permission of the Commonwealth Information Services. It appeared as National Health and Medical Research Council, (1992) *MHMRC Statement on Human Experimentation and Supplementary Notes*, Canberra: The Council (pp. 2–22). Commonwealth of Australia copyright reproduced by permission.

Appendix 4.13 is reproduced with the permission of The World Health Organization. It appeared in *The International Digest of Health Legislation* (1995) pp. 560–63.

INDEX